Asymptotic and Analytic Methods
in Stochastic Evolutionary Systems

"Nos esse quasi nanos gigantium humeris insidentes,
ut possimus plura eis et remotiora videre,
non utique proprii visus acumine, aut eminentia corporis,
sed quia in altum subvehimur et extollimur magnitudine gigantea"
(dicebat Bernardus Carnotensis)

In memory of our Teacher and Mentor,
Vladimir Semenovich Koroliuk

Series Editor
Nikolaos Limnios

Asymptotic and Analytic Methods in Stochastic Evolutionary Systems

Dmitri Koroliouk
Igor Samoilenko

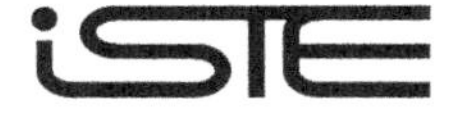

WILEY

First published 2023 in Great Britain and the United States by ISTE Ltd and John Wiley & Sons, Inc.

ISTE Ltd
27-37 St George's Road
London SW19 4EU
UK

www.iste.co.uk

John Wiley & Sons, Inc.
111 River Street
Hoboken, NJ 07030
USA

www.wiley.com

Library of Congress Control Number: 2023937508

British Library Cataloguing-in-Publication Data
A CIP record for this book is available from the British Library
ISBN 978-1-78630-911-2

Contents

Preface ix

Introduction xi

Chapter 1. Multidimensional Models of Kac Type 1

1.1. Definitions and basic properties 1
1.2. Moments of evolutionary process 8
1.3. Systems of Kolmogorov equations 17
1.4. Evolutionary operator and theorem about weak convergence to the measure of the Wiener process 23

Chapter 2. Symmetry of Markov Random Evolutionary Processes in R^n . . 29

2.1. Symmetrization: definition and properties 29
2.2. Examples of symmetric distributions in R^n and distributions on $n+1$-hedra 32
2.2.1. Symmetric distributions 32
2.2.2. Distributions on $n+1$-hedra 35

Chapter 3. Hyperparabolic Equations, Integral Equation and Distribution for Markov Random Evolutionary Processes 39

3.1. Hyperparabolic equations and methods of solving Cauchy problems 39
3.2. Analytical solution of a hyperparabolic equation with real-analytic initial conditions 46
3.3. Integral representation of the hyperparabolic equation 57
3.4. Distribution function of evolutionary process 67

Chapter 4. Fading Markov Random Evolutionary Process 77

4.1. Definition of fading Markov random evolutionary process, its moments and limit distribution 77
4.2. Integral equation for a function from the fading random evolutionary process 89
4.3. Equations in partial derivatives for a function of the fading random evolutionary process 93

Chapter 5. Two Models of the Evolutionary Process 99

5.1. Evolution on a complex plane 99
5.2. Evolution with infinitely many directions 109
5.2.1. Symmetric case 110
5.2.2. Non-symmetric case 119

Chapter 6. Diffusion Process with Evolution and Its Parameter Estimation 125

6.1. Asymptotic diffusion environment 125
6.2. Approximation of a discrete Markov process in asymptotic diffusion environment 127
6.3. Parameter estimation of the limit process 132

Chapter 7. Filtration of Stationary Gaussian Statistical Experiments 135

7.1. Introduction 135
7.2. Stochastic difference equation of the process of filtration 137
7.3. Coefficient of filtration 138
7.4. Equation of optimal filtration 139
7.5. Characterization of a filtered signal 141

Chapter 8. Adapted Statistical Experiments with Random Change of Time 143

8.1. Introduction 143
8.2. Statistical experiments and evolutionary processes 144
8.3. Stochastic dynamics of statistical experiments 145
8.4. Adapted statistical experiments in series scheme 147
8.5. Convergence of the adapted statistical experiments 149
8.6. Scaling parameter estimation 154
8.7. Statistical estimations of the renewal intensity parameter 155
8.7.1. Poisson's renewal process with parameter $q = 2$ 156
8.7.2. Stationary renewal process with delay, determined by the initial distribution function of the limit overjumps 156
8.7.3. Renewal processes with arbitrarily distributed renewal intervals 157

Chapter 9. Filtering of Stationary Gaussian Statistical Experiments 159

9.1. Stationary statistical experiments 159
9.2. Filtering of discrete Markov diffusion 161
9.3. The filtering error 164
9.4. The filtering empirical estimation 166

Chapter 10. Asymptotic Large Deviations for Markov Random Evolutionary Process 171

10.1. Asymptotic large deviations 171
10.2. Asymptotically stopped Markov random evolutionary process 191
10.3. Explicit representation for the normalizing function 206

Chapter 11. Asymptotic Large Deviations for Semi-Markov Random Evolutionary Processes 209

11.1. Recurrent semi-Markov random evolutionary processes 209
11.2. Asymptotic large deviations 212

Chapter 12. Heuristic Principles of Phase Merging in Reliability Analysis 221

12.1. The duplicated renewal system 221
12.2. The duplicated renewal system in the series scheme 222
12.3. Heuristic principles of the phase merging 223
12.4. The duplicated renewal system without failure 225

References 227

Index 233

Preface

This book is devoted to the study of Markov and semi-Markov random evolutionary processes.

The material presented in this book is classified by the authorship as follows:

– Chapters 1–5 were written by Igor Samoilenko;

– Chapters 6–12 were written by Dmitri Koroliouk.

This book is devoted to analytical methods for studying Markov and semi-Markov random evolutionary processes, in particular the derivation and solving of corresponding differential and integral equations, constructing new models, like fading evolution, etc.

The statistics of random evolutionary processes considers the problem of estimating parameters, as well as optimal filtering of stationary Gaussian evolutions.

Particular attention is paid to the problems of asymptotically large deviations for Markov and semi-Markov random evolutionary processes, in the sense of the random time of entering a region with the asymptotically decreasing probability of hitting it.

Dmitri Koroliouk expresses his appreciation and gratitude to the mathematical department of the University of Rome II – Tor Vergata, in particular to Professor Filippo Bracci for partially supporting the contents of this book.

Dmitri KOROLIOUK
NTUU Igor Sikorsky Kyiv Polytechnic Institute
Institute of Mathematics NAS
Institute of Telecommunications and Global Information Space NAS
Kyiv
Ukraine
and
University of Rome II – Tor Vergata
UNESCO Interdisciplinary Chair in Biotechnology and Bioethics
Rome
Italy

Igor SAMOILENKO
Taras Shevchenko National University of Kyiv
Institute for Applied System Analysis of
NTUU Igor Sikorsky Kyiv Polytechnic Institute
Kyiv
Ukraine

March 2023

Introduction

This book continues with the studies found in our previous book *Random Evolutionary Systems: Asymptotic Properties and Large Deviations* in the Mathematics and Statistics series, edited by Nikolaos Limnios.

Here, we study some important aspects of random evolutionary systems, considering typical problems on some specific examples.

Numerous monographs have been devoted to the study and description of the Wiener process, in particular the fundamental works of Hida (1980) and Knight (1981). But such a process does not in fact exist in nature. In particular, Brownian motion is not a Wiener process, because the latter is only a mathematical idealization of physical Brownian motion. It is sufficient to indicate that when the property of continuous trajectories of the Wiener process is indifferentiable, a particle has no free run between two successive collisions; otherwise, it would have an infinite number of collisions per unit of time, which is unrealistic. Here, we examine models in which a particle has some free distance between two consecutive collisions. At the same time, we investigate two cases: Markov evolution, when the time during which the particle moves towards some direction is distributed exponentially with the parameter λ; semi-Markov evolution with an arbitrary distribution of the switching process. A similar example can be given by considering the process of heat distribution from a source in some environment. It is known that such a process in mathematical physics is described by a parabolic thermal conductivity equation, where parameters depend on the properties of the environment, and the initial conditions are determined by the initial position of the source or the initial distribution of heat in the medium. The classical theory proposes a model where the propagation of heat from the source occurs instantaneously, with an arbitrarily high speed, which is an analogue of the Wiener process. It is not difficult to note the analogy between the process of heat propagation, as a process of heat transfer by particles, and the process of Brownian motion. In both cases, we have diffusion with an infinite propagation speed. What distinguishes natural physical processes from their mathematical idealizations, which are the Wiener process and the classical model of heat conduction, is precisely the finiteness of the propagation speed. Many authors have studied various physical aspects of such models. The models investigated here describe the motion of a particle with a finite speed. Thus, the proposed random evolutionary process has the characteristics of a natural physical process: free run and finiteness propagation speed. In the proposed models, the number of possible directions of evolution can be both finite and infinite. In the theory of random evolutions (TRE), an asymptotic technique has been developed, which is based on the well-developed apparatus of the theory of random products of matrices and operators (Furstenberg 1963; Grenander 1963; Tutubalin 1965; Hannan 1965) and the theory of singularly perturbed semigroups of operators. The main goal of these studies is the proof of various limit theorems. In this aspect, it is necessary to mention the works of American mathematicians Griego and Hersh (1969, 1971), Papanicolaou (1971a), Papanicolaou and Kellek (1971), Gorostiza (1972, 1973b), Hersh and Pinsky (1972), Hersh (1974), Pinsky (1991) and others. An effective means of proving limit theorems in TRE is the theory of phase merging of complex systems developed by Korolyuk and Turbin (1993) and by Korolyuk and Limnios (2005). Thanks to their methods, many authors have proven important limit theorems on regular approximations to solutions of singularly perturbed differential equations for various stochastic models, as well as for dynamic systems with coefficients dependent on Markov processes, for example, Skorokhod (1989). Korolyuk and Swishchuk (1995a, 1995b) developed the theory of semi-Markov random evolutions based on the theory of martingales. But at the same time, it is not only the limit theorems which lead to Wiener or diffusion processes which are of interest, but also the equation and systems of equations describing the limit behavior of one or another characteristics of a random evolutionary system. Thanks to this, it is possible to get various limit theorems, based on the equation by the limit transition. This work is dedicated to this topic. The boundary behavior of the Markov random evolutionary process was studied, equations describing this process were found and methods for solving these equations were proposed. It should be noted that the first work in this particular field was the work of Goldstein (1951). By studying the simplest model – one-dimensional random evolution governed by a Poisson process – he obtained the equation

$$\frac{\partial^2}{\partial t^2}u(t,x) + 2\lambda\frac{\partial}{\partial t}u(t,x) = v^2\frac{\partial^2}{\partial x^2}u(t,x)$$

$$u(0,x) = f(x),\ \frac{\partial}{\partial t}\ u(t,x)|_{t=0} = g(x) \qquad [I.1]$$

which is known as a damped wave or telegraph equation. In this case, the constants v and λ refer to the speed of the particle and the intensity of the switching process in accordance. Goldstein proved that the density of the probability distribution of the coordinate of a particle on a straight line satisfies the equation found and, with the correspondingly given initial conditions, a solution to the Cauchy problem can also be found. Further research in this direction was carried out by Kac, who in 1956 showed that not only the density distribution, but also any measurable functional of the particle trajectory (Kac 1957, 1974) satisfy this equation. He also found the solution of the Cauchy problem in the form of expectation functions from a random process and proved the validity of such a formula for more general equations. Here, we describe some generalizations of the Goldstein–Katz model to the case of the space R^n. Kac was also the first to notice that if $v \to \infty$ and $\lambda \to \infty$ so that $\frac{v^2}{\lambda} \to \sigma^2$, then such a model is an asymptotically Wiener process with zero drift and the diffusion coefficient σ^2. We have proven the theorem about weak convergence of measures generated by a Markov random evolutionary process in R^n to the measure of a Wiener process. Subsequently, the Goldstein–Katz model was generalized to the case of the different intensity of the controlling Poisson process when moving in the positive and negative directions. Bartlett (1957, 1978), Kaplan (1964), Cane (1967, 1975), Griego and Hersh (1969, 1971) generalized probabilistic Kac's formula for the solution of the abstract telegraph equation $\frac{\partial^2}{\partial t^2}u(t,x) + 2a\frac{\partial}{\partial t}u(t,x) = A^2u(t,x)$, where $a > 0$ is some constant, and A is the infinitesimal operator of the semigroup of compressions of the class C_0 of operators in some Banach space. Kisinski (1974) and other authors further strengthened this result by generalizing Kac's probabilistic formula to the solution of the equation $\frac{\partial^n}{\partial t^n}u(t,x) + 2a\frac{\partial^{n-1}}{\partial t^{n-1}}u(t,x) = A^2u(t,x)$, where $n \geq 2$ is any integer.

It is also necessary to mention numerous works of the Italian mathematician Orsingher that were devoted to the equations arising in various one-dimensional model random evolutions (Orsingher 1986; Orsingher and Sommella 2004), some models on the plane (Orsingher 1985, 1990b; Orsingher and Kolesnik 1994) and on the sphere (Orsingher 1987c), etc., as well as their solution and physical interpretation of solutions. However, it should be noted that the works of Orsingher are mostly devoted to the study of processes described by equations that can be factored. The solutions of such equations are written down as a linear combination of known solutions of factorization elements. We get equations that are not factorable, and two solution methods are proposed for them.

In particular, when studying the Markov random evolutionary process, integral equations are applied, which makes it possible to describe processes governed by a non-exponential distribution (semi-Markov evolutionary process), as well as write down equations for processes for which it is impossible to find differential equations directly (fading evolutionary process).

Other works on this topic should also be noted: Jenssen (1990), Pinsky (1991), Foong (1992) and Foong and Kanno (1994).

In Chapter 1, we define multidimensional models of the Kac type, describe corresponding moments, systems of Kolmogorov equations and some results on their convergence of the Wiener process.

Chapter 2 describes some symmetric properties of the Markov random evolutionary processes in R^n and implies some generalizations of well-known symmetric distributions.

Chapter 3 is devoted to the description of hyperparabolic equations and the integral equation for Markov random evolutionary processes in R^n, methods of their solutions for specific initial conditions. An obvious view of the corresponding distribution is also presented.

Chapter 4 deals with a special case, model of the fading Markov random evolutionary process, which cannot be studied with the use of differential equations only. At the same time, it is interesting because of the existence of the limit distribution at $t \to \infty$, which is impossible in the classical model.

Chapter 5 presents two models of evolutionary processes, namely the evolution of Kac's type on a complex plane, in which moments define solutions of the Cauchy problem for a Schrödinger-type equation, and the evolutionary process in R^n with infinitely many directions, for which methods of our previous book *Random Evolutionary Systems: Asymptotic Properties and Large Deviations* are applied to obtain the limit process in the sense of the Kac-type hydrodynamic limit.

In Chapter 6, we consider a random evolution $\zeta(t)$, $t \geq 0$, which depends on a random environment $Y(t)$, $t \geq 0$, which, in turn, is switched by an embedded Markov chain X_k, $k \geq 0$, considering a specific relation between the continuous-time $t \geq 0$ and the discrete-time $k \geq 0$. The purpose is to prove the convergence (in distribution) of the process $\zeta(t)$, $t \geq 0$ to the Ornstein–Uhlenbeck process under some scaling of the process and its time parameter. The limit will be considered by a small series parameter $\varepsilon > 0$, $\varepsilon \to 0$.

Chapter 7 is devoted to the filtration of random Gaussian–Markov evolutionary processes represented by stationary Gaussian statistical experiments, determined by the solution of the optimal filtration equation. It is characterized by a two-dimensional matrix of covariances. The parameters of the filtered signal are set by empirical covariances.

In Chapter 8, we study a random evolutionary process, represented as statistical experiments with the random change of time, which transforms a discrete stochastic basis in a continuous one. The adapted stochastic experiments are studied in the continuous stochastic basis in the series scheme. The transition to limit by the series parameter generates an approximation of adapted statistical experiments by a diffusion process with evolution.

The average intensity parameter of renewal times is estimated in three different cases: the Poisson renewal process, a stationary renewal process with delay and the general renewal process with the Weibull–Gnedenko renewal time distribution.

Chapter 9 repeats the statement of the filtering problem discussed in Chapter 7. However, the analysis of this problem differs significantly from the previous one. This chapter is placed separately from Chapter 7 intentionally, in order to separate the analytical approach to the problem. The performed analysis casts doubt on the well-known fact about the equivalence of the independence and non-correlation conditions for Gaussian random sequences and processes, despite the indisputable proof of the equivalence theorem.

In Chapter 10, we discuss the necessary and sufficient conditions for the convergence of the distributions of normalized first entry times into asymptotically receding domains for asymptotic large deviations for Markov random evolutionary processes.

In Chapter 11, we discuss the necessary and sufficient conditions for the convergence of the distributions of normalized first entry times into asymptotically large deviations for semi-Markov random evolutionary processes.

Chapter 12 deals with some analytical methods in reliability theory that stimulate the consideration of the principles of merging subsets of states (phases) for Markov and semi-Markov processes. The peculiarity of the algorithm is that the heuristic principles of phase merging can be constructively used to analyze the reliability of stochastic systems. In particular, the stationary phase merging algorithm can be used to simplify the analysis of the reliability of a redundant recovery system.

1

Multidimensional Models of Kac Type

1.1. Definitions and basic properties

In this section, the Goldstein–Kac model of the motion of a particle in a straight line is generalized to the case of the space $R^n (n > 1)$. The analytical characteristics of this process have been studied.

Unlike the Goldstein–Kac model (Goldstein 1951; Kac 1957), where the evolution had two possible directions that changed sequentially, in the case of the $R^n (n > 1)$ space, we are faced with the problem of determining the possible directions of movement and the order of their change.

We study random evolutionary processes in $R^n (n > 1)$ in which the number of directions of movement is $n + 1$. Two cases are considered where the direction of movement changes uniformly and cyclically. Examples of such evolutions in the spaces R^1, R^2 were studied in works Orsingher (1986) and Orsingher and Kolesnik (1994). Let us set the directions of movement in a way that was not used in the mentioned works, namely: the particle can move in the directions of the vectors, with the beginning in the center of the regular $n + 1$-hedron inscribed in the unit sphere (generalization of tetrahedron) and the ends at its vertices.

Here, we call a regular $n + 1$-hedron in R^n inscribed in the unit sphere a convex polyhedron, which is given by the formula

$$Tetr_{n+1}(0,1) = \{\overline{x} = x_1\overline{\tau_1} + \cdots + x_n\overline{\tau_n} \in R^n : \gamma(\overline{x}) \leq 1\},$$

where the vectors $\overline{\tau}_0, \ldots, \overline{\tau}_n$ have coordinates $(k = \overline{0,n}, i = \overline{1,n})$

$$\tau_k^{(i)} = \begin{cases} -\frac{1}{n}\sqrt{\frac{n(n+1)}{(n-i+1)(n-i+2)}}, i \leq k, \\ \sqrt{\frac{(n-k)(n+1)}{n(n-k+1)}}, i = k+1, \\ 0, i > k+1. \end{cases}$$

These vectors determine the direction of movement of the Markov random evolutionary process in R^n.

DEFINITION 1.1.– *A Markov random evolutionary process in R^n with a cyclic (uniform) change in the directions of movement is a process that satisfies the following conditions:*

1) the process starts at the point $\overline{x} = (x_1, \ldots, x_n)$;

2) initial direction of movement $\overline{\tau}_i, i = \overline{0, n}$;

3) if θ is the time during which the process moves in some direction, then $P(\theta > t) = e^{-\lambda t}$;

4) k-th direction is followed by $k+1$-th, n-th by 0-th (k-th is followed by any of the others with probability $\frac{1}{n}$);

5) the speed of movement is constant and is equal to v.

REMARK 1.1.– *By analogy with the Goldstein–Kac process, we can write the formula for the process coordinate: $S(t) = \overline{x} + v\int_0^t \overline{\tau}_{\xi(u)}du$, where $\xi(u)$ is a Markov chain with values from the set $S = \{0, 1, 2, \ldots, n\}$, which conducts in each state exponentially distributed with parameter λ time, and then passes into the next state in the case of cyclic evolution and into one of the remaining states in uniform evolution with probability $\frac{1}{n}$.*

Hereinafter, we call $S(t)$ the Markov random evolutionary process in R^n; $\overline{\tau}_{\xi(t)}$ is a multidimensional homogeneous alternating process (an analogue of the telegraphic process).

In the following, we use hyperbolic functions of the n-th order $ch_{n,i}(x), i = \overline{0, n}$ given by the equalities (see Bateman and Erdelyi (1953a, 1953b, 1955)):

$$ch_{n,0}(x) = 1 + \frac{x^n}{n!} + \frac{x^{2n}}{(2n)!} + \ldots$$

$$ch_{n,1}(x) = \frac{x^{n-1}}{(n-1)!} + \frac{x^{2n-1}}{(2n-1)!} + \ldots$$

$$\ldots$$

$$ch_{n,n-1}(x) = \frac{x}{1!} + \frac{x^{n+1}}{(n+1)!} + \ldots$$

Note that these functions are obtained by multisectioning the exponent.

The function $ch_{n,i}x, i = \overline{0, n-1}$ can also be defined as the derivative of the i-th order of the hyperbolic cosine of the n-th order.

Let us indicate some properties of high-order hyperbolic functions.

a) $ch_{n,0}(0) = 1$;

b) $ch_{n,i}(0) = 0, i = \overline{1, n-1}$;

c) the functions $ch_{n,i}x, i = \overline{0, n-1}$ are solutions of the differential equation $f^{(n)}(x) = f(x)$.

Note that the set of solutions of this equation with the initial conditions a) and b) coincides with the set of functions $ch_{n,i}x, i = \overline{0, n-1}$.

In order to determine the transition probability matrices of the above process, it is necessary to express high-order hyperbolic functions through elementary functions. Let us use the obvious ratio:

$$ch_{n,0}x = \frac{1}{n}(e^{x} + e^{(\cos\frac{2\pi}{n} + i\sin\frac{2\pi}{n})x} + \dots + e^{(\cos\frac{2(n-1)\pi}{n} + i\sin\frac{2(n-1)\pi}{n})x}) \quad [1.1]$$

THEOREM 1.1.– *Transition probability matrices of Markov random evolutionary process in R^n in cases of cyclic and uniform changes in the direction of movement, respectively, have the form:*

$$P(t) = \begin{pmatrix} e^{-\lambda t}ch_{n+1,0}(\lambda t) & e^{-\lambda t}ch_{n+1,n}(\lambda t) & \dots & e^{-\lambda t}ch_{n+1,1}(\lambda t) \\ e^{-\lambda t}ch_{n+1,1}(\lambda t) & e^{-\lambda t}ch_{n+1,0}(\lambda t) & \dots & e^{-\lambda t}ch_{n+1,2}(\lambda t) \\ \dots & \dots & \dots & \dots \\ e^{-\lambda t}ch_{n+1,n}(\lambda t) & e^{-\lambda t}ch_{n+1,n-1}(\lambda t) & \dots & e^{-\lambda t}ch_{n+1,0}(\lambda t) \end{pmatrix} \quad [1.2]$$

$$P(t) = \begin{pmatrix} A & B & B & \dots \\ B & A & B & \dots \\ \dots & \dots & \dots & \dots \end{pmatrix}, \quad [1.3]$$

where $A = \frac{1}{n+1} + \frac{n}{n+1}e^{-\frac{n+1}{n}\lambda t}$, $B = \frac{1}{n+1} - \frac{1}{n+1}e^{-\frac{n+1}{n}\lambda t}$.

Moreover, in both cases, we have: $\lim_{t\to\infty} P(t) = \frac{1}{n+1}\begin{pmatrix} 1 & 1 & \dots & 1 \\ 1 & 1 & \dots & 1 \\ \dots & \dots & \dots & \dots \\ 1 & 1 & \dots & 1 \end{pmatrix}$.

PROOF.– It is known (Chung 2012) that the transition probability matrix of the Markov chain described in Remark 1.1 can be written in the form $P(t) = e^{tQ}$, where $Q = \lambda(P - I)$, $P = \begin{pmatrix} 0 & 1 & 0 & \dots \\ 0 & 0 & 1 & \dots \\ 0 & 0 & 0 & \dots \\ \dots & \dots & \dots & \dots \\ 1 & 0 & 0 & \dots \end{pmatrix}$ in the case of a cyclical change in the direction of movement and $P = \begin{pmatrix} 0 & \frac{1}{n} & \frac{1}{n} & \dots \\ \frac{1}{n} & 0 & \frac{1}{n} & \dots \\ \frac{1}{n} & \frac{1}{n} & 0 & \dots \\ \dots & \dots & \dots & \dots \end{pmatrix}$ in the case of a uniform change in the direction of movement.

We have for the cyclic change in the direction of movement: $P(t) = e^{Qt} = e^{-\lambda It}e^{\lambda\Gamma_1 t}$, where $\Gamma_1 = \begin{pmatrix} 0 & 1 & 0 & \dots & 0 \\ 0 & 0 & 1 & \dots & 0 \\ \dots & \dots & \dots & \dots & \dots \\ 0 & 0 & 0 & \dots & 1 \\ 1 & 0 & 0 & \dots & 0 \end{pmatrix}$. Γ_1 satisfies the relation: $\Gamma_1^{n+1} = I$.

Let us denote $\Gamma_i = \Gamma_1^i, i = \overline{2, n}$. Then

$$P(t) = e^{-\lambda It}\left(I + \frac{\lambda t}{1!}\Gamma_1 + \frac{(\lambda t)^2}{2!}\Gamma_2 + \dots + \frac{(\lambda t)^n}{n!}\Gamma_n + \frac{(\lambda t)^{n+1}}{(n+1)!}I + \dots\right)$$
$$= e^{-\lambda It}(ch_{n+1,0}xI + ch_{n+1,1}x\Gamma_n + ch_{n+1,2}x\Gamma_{n-1} + \dots + ch_{n+1,n}x\Gamma_1).$$

Thus, equality [1.2] is proven.

Using relation [1.1], we have:

$$P(t) = \left(I - \frac{\lambda t}{1!}I + \frac{(\lambda t)^2}{2!}I - \dots\right)\left(\frac{1}{n+1}[e^{\lambda t} + e^{\omega_{n+1}\lambda t} + \dots + e^{\omega_{n+1}^n\lambda t}]I + \right.$$
$$\frac{1}{n+1}[e^{\lambda t} + \omega_{n+1}e^{\omega_{n+1}\lambda t} + \dots + \omega_{n+1}^n e^{\omega_{n+1}^n\lambda t}]\Gamma_n + \dots + \frac{1}{n+1}[e^{\lambda t} + \omega_{n+1}^n \times$$
$$\left. e^{\omega_{n+1}\lambda t} + \dots + \omega_{n+1}^{n^2}e^{\omega_{n+1}^n\lambda t}]\Gamma_1\right) = \frac{1}{n}e^{-\lambda t}I\left([e^{\lambda t} + e^{\omega_{n+1}\lambda t} + \dots + e^{\omega_{n+1}^n\lambda t}]I + \right.$$
$$\frac{1}{n+1}[e^{\lambda t}+\omega_{n+1}e^{\omega_{n+1}\lambda t}+\dots+\omega_{n+1}^n e^{\omega_{n+1}^n\lambda t}]\Gamma_n+\dots+\frac{1}{n+1}[e^{\lambda t}+\omega_{n+1}^n e^{\omega_{n+1}\lambda t}+$$
$$\left.\dots+\omega_{n+1}^{n^2}e^{\omega_{n+1}^n\lambda t}]\Gamma_1\right) = \frac{1}{n+1}([1+e^{-\lambda t(1-\omega_{n+1})}+\dots+e^{-\lambda t(1-\omega_{n+1}^n)}]I+\dots+[1+$$
$$\omega_{n+1}^n e^{-\lambda t(1-\omega_{n+1})} + \dots + \omega_{n+1}^{n^2}e^{-\lambda t(1-\omega_{n+1}^n)}]\Gamma_1) = \frac{1}{n+1}([1 + e^{-\lambda t(1-Re\omega_{n+1})}\times$$
$$(\cos(Im\omega_{n+1}\lambda t) + i\sin(Im\omega_{n+1}\lambda t)) + \dots + e^{-\lambda t(1-Re\omega_{n+1}^n)}(\cos(Im\omega_{n+1}^n\lambda t)+$$
$$i\sin(Im\omega_{n+1}^n\lambda t))]I+\dots+[1+\omega_{n+1}^n e^{-\lambda t(1-Re\omega_{n+1})}(\cos(Im\omega_{n+1}\lambda t)+i\sin(Im\omega_{n+1}\times$$
$$\lambda t)) + \dots + \omega_{n+1}^{n^2}e^{-\lambda t(1-Re\omega_{n+1}^n)}(\cos(Im\omega_{n+1}^n\lambda t) + i\sin(Im\omega_{n+1}^n\lambda t))]\Gamma_1).$$

Since $0 < \frac{2\pi}{n} < 2\pi, n > 1$, then $-1 \leq Re\omega_{n+1} < 1$, and moreover $-1 \leq Re\omega_{n+1}^n < 1$. Directing t to ∞ in the last ratio, we get $\lim_{t\to\infty} P(t) = \frac{1}{n+1}(I + \Gamma_n + \dots + \Gamma_1)$ or $\lim_{t\to\infty} P(t) = \frac{1}{n+1}\begin{pmatrix} 1 & 1 & \dots & 1 \\ 1 & 1 & \dots & 1 \\ \dots & \dots & \dots & \dots \\ 1 & 1 & \dots & 1 \end{pmatrix}$.

For a uniform change of movement directions, we have:

$$Q = -\lambda I + \lambda \begin{pmatrix} 0 & \frac{1}{n} & \frac{1}{n} & \dots \\ \frac{1}{n} & 0 & \frac{1}{n} & \dots \\ \frac{1}{n} & \frac{1}{n} & 0 & \dots \\ \dots & \dots & \dots & \dots \end{pmatrix} = \lambda \begin{pmatrix} -1 & \frac{1}{n} & \frac{1}{n} & \dots \\ \frac{1}{n} & -1 & \frac{1}{n} & \dots \\ \frac{1}{n} & \frac{1}{n} & -1 & \dots \\ \dots & \dots & \dots & \dots \end{pmatrix} =$$

$$= \frac{n+1}{n}\lambda \begin{pmatrix} -\frac{n}{n+1} & \frac{1}{n+1} & \frac{1}{n+1} & \dots \\ \frac{1}{n+1} & -\frac{n}{n+1} & \frac{1}{n+1} & \dots \\ \frac{1}{n+1} & \frac{1}{n+1} & -\frac{n}{n+1} & \dots \\ \dots & \dots & \dots & \dots \end{pmatrix} = \frac{n+1}{n}\lambda(\Pi - I).$$

$$\text{Here, } \Pi = \begin{pmatrix} \frac{1}{n+1} & \frac{1}{n+1} & \frac{1}{n+1} & \dots \\ \frac{1}{n+1} & \frac{1}{n+1} & \frac{1}{n+1} & \dots \\ \frac{1}{n+1} & \frac{1}{n+1} & \frac{1}{n+1} & \dots \\ \dots & \dots & \dots & \dots \end{pmatrix}, \Pi^k = \Pi, k = 2, 3, \dots$$

Then, $P(t) = \exp(tQ) = \exp(-\frac{n+1}{n}\lambda t)\exp(\frac{n+1}{n}\lambda \Pi t) = e^{-\frac{n+1}{n}\lambda t}(I + \frac{1}{1!}\frac{n+1}{n}\lambda t\Pi + \frac{1}{2!}(\frac{n+1}{n}\lambda t)^2\Pi + \dots) = e^{-\frac{n+1}{n}\lambda t}(I - \Pi + e^{\frac{n+1}{n}\lambda t}\Pi) = \Pi + e^{-\frac{n+1}{n}\lambda t}(I - \Pi) = \begin{pmatrix} A & B & B & \dots \\ B & A & B & \dots \\ B & B & A & \dots \\ \dots & \dots & \dots & \dots \end{pmatrix}$, where $A = \frac{1}{n+1} + \frac{n}{n+1}e^{-\frac{n+1}{n}\lambda t}$, $B = \frac{1}{n+1} - \frac{1}{n+1}e^{-\frac{n+1}{n}\lambda t}$,

and thus $\lim_{t\to\infty} P(t) = \frac{1}{n+1}\begin{pmatrix} 1 & 1 & \dots & 1 \\ 1 & 1 & \dots & 1 \\ \dots & \dots & \dots & \dots \\ 1 & 1 & \dots & 1 \end{pmatrix}$.

The theorem is proven.

Note that the Kubo–Anderson process (Anderson 1954) has many properties of the telegraphic process: its moments, equations for characteristic functional, etc.

It turns out that the presence of these properties in the Kubo–Anderson process is due to the fact that the Kubo–Anderson process is a trace of a multidimensional homogeneous alternating process, which it leaves on a one-dimensional subspace. Accordingly, the Kubo–Anderson process inherits all the properties of the multidimensional homogeneous alternating process.

THEOREM 1.2.– *The Kubo–Anderson process is a projection onto the axis OX of a multidimensional homogeneous alternating process.*

PROOF.– Consider a multidimensional homogeneous alternating process in R^n ($n+1$ – number of different a_i) $\eta_t = \overline{\tau}_{\vartheta(0,t)}$, where $\overline{\tau} = (\tau^{(1)}, \ldots, \tau^{(n)})$. Then, $\tau^{(1)}_{\vartheta(0,t)}$ is a multidimensional projection of a homogeneous alternating process on OX, and by means of selection of $\overline{\tau}_i$ or the coordinate system, we establish the equality $\tau^{(1)}_{\vartheta(0,t)} = a_{\vartheta(0,t)}$.

The theorem is proven.

It is also interesting to study the front of random evolutionary processes and the probabilities associated with evolution being on the edge of the front or inside the front. The answer to the question about the evolution front is given in the works of Kolesnik (see some of these results in Orsingher and Kolesnik (1994)), where it is proven that at the moment of time t, the evolution front in R^n space, which has m directions of movement ($m > n$), will be a regular m-angle inscribed in a sphere of radius vt, and with the center at the point from which the evolution starts (we will assume that this is the origin of the coordinates). Thus, in the Markovian case of a random evolutionary process in R^n at the moment of time t, the evolution front is an $n+1$-hedron inscribed in a sphere of radius vt, with the center at the origin of the coordinates.

Let $S(t) = v\int_0^t \overline{\tau}_{\xi(u)} du$ be the coordinate of the evolutionary process at the moment of time t, $Tetr_{n+1}(0, vt)$ – an $n+1$-hedron inscribed in a sphere of radius vt, $\overline{Tetr}_{n+1}(0, vt)$ – its boundary.

THEOREM 1.3.– *For a Markov random evolutionary process in R^n with a cyclical change in the direction of movement, the following relations are true:*

$$P(S(t) \in Tetr_{n+1}(0, vt)) = 1,$$

$$P(S(t) \in \overline{Tetr}_{n+1}(0, vt)) = e^{-\lambda t}\left(1 + \frac{\lambda t}{1!} + \cdots + \frac{(\lambda t)^{n-1}}{(n-1)!}\right),$$

$$P(S(t) \in (Tetr_{n+1}(0, vt) - \overline{Tetr}_{n+1}(0, vt))) = 1 - e^{-\lambda t}\left(1 + \frac{\lambda t}{1!} + \ldots + \frac{(\lambda t)^{n-1}}{(n-1)!}\right).$$

For the evolutionary process with a uniform change of directions:

$$P(S(t) \in Tetr_{n+1}(0, vt)) = 1,$$

$$P(S(t) \in \overline{Tetr}_{n+1}(0, vt)) = ne^{-\lambda t}\left(\frac{1-n}{n} + e^{\frac{\lambda t}{n}}\right),$$

$$P(S(t) \in (Tetr_{n+1}(0, vt) - \overline{Tetr}_{n+1}(0, vt))) = 1 - ne^{-\lambda t}\left(\frac{1-n}{n} + e^{\frac{\lambda t}{n}}\right).$$

PROOF.– Consider the case of the space R^2. The first ratio in both cases follows from the results of Orsingher and Kolesnik (1994). The last ratio is an obvious consequence of the previous two. Therefore, it is necessary to prove only the second relation.

The probability that the evolutionary process will end up at the top of the triangle is equal to the probability that the evolution during time t will not change the direction of movement, and is equal to $e^{-\lambda t}$.

The sides of a triangle are sets of vector ends $vtk\overline{\tau}_0 + vt(1-k)\overline{\tau}_1, vtk\overline{\tau}_1 + vt(1-k)\overline{\tau}_2, vtk\overline{\tau}_2 + vt(1-k)\overline{\tau}_0, 0 \leq k \leq 1$. At the same time, if one more vector is added to any of the sums, the end of the sum-vector will not belong to the side of the triangle.

Thus, in the case of a cyclical change of directions, only $S(t) = vt_0\overline{\tau}_0 + vt_1\overline{\tau}_1 = vt_0\overline{\tau}_0 + v(t-t_0)\overline{\tau}_1$, $S(t) = vt_0\overline{\tau}_1 + v(t-t_0)\overline{\tau}_2$ or $S(t) = vt_0\overline{\tau}_2 + v(t-t_0)\overline{\tau}_0$, respectively, will belong to the side of the triangle. The probability of one change in the direction of movement during time t is equal to $e^{-\lambda t}\frac{\lambda t}{1!}$. We have $P(S(t) \in \overline{Tp_3}(0, vt)) = e^{-\lambda t}(1 + \frac{\lambda t}{1!})$.

In the case of uniform evolution, sums of the form belong to the sides of the triangle: $S(t) = vt_0\overline{\tau}_0 + vt_1\overline{\tau}_1 + vt_2\overline{\tau}_0 + vt_3\overline{\tau}_1 + \ldots$, i.e. evolutionary process moves in the time interval t in only two of three possible directions. The probability of this event is equal to $e^{-\lambda t}\frac{\lambda t}{1!} + e^{-\lambda t}\frac{1}{2}\frac{(\lambda t)^2}{2!} + \cdots + e^{-\lambda t}\frac{1}{2^{n-1}}\frac{(\lambda t)^n}{n!} + \ldots$. Then, $P(S(t) \in \overline{Tetr_3}(0, vt)) = e^{-\lambda t}(1 + \frac{\lambda t}{1!} + \frac{1}{2}\frac{(\lambda t)^2}{2!} + \cdots + \frac{1}{2^{n-1}}\frac{(\lambda t)^n}{n!} + \ldots) = 2e^{-\lambda t}(-\frac{1}{2} + e^{\frac{\lambda t}{2}})$.

Note that $(1 + \frac{\lambda t}{1!} + \frac{1}{2}\frac{(\lambda t)^2}{2!} + \cdots + \frac{1}{2^{n-1}}\frac{(\lambda t)^n}{n!} + \ldots) < e^{\lambda t}$, thus $P(S(t) \in \overline{Tetr_3}(0, vt)) < 1$, $P(S(0) \in \overline{Tetr_3}(0, 0)) = 1$.

In the case of the R^n space, the one-dimensional faces of the $n+1$-hedron are defined by the sum of two vectors, as in the previous case; two-dimensional faces are the sum of three vectors; $n-1$-dimensional faces are the sum of n vectors. Writing similar ratios to the previous ones, we will have:

– for a cyclical change of movement directions $P(S(t) \in \overline{Tetr_{n+1}}(0, vt)) = e^{-\lambda t}(1 + \frac{\lambda t}{1!} + \cdots + \frac{(\lambda t)^{n-1}}{(n-1)!})$;

– for a uniform change in the direction of movement $P(S(t) \in \overline{Tetr_{n+1}}(0, vt)) = e^{-\lambda t}(1 + \frac{\lambda t}{1!} + \frac{1}{n}\frac{(\lambda t)^2}{2!} + \cdots + \frac{1}{n^{k-1}}\frac{(\lambda t)^k}{k!} + \ldots) = ne^{-\lambda t}(\frac{1-n}{n} + e^{\frac{\lambda t}{n}})$.

The theorem is proven.

It is also interesting to study the probabilities of getting into some limited area which lies inside the front of the evolutionary process. The answer to this question in the case of the space R^1 is given by the following theorem.

THEOREM 1.4.– *In the case of evolutionary process in R^1, the probability to get to some point of the segment $[-vs, vs]$, $s < t$, in time t is equal to:*

$$F(s,t) = e^{-\frac{3}{2}\lambda t}\left[\left(\frac{\lambda t}{1!} + \frac{(\lambda t)^2}{2!}\right)\frac{e^{\frac{s}{2}\lambda} - e^{-\frac{s}{2}\lambda}}{1 - e^{-\lambda t}} + \left(\frac{(\lambda t)^3}{3!} + \frac{(\lambda t)^4}{4!}\right) \times\right.$$

$$\frac{e^{\frac{s}{2}\lambda}(1 + \lambda\frac{t-s}{2}) - e^{-\frac{s}{2}\lambda}(1 + \lambda\frac{t+s}{2})}{1 - e^{-\lambda t}(1 + \lambda t)} + \cdots + \left(\frac{(\lambda t)^{2k+1}}{(2k+1)!} + \frac{(\lambda t)^{2k+2}}{(2k+2)!}\right) \times$$

$$\left.\frac{e^{\frac{s}{2}\lambda}(1 + \lambda\frac{t-s}{2} + \cdots + (\lambda\frac{t-s}{2})^k\frac{1}{k!}) - e^{-\frac{s}{2}\lambda}(1 + \lambda\frac{t+s}{2} + \cdots + (\lambda\frac{t+s}{2})^k\frac{1}{k!})}{1 - e^{-\lambda t}(1 + \lambda t + \cdots + \frac{(\lambda t)^k}{k!})} + \cdots\right]. \quad [1.4]$$

Note that if $s = t - 0$, we have $F(t-0,t) = 1 - e^{-\lambda t} = P(S(t) < vt)$.

PROOF.– If no change of direction occurs during time t movement, then at the moment t, the evolutionary process is at the point vt or $-vt$ which do not belong to the segment $[-vs, vs]$.

If there was one change in the direction of movement, then we have $S(t) = v(\theta_1 - \theta_2)$, where $\theta_2 = t - \theta_1, \theta_1 < t$ exponentially distributed with parameter λ. Let us find out when $S(t) \in [-vs, vs]$. We have $-vs \leq S(t) \leq vs; -s \leq \theta_1 - \theta_2 \leq s; -s \leq \theta_1 - (t - \theta_1) \leq s$, where $\frac{t-s}{2} \leq \theta_1 \leq \frac{t+s}{2}$.

The probability of this event is $P(\frac{t-s}{2} \leq \theta_1 \leq \frac{t+s}{2} | \theta_1 < t) = \frac{e^{-\frac{t-s}{2}\lambda} - e^{-\frac{t+s}{2}\lambda}}{1 - e^{-\lambda t}}$.

Similarly, in the case of two changes of direction.

If there were $2k+1$ or $2k+2$ changes in the direction of movement, then: $S(t) = v(\theta_1 - \theta_2 + \cdots - \theta_{2k+2})$, where $\theta_{2k+2} = t - \theta_1 - \cdots - \theta_{2k+1}$, the rest $\theta_i < t, i = \overline{1, 2k+1}$, and are exponentially distributed with a parameter λ. We have $-vs \leq S(t) \leq vs$, from where $\frac{t-s}{2} \leq (\theta_1 + \theta_3 + \cdots + \theta_{2k+1}) \leq \frac{t+s}{2}$, where $(\theta_1 + \theta_3 + \cdots + \theta_{2k+1})$ has an Erlang distribution with parameters k, λ.

Now, using the full probability formula, we obtain [1.4].

The theorem is proven.

1.2. Moments of evolutionary process

In this section, we find the moments of a multidimensional homogeneous alternating process and, accordingly, the moments of the Markov random evolutionary process in R^n. In the following, these moments are used to find the solution of hyperparabolic equations, which are satisfied by the functions from the evolutionary process.

Let us first consider the case of the space R^1. Let the initial distribution of $\xi(t)$ be: $P(\xi(0)=0)=p$, $P(\xi(0)=1)=q, p+q=1, p-q=r$.

THEOREM 1.5.– *Moments of the telegraphic process are equal*

$$E[(-1)^{\xi(u_1)}\dots(-1)^{\xi(u_k)}]=\begin{cases} re^{-2\lambda(u_k+u_{k-2}+\dots+u_1-u_{k-1}-u_{k-3}-\dots-u_2)}, k=2n+1\\ e^{-2\lambda(u_k+u_{k-2}+\dots+u_2-u_{k-1}-u_{k-3}-\dots-u_1)}, k=2n,\end{cases}$$

where $u_1<\dots<u_k$.

PROOF.–

$$E[(-1)^{\xi(u_1)}\dots(-1)^{\xi(u_k)}]=p\sum_{n_1=0}^{\infty}(-1)^{n_1}P(\xi(u_1)=n_1)\sum_{n_2=n_1}^{\infty}(-1)^{n_2}\times$$

$$P(\xi(u_2-u_1)=n_2-n_1)\cdots\sum_{n_{k-1}=n_{k-2}}^{\infty}(-1)^{n_{k-1}}P(\xi(u_{k-1}-u_{k-2})=n_{k-1}-n_{k-2})\times$$

$$\sum_{n_k=n_{k-1}}^{\infty}(-1)^{n_k}P(\xi(u_k-u_{k-1})=n_k-n_{k-1})+q\sum_{n_1=0}^{\infty}(-1)(-1)^{n_1}P(\xi(u_1)=n_1)\times$$

$$\sum_{n_2=n_1}^{\infty}(-1)(-1)^{n_2}P(\xi(u_2-u_1)=n_2-n_1)\cdots\sum_{n_{k-1}=n_{k-2}}^{\infty}(-1)(-1)^{n_{k-1}}\times$$

$P(\xi(u_{k-1}-u_{k-2})=n_{k-1}-n_{k-2})\sum_{n_k=n_{k-1}}^{\infty}(-1)\ (-1)^{n_k}P(\xi(u_k-u_{k-1})=n_k-n_{k-1})=p\sum_{n_1=0}^{\infty}(-1)^{n_1}P(\xi(u_1)=n_1)\sum_{n_2=n_1}^{\infty}(-1)^{n_2}P(\xi(u_2-u_1)=n_2-$

$$n_1)\cdots\sum_{n_{k-1}=n_{k-2}}^{\infty}(-1)^{n_{k-1}}P(\xi(u_{k-1}-u_{k-2})=n_{k-1}-n_{k-2})(-1)^{n_{k-1}}\times$$

$$e^{-2\lambda(u_k-u_{k-1})}+(-1)^kq\sum_{n_1=0}^{\infty}(-1)^{n_1}P(\xi(u_1)=n_1)\sum_{n_2=n_1}^{\infty}(-1)^{n_2}P(\xi(u_2-u_1)=n_2-$$

$$n_1)\dots\sum_{n_{k-1}=n_{k-2}}^{\infty}(-1)^{n_{k-1}}P(\xi(u_{k-1}-u_{k-2})=n_{k-1}-n_{k-2})(-1)^{n_{k-1}}e^{-2\lambda(u_k-u_{k-1})}=$$

$pe^{-2\lambda(u_k-u_{k-1})}\sum_{n_1=0}^{\infty}(-1)^{n_1}P(\xi(u_1)=n_1)\sum_{n_2=n_1}^{\infty}(-1)^{n_2}P(\xi(u_2-u_1)=n_2-n_1)\cdots\sum_{n_{k-1}=n_{k-2}}^{\infty}(-1)^{2n_{k-1}}P(\xi(u_{k-1}-u_{k-2})=n_{k-1}-n_{k-2})+$

$(-1)^k q e^{-2\lambda(u_k-u_{k-1})} \sum_{n_1=0}^{\infty}(-1)^{n_1} P(\xi(u_1) = n_1) \sum_{n_2=n_1}^{\infty}(-1)^{n_2} P(\xi(u_2 - u_1) = n_2 - n_1) \cdots \sum_{n_{k-1}=n_{k-2}}^{\infty}(-1)^{2n_{k-1}} P(\xi(u_{k-1} - u_{k-2}) = n_{k-1} - n_{k-2}) =$

$\cdots = pe^{-\lambda[2(u_k-u_{k-1})+2(u_{k-2}-u_{k-3})+\cdots+(1-(-1)^k)u_1]}+$

$(-1)^k q e^{-\lambda[2(u_k-u_{k-1})+2(u_{k-2}-u_{k-3})]} \ldots e^{-\lambda[(1-(-1)^k)u_1]} =$

$$\begin{cases} re^{-2\lambda(u_k+u_{k-2}+\cdots+u_1-u_{k-1}-u_{k-3}-\cdots-u_2)}, k = 2n+1 \\ e^{-2\lambda(u_k+u_{k-2}+\cdots+u_2-u_{k-1}-u_{k-3}-\cdots-u_1)}, k = 2n, \end{cases}$$

The theorem is proven.

EXAMPLE 1.1.– *Using the transition probability matrix* [1.3], *we have:*

1) $E[(-1)^{\xi(t)}] = 1(p(\frac{1}{2} + \frac{1}{2}e^{-2\lambda t}) + q(\frac{1}{2} - \frac{1}{2}e^{-2\lambda t})) + (-1)(p(\frac{1}{2} - \frac{1}{2}e^{-2\lambda t}) + q(\frac{1}{2} + \frac{1}{2}e^{-2\lambda t})) = \frac{1}{2} + \frac{1}{2}re^{-2\lambda t} - \frac{1}{2} + \frac{1}{2}re^{-2\lambda t} = re^{-2\lambda t}$,

2) $E[(-1)^{\xi(u)}(-1)^{\xi(t)}] = 1(p(\frac{1}{2}+\frac{1}{2}e^{-2\lambda u})+q(\frac{1}{2}-\frac{1}{2}e^{-2\lambda u}))[1(\frac{1}{2}+\frac{1}{2}e^{-2\lambda(t-u)})+(-1)(\frac{1}{2}-\frac{1}{2}e^{-2\lambda(t-u)})](-1)(p(\frac{1}{2}-\frac{1}{2}e^{-2\lambda u})+q(\frac{1}{2}+\frac{1}{2}e^{-2\lambda u}))[1(\frac{1}{2}-\frac{1}{2}e^{-2\lambda(t-u)})+(-1)(\frac{1}{2}+\frac{1}{2}e^{-2\lambda(t-u)})] = (\frac{1}{2}+\frac{1}{2}re^{-2\lambda u})[e^{-2\lambda(t-u)}]-(\frac{1}{2}-\frac{1}{2}re^{-2\lambda u})[-e^{-2\lambda(t-u)}] = e^{-2\lambda(t-u)}, t > u$.

THEOREM 1.6.– *Moments of the Markov random evolutionary process in* R^1 *satisfy the recurrence relations:*

$$m_{2k}(v,\lambda,t) = E\left(v\int_0^t(-1)^{\xi(u)}du\right)^{2k} = 2kv\int_0^t e^{-2\lambda u_{2k}} \frac{m_{2k-1}(v,-\lambda,u_{2k})}{r} du_{2k},$$

$$m_{2k+1}(v,\lambda,t) = E\left(v\int_0^t(-1)^{\xi(u)}du\right)^{2k+1} = (2k+1)rv\int_0^t e^{-2\lambda u_{2k+1}} \times$$

$$m_{2k}(v,-\lambda,u_{2k+1})du_{2k+1},$$

where $m_0(v,\lambda,t) = 1$.

PROOF.– Using the methods proposed in Kac (1957) and the relations established in the previous theorem, we find

$$E\left(v\int_0^t(-1)^{\xi(u)}du\right)^k = k!v^k\int_0^t\cdots\int_0^{u_2} E\left[(-1)^{\xi(u_1)}\ldots(-1)^{\xi(u_k)}\right]du_1\ldots du_k =$$

$$= \begin{cases} k!v^k\int_0^t\cdots\int_0^{u_2} re^{-2\lambda(u_k+u_{k-2}+\cdots+u_1-u_{k-1}-u_{k-3}-\cdots-u_2)}du_1\ldots du_k, k = 2n+1 \\ k!v^k\int_0^t\cdots\int_0^{u_2} e^{-2\lambda(u_k+u_{k-2}+\cdots+u_2-u_{k-1}-u_{k-3}-\cdots-u_1)}du_1\ldots du_k, k = 2n, \end{cases}$$

$$= \begin{cases} (2n+1)!v^{2n+1}\int_0^t\ldots\int_0^{u_2} re^{-2\lambda(u_{2n+1}+u_{2n-1}+\cdots+u_1-u_{2n}-u_{2n-2}-\cdots-u_2)}du_1\ldots du_{2n+1} \\ (2n)!v^{2n}\int_0^t\cdots\int_0^{u_2} e^{-2\lambda(u_{2n}+u_{2n-2}+\cdots+u_2-u_{2n-1}-u_{2n-3}-\cdots-u_1)}du_1\ldots du_{2n} \end{cases}$$

$$= \begin{cases} m_{2n+1}(v, \lambda, t) \\ m_{2n}(v, \lambda, t) \end{cases}$$

Obviously,

$m_{2n+1}(v, \lambda, t) = (2n+1)! v^{2n+1} \int_0^t \cdots \int_0^{u_2} r e^{-2\lambda(u_{2n+1}+\cdots+u_1-u_{2n}-\cdots-u_2)} du_1 \ldots du_{2n+1} = (2n+1)! r v^{2n+1} \int_0^t e^{-2\lambda u_{2n+1}} \int_0^{u_{2n+1}} \cdots \int_0^{u_2} e^{-2\lambda(u_{2n-1}+\cdots+u_1-u_{2n}-\cdots-u_2)} du_1 \ldots du_{2n+1} = (2n+1)! r v^{2n+1} \int_0^t e^{-2\lambda u_{2n+1}} \int_0^{u_{2n+1}} \cdots \int_0^{u_2} e^{2\lambda(u_{2n}+\cdots+u_2-u_{2n-1}-\cdots-u_1)} du_1 du_2 \ldots du_{2n+1} = (2n+1) r v \int_0^t e^{-2\lambda u_{2n+1}} m_{2n}(v, -\lambda, u_{2n+1}) du_{2n+1}$, and $m_1(v, \lambda, t) = E(v \int_0^t (-1)^{\xi(u_1)} du_1) = rv \int_0^t e^{-2\lambda u_1} du_1$, thus we put $m_0(v, \lambda, t) = 1$.

By analogy,

$m_{2n}(v, \lambda, t) = (2n)! v^{2n} \int_0^t \cdots \int_0^{u_2} e^{-2\lambda(u_{2n}+\cdots+u_2-u_{2n-1}-\cdots-u_1)} du_1 \ldots du_{2n} = (2n)! v^{2n} \int_0^t e^{-2\lambda u_{2n}} \int_0^{u_{2n}} \cdots \int_0^{u_2} e^{-2\lambda(u_{2n-2}+\cdots+u_2-u_{2n-1}-\cdots-u_1)} du_1 \ldots du_{2n} = (2n)! v^{2n} \int_0^t e^{-2\lambda u_{2n}} \int_0^{u_{2n}} \cdots \int_0^{u_2} e^{2\lambda(u_{2n-1}+\cdots+u_1-u_{2n-2}-\cdots-u_2)} du_1 \ldots du_{2n} = 2nv \int_0^t e^{-2\lambda u_{2n}} \frac{m_{2n-1}(v, -\lambda, u_{2n})}{r} du_{2n}$.

The theorem is proven.

EXAMPLE 1.2.–

$$E\left(v \int_0^t (-1)^{\xi(u)} du\right) = vr \int_0^t e^{-2\lambda u} du = r\frac{v}{2\lambda}(1 - e^{-2\lambda t}),$$

$$E\left(v \int_0^t (-1)^{\xi(u)} du\right)^2 = 2v \int_0^t e^{-2\lambda u} \left(-\frac{v}{2\lambda}(1 - e^{2\lambda u})\right) du - \frac{v^2}{2\lambda^2}(1 - e^{-2\lambda t}) + \frac{v^2}{\lambda} t.$$

In the following, we will consider functions from Markov random evolutionary processes of the form $u(x, t) = Ef(x + v \int_0^t (-1)^{\xi(u)} du)$, where the conditions on the function f are given below. In the case $f(x) = x^k$, we have:

$$k = 1 : u(x, t) = E\left(x + v \int_0^t (-1)^{\xi(u)} du\right) = x + r\frac{v}{2\lambda}(1 - e^{-2\lambda t})$$

$$k = 2 : u(x, t) = E\left(x + v \int_0^t (-1)^{\xi(u)} du\right)^2 = E(x^2 + 2xv \times$$

$$\int_0^t (-1)^{\xi(u)} du + v^2 \left[\int_0^t (-1)^{\xi(u)} du\right]^2\Bigg) = x^2 + 2xr\frac{v}{2\lambda}(1 - e^{-2\lambda t}) +$$

$$\frac{v^2}{\lambda} t - \frac{v^2}{2\lambda^2}(1 - e^{-2\lambda t}) = x^2 + \frac{v^2}{\lambda} t + \left(xr\frac{v}{\lambda} - \frac{v^2}{2\lambda^2}\right)(1 - e^{-2\lambda t}),$$

$$k > 2 : u(x, t) = E\left(x + v \int_0^t (-1)^{\xi(u)} du\right)^k = \sum_{i=0}^{k} C_k^i x^i m_{k-i}(v, \lambda, t) \quad [1.5]$$

by Newton's binomial formula.

EMARK 1.2.– *Passing the hydrodynamic limit (Kac 1957; Korolyuk and Turbin 993) in relations* [1.5]*: $v \to \infty$, $\lambda \to \infty$, $\frac{v^2}{\lambda} \to \sigma^2$, we obtain the moments of the Viener process: $x, x^2 + \sigma^2 t, \dots$*

Let us move on to the study of the multidimensional case: Markov random volutionary processes in R^n. In order to write the corresponding moments, we use ansition probability matrices [1.2] and [1.3]. We have $n+1$ possible directions of novement, which are specified by vectors $\overline{\tau}_0, \dots, \overline{\tau}_n$. Let the initial direction of novement have the distribution $P(\xi(0) = 0) = r_0, \dots, P(\xi(0) = n) = r_n$. A nultivariate alternating process at time t has a value $\overline{\tau}_{\xi(t)} = (\tau^{(1)}_{\xi(t)}, \dots, \tau^{(n)}_{\xi(t)})$. Let us nd the moments of each individual component of the vector.

The moments of a multidimensional homogeneous alternating process with a niform change in the directions of motion have the following form, provided that ney begin in the direction $\overline{\tau}_0$ $(i = \overline{1,n})$:

$$m_0^{(i)}(u_1) = E[\tau^{(i)}_{\xi(u_1)}] = \left[\tau_0^{(i)}\left(\frac{1}{n+1} + \frac{n}{n+1}e^{-\frac{n+1}{n}\lambda u_1}\right) + \dots + \tau_n^{(i)} \times \left(\frac{1}{n+1} - \frac{1}{n+1}e^{-\frac{n+1}{n}\lambda u_1}\right)\right] = \left[\frac{1}{n+1}(\tau_0^{(i)} + \dots + \tau_n^{(i)}) + \tau_0^{(i)} e^{-\frac{n+1}{n}\lambda u_1}\right] = \tau_0^{(i)} e^{-\frac{n+1}{n}\lambda u_1},$$

s soon as the sum $\tau_0^{(i)} + \dots + \tau_n^{(i)} = 0, i = \overline{0,n}$.

In the case when the initial direction of movement is i-th with probability $r_i, \sum_{i=0}^n r_i = 1$, we have: $E[\tau^{(i)}_{\xi(u_1)}] = \sum_{j=0}^n r_j \tau_j^{(i)} e^{-\lambda u_1 \frac{n+1}{n}} = \sum_{j=0}^n r_j m_j^{(i)}(u_1)$.

For the mixed moment, we have:

$$E\left[\tau^{(i_1)}_{\xi(u_1)} \tau^{(i_2)}_{\xi(u_2)}\right] = r_0 \sum_{n_1=0}^{\infty} \tau_{n_1}^{(i_1)} P(\xi(u_1) = n_1) \sum_{n_2=n_1}^{\infty} \tau_{n_2}^{(i_2)} P(\xi(u_2 - u_1) = n_2 - n_1) + \dots + r_n \sum_{n_1=n}^{\infty} \tau_{n_1}^{(i_1)} P(\xi(u_1) = n_1) \sum_{n_2=n_1}^{\infty} \tau_{n_2}^{(i_2)} P(\xi(u_2 - u_1) = n_2 - n_1) = r_0 \times \sum_{n_1=0}^{\infty} \tau_{n_1}^{(i_1)} P(\xi(u_1) = n_1) m_{n_1}^{(i_2)}(u_2 - u_1) + \dots + r_n \sum_{n_1=n}^{\infty} \tau_{n_1}^{(i_1)} P(\xi(u_1) = n_1) \times m_{n_1}^{(i_2)}(u_2 - u_1) = \sum_{j=0}^{n} r_j m_j^{(i_1,i_2)}(u_1, u_2 - u_1).$$

From here, by induction, we conclude that:

$$E\left[\tau^{(i_1)}_{\xi(u_1)}\cdots\tau^{(i_k)}_{\xi(u_k)}\right]=\sum_{j=0}^{n} r_j m_j^{(i_1,\ldots,i_k)}(u_1,u_2-u_1,\ldots,u_k-u_{k-1})=\sum_{j=0}^{n} r_j\times$$

$$\sum_{n_1=j}^{\infty}\tau^{(i_1)}_{n_1}P(\xi(u_1)=n_1)m^{(i_2,\ldots,i_k)}_{n_1}(u_2-u_1,\ldots,u_k-u_{k-1}).$$

With a cyclical change: ($i=\overline{1,n}$):

$$m_0^{(i)}(u_1)=E[\tau^{(i)}_{\xi(u_1)}]=\tau_0^{(i)}e^{-\lambda u_1}ch_{n+1,0}(\lambda u_1)+\cdots+\tau_n^{(i)}e^{-\lambda u_1}ch_{n+1,1}(\lambda u_1)=$$

$$\left[\tau_0^{(i)}\frac{e^{-\lambda u_1}}{n+1}\{e^{\lambda u_1}+e^{\omega_{n+1}\lambda u_1}+\cdots+e^{\omega_{n+1}^n\lambda u_1}\}+\cdots+\tau_n^{(i)}\frac{e^{-\lambda u_1}}{n+1}\{\lambda e^{\lambda u_1}+\cdots+\right.$$

$$\left.\lambda\omega_{n+1}^n e^{\omega_{n+1}^n\lambda u_1}\}\right]=\frac{1}{n+1}[\tau_0^{(i)}\{1+e^{(\omega_{n+1}-1)\lambda u_1}+\ldots+e^{(\omega_{n+1}^n-1)\lambda u_1}\}+\ldots+\tau_n^{(i)}\{\lambda+$$

$$\cdots+\lambda\omega_{n+1}^n e^{(\omega_{n+1}^n-1)\lambda u_1}\}]=\frac{1}{n+1}[\{1+e^{(\omega_{n+1}-1)\lambda u_1}+\cdots+e^{(\omega_{n+1}^n-1)\lambda u_1}\}\tau_0^{(i)}+$$

$$\{\lambda+\lambda\omega_{n+1}e^{(\omega_{n+1}-1)\lambda u_1}+\cdots+\lambda\omega_{n+1}^n e^{(\omega_{n+1}^n-1)\lambda u_1}\}\tau_n^{(i)}+\cdots+\{\lambda^n+\lambda^n\omega_{n+1}^n\times$$

$$e^{(\omega_{n+1}-1)\lambda u_1}+\cdots+\lambda^n\omega_{n+1}^{n^2}e^{(\omega_{n+1}^n-1)\lambda u_1}\}\tau_1^{(i)}].$$

In the case where the initial direction of movement is i-th with probability $r_i, \sum_{i=0}^n r_i=1$, we have:

$$E[\tau^{(i)}_{\xi(u_1)}]=[\tau_0^{(i)}(r_0e^{-\lambda u_1}ch_{n+1,0}(\lambda u_1)+\cdots+r_ne^{-\lambda u_1}ch_{n+1,n}(\lambda u_1))]+\cdots+[\tau_n^{(i)}\times$$

$$(r_0e^{-\lambda u_1}ch_{n+1,1}(\lambda u_1)+\cdots+r_ne^{-\lambda u_1}ch_{n+1,0}(\lambda u_1)]=\left[\tau_0^{(i)}\frac{e^{-\lambda u_1}}{n+1}(r_0\{e^{\lambda u_1}+e^{\omega_{n+1}\lambda u_1}+\right.$$

$$\cdots+e^{\omega_{n+1}^n\lambda u_1}\}+\cdots+r_n\{\lambda^n e^{\lambda u_1}+\cdots+\lambda^n\omega_{n+1}^{n^2}e^{\omega_{n+1}^n\lambda u_1}\})+\cdots+\tau_n^{(i)}\frac{e^{-\lambda u_1}}{n+1}(r_0\times$$

$$\left.\{\lambda e^{\lambda u_1}+\cdots+\lambda\omega_{n+1}^n e^{\omega_{n+1}^n\lambda u_1}\}+\cdots+r_n\{e^{\lambda u_1}+\cdots+e^{\omega_{n+1}^n\lambda u_1}\})\right]=\frac{1}{n+1}[\tau_0^{(i)}(r_0\{1+$$

$$e^{(\omega_{n+1}-1)\lambda u_1}+\cdots+e^{(\omega_{n+1}^n-1)\lambda u_1}\}+\cdots+r_n\{\lambda^n+\cdots+\lambda^n\omega_{n+1}^{n^2}e^{(\omega_{n+1}^n-1)\lambda u_1}\})+$$

$$\cdots+\tau_n^{(i)}(r_0\{\lambda+\cdots+\lambda\omega_{n+1}^n e^{(\omega_{n+1}^n-1)\lambda u_1}\}+\cdots+r_n\{1+\cdots+e^{(\omega_{n+1}^n-1)\lambda u_1}\})]=\frac{1}{n+1}\times$$

$$[\{1+e^{(\omega_{n+1}-1)\lambda u_1}+\cdots+e^{(\omega_{n+1}^n-1)\lambda u_1}\}(r_0\tau_0^{(i)}+r_1\tau_1^{(i)}+\cdots+r_n\tau_n^{(i)})+\{\lambda+$$

$$\lambda\omega_{n+1}e^{(\omega_{n+1}-1)\lambda u_1}+\cdots+\lambda\omega_{n+1}^n e^{(\omega_{n+1}^n-1)\lambda u_1}\}(r_0\tau_n^{(i)}+r_1\tau_0^{(i)}+\cdots+r_n\tau_{n-1}^{(i)})+\cdots+$$

$$\{\lambda^n+\lambda^n\omega_{n+1}^n e^{(\omega_{n+1}-1)\lambda u_1}+\cdots+\lambda^n\omega_{n+1}^{n^2}e^{(\omega_{n+1}^n-1)\lambda u_1}\}(r_0\tau_1^{(i)}+r_1\tau_2^{(i)}+\cdots+r_n\tau_0^{(i)})]=$$

$$\sum_{j=0}^{n} r_j m_j^{(i)}(u_1),$$

from where, like above,

$$E\left[\tau^{(i_1)}_{\xi(u_1)}\cdots\tau^{(i_k)}_{\xi(u_k)}\right]=\sum_{j=0}^{n}r_j m_j^{(i_1,\ldots,i_k)}(u_1,u_2-u_1,\ldots,u_k-u_{k-1})=\sum_{j=0}^{n}r_j\times$$

$$\sum_{n_1=j}^{\infty}\tau^{(i_1)}_{n_1}P(\xi(u_1)=n_1)m_{n_1}^{(i_2,\ldots,i_k)}(u_2-u_1,\ldots,u_k-u_{k-1}).$$

From these ratios, using the method from Kac (1957), we deduce the following theorem.

THEOREM 1.7.– *Moments of a multidimensional alternating process have the form:*

$$E\left[\tau^{(i_1)}_{\xi(u_1)}\cdots\tau^{(i_k)}_{\xi(u_k)}\right]=\sum_{j=0}^{n}r_j m_j^{(i_1,\ldots,i_k)}(u_1,u_2-u_1,\ldots,u_k-u_{k-1})=\sum_{j=0}^{n}r_j\times$$

$$\sum_{n_1=j}^{\infty}\tau^{(i_1)}_{n_1}P(\xi(u_1)=n_1)m_{n_1}^{(i_2,\ldots,i_k)}(u_2-u_1,\ldots,u_k-u_{k-1}), \qquad [1.6]$$

where in the case of uniform change in the direction of movement:

$$m_j^{(i)}(u_1)=\tau_j^{(i)}e^{-\frac{n+1}{n}\lambda u_1}.$$

With the cyclic change:

$$m_j^{(i)}(u_1)=\frac{1}{n+1}[\{1+e^{(\omega_{n+1}-1)\lambda u_1}+\cdots+e^{(\omega_{n+1}^n-1)\lambda u_1}\}\tau_j^{(i)}+\{\lambda+$$

$$+\lambda\omega_{n+1}e^{(\omega_{n+1}-1)\lambda u_1}+\cdots+\lambda\omega_{n+1}^n e^{(\omega_{n+1}^n-1)\lambda u_1}\}\tau_{j+n}^{(i)}+\cdots+$$

$$+\{\lambda^n+\lambda^n\omega_{n+1}^n e^{(\omega_{n+1}-1)\lambda u_1}+\cdots+\lambda^n\omega_{n+1}^{n^2}e^{(\omega_{n+1}^n-1)\lambda u_1}\}\tau_{j+1}^{(i)}].$$

The moments of the Markov random evolutionary process in R^n have the form:

– with the uniform change of direction of movement

$$E\left(v\int_0^t\tau^{(i)}_{\xi(u)}du\right)=-v\left[\frac{n}{n+1}\frac{1}{\lambda}\right](\tau_0^{(i)}r_0+\ldots+\tau_n^{(i)}r_n)(e^{-\frac{n+1}{n}\lambda t}-1), \quad [1.7]$$

$$\ldots$$

$$E\left(v\int_0^t\tau^{(1)}_{\xi(u_1)}du_1\right)^{k_1}\cdots\left(v\int_0^t\tau^{(n)}_{\xi(u_n)}du_n\right)^{k_n}=v^{k_1+\cdots+k_n}\times$$

$$\sum\int_0^t\int_0^{\theta_2}\cdots\int_0^{\theta_{k_1+\cdots+k_n}}E[\tau^{(1)}_{\xi(\theta_1)}\cdots\tau^{(n)}_{\xi(\theta_{k_1+\cdots+k_n})}]d\theta_1\ldots d\theta_{k_1+\cdots+k_n},$$

$$0\le\theta_1<\cdots<\theta_{k_1+\cdots+k_n}\le t,$$

where the sum is taken over all possible permutations of $\tau_j^{(i)}$ ($(k_1+\cdots+k_n)!$ in total);

– *with the cyclic change of direction of movement*

$$E\left(v\int_0^t \tau_{\xi(u)}^{(i)}du\right) = \frac{v}{n+1}\left[\left\{t+\frac{1}{(\omega_{n+1}-1)\lambda}(e^{(\omega_{n+1}-1)\lambda t}-1)+\cdots+\right.\right.$$
$$\left.\frac{1}{(\omega_{n+1}^n-1)\lambda}(e^{(\omega_{n+1}^n-1)\lambda t}-1)\right\}(r_0\tau_0^{(i)}+r_1\tau_1^{(i)}+\cdots+r_n\tau_n^{(i)})+\left\{\lambda t+\frac{\lambda\omega_{n+1}}{(\omega_{n+1}-1)\lambda}\times\right.$$
$$\left.(e^{(\omega_{n+1}-1)\lambda t}-1)+\cdots+\frac{\lambda\omega_{n+1}^n}{(\omega_{n+1}^n-1)\lambda}(e^{(\omega_{n+1}^n-1)\lambda t}-1)\right\}(r_0\tau_n^{(i)}+r_1\tau_0^{(i)}+$$
$$\cdots+r_n\tau_{n-1}^{(i)})+\cdots+\left\{\lambda^n t+\frac{\lambda^n\omega_{n+1}^n}{(\omega_{n+1}-1)\lambda}(e^{(\omega_{n+1}-1)\lambda t}-1)+\cdots+\right.$$
$$\left.\left.\frac{\lambda^n\omega_{n+1}^{n^2}}{(\omega_{n+1}^n-1)\lambda}(e^{(\omega_{n+1}^n-1)\lambda t}-1)\right\}(r_0\tau_1^{(i)}+r_1\tau_2^{(i)}+\cdots+r_n\tau_0^{(i)})\right], \qquad [1.8]$$

...

$$E\left(v\int_0^t \tau_{\xi(u_1)}^{(1)}du_1\right)^{k_1}\cdots\left(v\int_0^t \tau_{\xi(u_n)}^{(n)}du_n\right)^{k_n} = v^{k_1+\cdots+k_n}\times$$
$$\sum\int_0^t\int_0^{\theta_2}\cdots\int_0^{\theta_{k_1+\cdots+k_n}} E[\tau_{\xi(\theta_1)}^{(1)}\cdots\tau_{\xi(\theta_{k_1+\cdots+k_n})}^{(n)}]d\theta_1\ldots d\theta_{k_1+\cdots+k_n},$$
$$0\le\theta_1<\cdots<\theta_{k_1+\cdots+k_n}\le t,$$

where the sum is taken over all possible permutations of $\tau_j^{(i)}$ *(*$(k_1+\cdots+k_n)!$ *in total).*

The integral expressions are found according to the formula [1.6].

EXAMPLE 1.3.– $n=2$

1) $P(t) = \begin{pmatrix} \frac{1}{3}+\frac{2}{3}e^{-\frac{3}{2}\lambda t} & \frac{1}{3}-\frac{1}{3}e^{-\frac{3}{2}\lambda t} & \frac{1}{3}-\frac{1}{3}e^{-\frac{3}{2}\lambda t} \\ \frac{1}{3}-\frac{1}{3}e^{-\frac{3}{2}\lambda t} & \frac{1}{3}+\frac{2}{3}e^{-\frac{3}{2}\lambda t} & \frac{1}{3}-\frac{1}{3}e^{-\frac{3}{2}\lambda t} \\ \frac{1}{3}-\frac{1}{3}e^{-\frac{3}{2}\lambda t} & \frac{1}{3}-\frac{1}{3}e^{-\frac{3}{2}\lambda t} & \frac{1}{3}+\frac{2}{3}e^{-\frac{3}{2}\lambda t} \end{pmatrix}$

$$f(x_1,x_2)=x_i, i=1,2: u(t,x_1,x_2)=E\left(x_i+v\int_0^t\tau_{\xi(u)}^{(i)}du\right)=$$
$$=x_i+\frac{3}{2}\frac{v}{\lambda}(\tau_0^{(i)}r_0+\tau_1^{(i)}r_1+\tau_2^{(i)}r_2)(1-e^{-\frac{3}{2}\lambda t});$$

$$f(x_1,x_2)=x_1x_2: u(t,x_1,x_2)=E\left(x_1+v\int_0^t\tau_{\xi(u_1)}^{(1)}du_1\right)(x_2+$$
$$\left.v\int_0^t\tau_{\xi(u_2)}^{(2)}du_2\right)=x_1x_2+\frac{3}{2}\frac{v}{\lambda}(1-e^{-\frac{3}{2}\lambda t})(x_1[\tau_0^{(2)}r_0+\cdots+\tau_2^{(2)}r_2]+$$

$$x_2[\tau_0^{(1)}r_0+\cdots+\tau_2^{(1)}r_2])+v^2\left[\int_0^t\int_0^{\theta_2}E(\tau^{(1)}_{\xi(\theta_1)}\tau^{(2)}_{\xi(\theta_2)})d\theta_1 d\theta_2+\right.$$
$$\left.\int_0^t\int_0^{\theta_2}E(\tau^{(2)}_{\xi(\theta_1)}\tau^{(1)}_{\xi(\theta_2)})d\theta_1 d\theta_2\right].$$

The penultimate and last terms are equal to:

$$v^2\int_0^t\int_0^{\theta_2}1\left\{r_0\left(\frac{1}{3}+\frac{2}{3}e^{-\frac{3}{2}\lambda\theta_1}\right)+r_1\left(\frac{1}{3}-\frac{1}{3}e^{-\frac{3}{2}\lambda\theta_1}\right)+r_2\left(\frac{1}{3}-\frac{1}{3}e^{-\frac{3}{2}\lambda\theta_1}\right)\right\}\times$$
$$\left\{0\left(\frac{1}{3}+\frac{2}{3}e^{-\frac{3}{2}\lambda(\theta_2-\theta_1)}\right)+\frac{\sqrt{3}}{2}\left(\frac{1}{3}-\frac{1}{3}e^{-\frac{3}{2}\lambda(\theta_2-\theta_1)}\right)-\frac{\sqrt{3}}{2}\left(\frac{1}{3}-\frac{1}{3}e^{-\frac{3}{2}\lambda(\theta_2-\theta_1)}\right)\right\}+$$
$$\left(-\frac{1}{2}\right)\left\{r_0\left(\frac{1}{3}-\frac{1}{3}e^{-\frac{3}{2}\lambda\theta_1}\right)+r_1\left(\frac{1}{3}+\frac{2}{3}e^{-\frac{3}{2}\lambda\theta_1}\right)+r_2\left(\frac{1}{3}-\frac{1}{3}e^{-\frac{3}{2}\lambda\theta_1}\right)\right\}\left\{0\left(\frac{1}{3}-\right.\right.$$
$$\left.\left.\frac{1}{3}e^{-\frac{3}{2}\lambda(\theta_2-\theta_1)}\right)+\frac{\sqrt{3}}{2}\left(\frac{1}{3}+\frac{2}{3}e^{-\frac{3}{2}\lambda(\theta_2-\theta_1)}\right)-\frac{\sqrt{3}}{2}\left(\frac{1}{3}-\frac{1}{3}e^{-\frac{3}{2}\lambda(\theta_2-\theta_1)}\right)\right\}+\left(-\frac{1}{2}\right)\times$$
$$\left\{r_0\left(\frac{1}{3}-\frac{1}{3}e^{-\frac{3}{2}\lambda\theta_1}\right)+r_1\left(\frac{1}{3}-\frac{1}{3}e^{-\frac{3}{2}\lambda\theta_1}\right)+r_2\left(\frac{1}{3}+\frac{2}{3}e^{-\frac{3}{2}\lambda\theta_1}\right)\right\}\left\{0\left(\frac{1}{3}-\right.\right.$$
$$\left.\left.\frac{1}{3}e^{-\frac{3}{2}\lambda(\theta_2-\theta_1)}\right)+\frac{\sqrt{3}}{2}\left(\frac{1}{3}-\frac{1}{3}e^{-\frac{3}{2}\lambda(\theta_2-\theta_1)}\right)-\frac{\sqrt{3}}{2}\left(\frac{1}{3}+\frac{2}{3}e^{-\frac{3}{2}\lambda(\theta_2-\theta_1)}\right)\right\}d\theta_1 d\theta_2=$$
$$\frac{\sqrt{3}}{4}(r_2-r_1)v^2\left[-\frac{2}{3\lambda}e^{-\frac{3}{2}\lambda t}t-\frac{4}{9\lambda^2}(e^{-\frac{3}{2}\lambda t}-1)\right].$$

$$2)\ P(t)=\begin{pmatrix}e^{-\lambda t}ch_{3,0} & e^{-\lambda t}ch_{3,2} & e^{-\lambda t}ch_{3,1}\\ e^{-\lambda t}ch_{3,1} & e^{-\lambda t}ch_{3,0} & e^{-\lambda t}ch_{3,2}\\ e^{-\lambda t}ch_{3,2} & e^{-\lambda t}ch_{3,1} & e^{-\lambda t}ch_{3,0}\end{pmatrix}$$

$$f(x_1,x_2)=x_i, i=1,2: u(t,x_1,x_2)=E\left(x_i+v\int_0^t\tau^{(i)}_{\xi(u)}du\right)=x_i+\frac{v}{3}\left[(\{t+\right.$$
$$\left.\frac{1}{(\omega_3-1)\lambda}(e^{(\omega_3-1)\lambda t}-1)+\frac{1}{(\omega_3^2-1)\lambda}(e^{(\omega_3^2-1)\lambda t}-1)\}\right)(r_0\tau_0^{(i)}+r_1\tau_1^{(i)}+r_2\tau_2^{(i)})+$$
$$\left(\left\{\lambda t+\frac{\lambda\omega_3}{(\omega_3-1)\lambda}(e^{(\omega_3-1)\lambda t}-1)+\frac{\lambda\omega_3^2}{(\omega_3^2-1)\lambda}(e^{(\omega_3^2-1)\lambda t}-1)\right\}\right)(r_0\tau_2^{(i)}+r_1\tau_0^{(i)}+$$
$$r_2\tau_1^{(i)})+\left(\left\{\lambda^2 t+\frac{\lambda^2\omega_3^2}{(\omega_3-1)\lambda}(e^{(\omega_3-1)\lambda t}-1)+\frac{\lambda^2\omega_3}{(\omega_3^2-1)\lambda}(e^{(\omega_3^2-1)\lambda t}-1)\right\}\right)\times$$
$$\left.(r_0\tau_1^{(i)}+r_1\tau_2^{(i)}+r_2\tau_0^{(i)})\right].$$

1.3. Systems of Kolmogorov equations

Let us write the systems of forward and backward Kolmogorov equations for Markov random evolutionary process.

We denote $\xi_i(u) := i + \xi(u)$, where $\xi(u)$ is a Markov chain with values from the set $\{0, 1, 2, \ldots, n\}$, which spends in each state exponentially distributed with the parameter λ time, and then moves to the next state in the case of cyclic evolution, and in the case of uniform evolution, to one of the remaining states with probability $\frac{1}{n}$.

Consider a function from a Markov random evolutionary process in R^n of the form:

$$u_i(\overline{x}, t) = Ef\left(\overline{x} + v\int_0^t \overline{\tau}_{\xi_i(u)} du\right) \qquad [1.9]$$

where $i = \overline{0, n}$ is the initial direction of movement. The conditions on $f(\overline{x})$ are described in the following theorem.

EXAMPLE 1.4.– *$f(x) = \overline{x}$, where $\overline{x} = (x_1, \ldots, x_n)$. Then, $u_i(\overline{x}, t) = E(\overline{x} + v\int_0^t \overline{\tau}_{\xi_i(u)} du)$, where in the case of the cyclic matrix* [1.2], *we have:*

$$E[\overline{\tau}_{\xi_0(t)}] = e^{-\lambda t}[\overline{\tau}_0 ch_{n+1,0}(\lambda t) + \overline{\tau}_1 ch_{n+1,n}(\lambda t) + \cdots + \overline{\tau}_n ch_{n+1,1}(\lambda t)],$$

$$\ldots,$$

$$E[\overline{\tau}_{\xi_n(t)}] = e^{-\lambda t}[\overline{\tau}_0 ch_{n+1,1}(\lambda t) + \overline{\tau}_1 ch_{n+1,2}(\lambda t) + \cdots + \overline{\tau}_n ch_{n+1,0}(\lambda t)],$$

and $u_i(\overline{x}, t) = \overline{x} + vE\left(\int_0^t \overline{\tau}_{\xi_i(u)} du\right)$.

Since the mathematical expectation is a finite sum, it can be carried under the integral, so: $u_0(\overline{x}, t) = \overline{x} + v\int_0^t E(\overline{\tau}_{\xi_0(u)})du = \overline{x} + v\int_0^t e^{-\lambda u}[\overline{\tau}_0 \times ch_{n+1,0}(\lambda u) + \overline{\tau}_1 ch_{n+1,n}(\lambda u) + \cdots + \overline{\tau}_n ch_{n+1,1}(\lambda u)]du = \overline{x} + \frac{v}{n+1}\int_0^t [e^{-\lambda u}[\overline{\tau}_0(e^{\lambda u} + \cdots + e^{\omega_{n+1}^n \lambda u}) + \overline{\tau}_1(\lambda^n e^{\lambda u} + \cdots + \lambda^n \omega_{n+1}^{n^2} e^{\omega_{n+1}^n \lambda u}) + \cdots + \overline{\tau}_n(\lambda e^{\lambda u} + \cdots + \lambda \omega_{n+1}^n e^{\omega_{n+1}^n \lambda u})] = \overline{x} + \frac{v}{n+1}\int_0^t [\overline{\tau}_0(1 + \cdots + e^{(\omega_{n+1}^n - 1)\lambda u}) + \overline{\tau}_1(\lambda^n + \cdots + \lambda^n \omega_{n+1}^{n^2} e^{(\omega_{n+1}^n - 1)\lambda u}) + \cdots + \overline{\tau}_n(\lambda + \cdots + \lambda\omega_{n+1}^n e^{(\omega_{n+1}^n - 1)\lambda u})] = \overline{x} + \frac{v}{n+1}[\overline{\tau}_0(t + \cdots + \frac{1}{(\omega_{n+1}^n - 1)\lambda}(e^{(\omega_{n+1}^n - 1)\lambda t} - 1)) + \overline{\tau}_1(\lambda^n t + \cdots + \frac{\lambda^n \omega_{n+1}^{n^2}}{(\omega_{n+1}^n - 1)\lambda}(e^{(\omega_{n+1}^n - 1)\lambda t} - 1)) + \cdots + \overline{\tau}_n(\lambda t + \cdots + \frac{\lambda\omega_{n+1}^n}{(\omega_{n+1}^n - 1)\lambda}(e^{(\omega_{n+1}^n - 1)\lambda t} - 1))]$, *and by analogy for the rest of $u_i(\overline{x}, t)$.*

In the case of matrix [1.3]*: $E[\overline{\tau}_{\xi_i(t)}] = e^{-\frac{n+1}{n}\lambda t}\overline{\tau}_i$, as soon as $\sum_0^n \overline{\tau}_i = 0$.*

For $u_i(\overline{x},t)$*, we have:*

$$u_i(\overline{x},t) = \overline{x} + v\int_0^t E[\overline{\tau}_{\xi_i(u)}]du = \overline{x} + v\int_0^t [e^{-\frac{n+1}{n}\lambda u}\overline{\tau}_i]du =$$
$$\overline{x} - v\overline{\tau}_i\frac{n}{\lambda(n+1)}(e^{-\frac{n+1}{n}\lambda t} - 1).$$

EXAMPLE 1.5.– *In the case of a linear function* $f(x) = \sum_{j=1}^n c_j x_j$*, we have:*

for the cyclic change of directions:

$$u_0(\overline{x},t) = \sum_{j=1}^n c_j x_j + \frac{v}{n+1}\left[\sum_{j=1}^n c_j\tau_0^{(j)}\left(t + \cdots + \frac{1}{(\omega_{n+1}^n - 1)\lambda}(e^{(\omega_{n+1}^n-1)\lambda t} - 1)\right) + \right.$$
$$\sum_{j=1}^n c_j\tau_1^{(j)}\left(\lambda^n t + \cdots + \frac{\lambda^n\omega_{n+1}^{n^2}}{(\omega_{n+1}^n - 1)\lambda}(e^{(\omega_{n+1}^n-1)\lambda t} - 1)\right) + \cdots + \sum_{j=1}^n c_j\tau_n^{(j)}\,(\lambda\times$$
$$\left. t + \cdots + \frac{\lambda\omega_{n+1}^n}{(\omega_{n+1}^n - 1)\lambda}(e^{(\omega_{n+1}^n-1)\lambda t} - 1)\right)\Bigg], \qquad [1.10]$$

for the uniform change:

$$u_i(\overline{x},t) = \sum_{j=1}^n c_j x_j - \sum_{j=1}^n c_j\tau_i^{(j)}\frac{vn}{\lambda(n+1)}(e^{-\frac{n+1}{n}\lambda t} - 1), \qquad [1.11]$$

where $\tau_i^{(j)}$ *is the* j*-th component of the vector* $\overline{\tau}_i$*.*

THEOREM 1.8.– *If* $f(x)$ *is continuously differentiable function, then* $u_i(\overline{x},t)$ *defined in* [1.9] *satisfies the system of backward Kolmogorov differential equations:*

– *when changing directions cyclically:*

$$\begin{cases} \frac{\partial}{\partial t}u_0(\overline{x},t) = -\lambda u_0(\overline{x},t) + v\frac{\partial}{\partial x_1}u_0(\overline{x},t) + \lambda u_1(\overline{x},t) \\ \frac{\partial}{\partial t}u_1(\overline{x},t) = -\lambda u_1(\overline{x},t) + v(-\frac{1}{n}\frac{\partial}{\partial x_1} + \sqrt{\frac{(n+1)(n-1)}{n^2}}\frac{\partial}{\partial x_2})u_1(\overline{x},t) + \\ +\lambda u_2(\overline{x},t) \\ \cdots \\ \frac{\partial}{\partial t}u_n(\overline{x},t) = -\lambda u_n(\overline{x},t) + v(-\frac{1}{n}\frac{\partial}{\partial x_1} - \sqrt{\frac{(n+1)(n-1)}{n^2}}\frac{\partial}{\partial x_2} - \cdots - \\ -\frac{1}{n}\sqrt{\frac{(n+1)n}{6}}\frac{\partial}{\partial x_{n-1}} - \frac{1}{n}\sqrt{\frac{(n+1)n}{2}}\frac{\partial}{\partial x_n})u_n(\overline{x},t) + \lambda u_0(\overline{x},t) \end{cases}$$

[1.12]

– *when changing directions uniformly:*

$$\begin{cases} \frac{\partial}{\partial t}u_0(\overline{x},t) = -\lambda u_0(\overline{x},t) + v\frac{\partial}{\partial x_1}u_0(\overline{x},t) + \frac{\lambda}{n}\sum_{i\neq 0}u_i(\overline{x},t) \\ \frac{\partial}{\partial t}u_1(\overline{x},t) = -\lambda u_1(\overline{x},t) + v(-\frac{1}{n}\frac{\partial}{\partial x_1} + \sqrt{\frac{(n+1)(n-1)}{n^2}}\frac{\partial}{\partial x_2})u_1(\overline{x},t) + \\ +\frac{\lambda}{n}\sum_{i\neq 1}u_i(\overline{x},t) \\ \dots \\ \frac{\partial}{\partial t}u_n(\overline{x},t) = -\lambda u_n(\overline{x},t) + v(-\frac{1}{n}\frac{\partial}{\partial x_1} - \sqrt{\frac{(n+1)(n-1)}{n^2}}\frac{\partial}{\partial x_2} - \dots - \\ -\frac{1}{n}\sqrt{\frac{(n+1)n}{6}}\frac{\partial}{\partial x_{n-1}} - \frac{1}{n}\sqrt{\frac{(n+1)n}{2}}\frac{\partial}{\partial x_n})u_n(\overline{x},t) + \frac{\lambda}{n}\sum_{i\neq n}u_i(\overline{x},t) \end{cases}$$

[1.13]

PROOF.– Consider the function $u_0(\overline{x},t)$:

$$u_0(\overline{x},t+\triangle t) = Ef\left(\overline{x} + v\int_0^{t+\triangle t}\overline{\tau}_{\xi_0(u)}du\right) = Ef\left(\overline{x} + v\int_0^{\triangle t}\overline{\tau}_{\xi_0(u)}du + v\int_{\triangle t}^{t+\triangle t}\overline{\tau}_{\xi(u)+0}du\right) = P(N(\triangle t)=0)Ef\left(\overline{x} + v\overline{\tau}_0\triangle t + v\int_{\triangle t}^{t+\triangle t}\overline{\tau}_{\xi_0(u)}du\right) + P(N(\triangle t)=1)Ef\left(\overline{x} + O(\triangle t) + v\int_{\triangle t}^{t+\triangle t}\overline{\tau}_{\xi_1(u)}du\right) + o(\triangle t), \triangle t \to 0,$$

where $N(t)$ is the number of Poisson events per time t.

$$u_0(\overline{x},t+\triangle t) - u_0(\overline{x},t) = (1-\lambda\triangle t)Ef\left(\overline{x} + v\overline{\tau}_0\triangle t + v\int_{\triangle t}^{t+\triangle t}\overline{\tau}_{\xi_0(u)}du\right) + \lambda\triangle t\times Ef\left(\overline{x} + O(\triangle t) + v\int_{\triangle t}^{t+\triangle t}\overline{\tau}_{\xi_1(u)}du\right) - Ef\left(\overline{x} + v\int_0^t\overline{\tau}_{\xi_0(u)}du\right) + o(\triangle t) = Ef\left(\overline{x} + v\overline{\tau}_0\triangle t + v\int_0^t\overline{\tau}_{\xi_0(u)}du\right) - Ef\left(\overline{x} + v\int_0^t\overline{\tau}_{\xi_0(u)}du\right) - \lambda\triangle t Ef\left(\overline{x} + v\overline{\tau}_0\triangle t + v\int_0^t\overline{\tau}_{\xi_0(u)}du\right) + \lambda\triangle t Ef\left(\overline{x} + O(\triangle t) + v\int_{\triangle t}^{t+\triangle t}\overline{\tau}_{\xi_1(u)}du\right) +$$

$o(\triangle t), \triangle t \to 0$, where the homogeneity of $\xi(u)$ is taken into account.

Dividing this expression by $\triangle t$ and directing $\triangle t$ to 0, we obtain

$$\frac{\partial}{\partial t}u_0(\overline{x},t) = -\lambda u_0(\overline{x},t) + v(\overline{\tau}_0,\nabla)u_0(\overline{x},t) + \lambda u_1(\overline{x},t), \qquad [1.14]$$

where $\nabla = (\frac{\partial}{\partial x_1},\dots,\frac{\partial}{\partial x_n})$. Here, $(\overline{\tau}_0,\nabla) = 1\frac{\partial}{\partial x_1} + 0\frac{\partial}{\partial x_2} + \dots + 0\frac{\partial}{\partial x_n} = \frac{\partial}{\partial x_1}$, similarly for other directions of movement.

It is necessary to substantiate the possibility of a limit transition, as a result of which [1.14] is obtained. For this, it is enough to justify the equality:

$$\lim_{\Delta t \to 0} \frac{Ef(\overline{x} + v\overline{\tau}_0 \Delta t + v\int_0^t \overline{\tau}_{\xi_0(u)} du) - Ef(\overline{x} + v\int_0^t \overline{\tau}_{\xi_0(u)} du)}{\Delta t} =$$

$$v(\overline{\tau}_0, \nabla)u_0(\overline{x}, t),$$

i.e. the possibility of passing the limit transition under the sign of mathematical expectation.

Really,

$$\lim_{\Delta t \to 0} \frac{Ef(\overline{x} + v\overline{\tau}_0 \Delta t + v\int_0^t \overline{\tau}_{\xi_0(u)} du) - Ef(\overline{x} + v\int_0^t \overline{\tau}_{\xi_0(u)} du)}{\Delta t} =$$

$$E \lim_{\Delta t \to 0} \frac{f(\overline{x} + v\overline{\tau}_0 \Delta t + v\int_0^t \overline{\tau}_{\xi_0(u)} du) - f(\overline{x} + v\int_0^t \overline{\tau}_{\xi_0(u)} du)}{\Delta t} =$$

$$E \lim_{\Delta t \to 0} \sum_{i=1}^{n} \frac{v\tau_0^{(i)} f'_{x_i}(\overline{x} + v\int_0^t \overline{\tau}_{\xi_0(u)} du)\Delta t + o(\Delta t)}{\Delta t} =$$

$$E(v \sum_{i=1}^{n} \tau_0^{(i)} f'_{x_i}) = v(\overline{\tau}_0, \nabla)u_0(\overline{x}, t) \qquad [1.15]$$

This follows from the theorem on the limit transition under the sign of the integral. A necessary condition is that $f(\overline{x})$ is integrable and uniform with respect to $\overline{x} + v\int_0^t \overline{\tau}_{\xi_0(u)} du$ convergence $\frac{f(\overline{x}+v\overline{\tau}_0\Delta t+v\int_0^t \overline{\tau}_{\xi_0(u)} du)-f(\overline{x}+v\int_0^t \overline{\tau}_{\xi_0(u)} du)}{\Delta t}$ to $v\sum_{i=1}^{n} \tau_0^{(i)} f'_{x_i}$.

Being continuous, the function $f(\overline{x})$ is integrable.

Consider $|\frac{f(\overline{x}+v\overline{\tau}_0\Delta t+v\int_0^t \overline{\tau}_{\xi_0(u)} du)-f(\overline{x}+v\int_0^t \overline{\tau}_{\xi_0(u)} du)}{\Delta t} - v(\overline{\tau}_0, \nabla)f(\overline{x})| =$

$$= |\frac{\begin{array}{l} f(x_1+v\tau_0^{(1)}\Delta t+v\int_0^t \tau_{\xi_0(u)}^{(1)} du, x_2+v\tau_0^{(2)}\Delta t+v\int_0^t \tau_{\xi_0(u)}^{(2)} du, \dots)-f(x_1+v\int_0^t \tau_{\xi_0(u)}^{(1)} du, x_2+v\tau_0^{(2)}\Delta t+ \\ v\int_0^t \tau_{\xi_0(u)}^{(2)} du, \dots)+f(x_1+v\int_0^t \tau_{\xi_0(u)}^{(1)} du, x_2+v\tau_0^{(2)}\Delta t+v\int_0^t \tau_{\xi_0(u)}^{(2)} du, \dots)-f(x_1+v\int_0^t \tau_{\xi_0(u)}^{(1)} du, x_2+v\int_0^t \tau_{\xi_0(u)}^{(2)} du, \\ \dots)+\dots-f(\overline{x}+v\int_0^t \overline{\tau}_{\xi_0(u)} du) \end{array}}{\Delta t} - v(\overline{\tau}_0, \nabla)f(\overline{x})| \leq |f'_{x_1}(x_1 + v\tau_0^{(1)}\theta_1 + v\int_0^t \tau_{\xi_0(u)}^{(1)} du, x_2 + v\tau_0^{(2)}\Delta t + v\int_0^t \tau_{\xi_0(u)}^{(2)} du, \dots)| + \dots + |f'_{x_n}(x_1 + v\tau_0^{(1)}\Delta t + v\int_0^t \tau_{\xi_0(u)}^{(1)} du, x_2 + v\tau_0^{(2)}\Delta t + v\int_0^t \tau_{\xi_0(u)}^{(2)} du, \dots, x_n + v\tau_0^{(1)}\theta_n + v\int_0^t \tau_{\xi_0(u)}^{(1)} du)| + |v\tau_0^{(1)} f'_{x_1}| + \dots + |v\tau_0^{(n)} f'_{x_n}| \leq k_1 + \dots + k_{2n}.$$

Since $\overline{x}$ is a fixed point of R^n, and f' is continuous, there exists K such that $|f'(\overline{x})| < K$. $v\int_0^t \overline{\tau}_{\xi(u)} du$ is computed on a finite interval, and the argument f' changes, thus, on the compact $[x_1, x_1 + v\tau_0^{(1)} + vt] \times \dots \times [x_n, x_n + v\tau_0^{(n)} + vt]$.

Continuous function f' is bounded on this compact. Uniform convergence is proven, i.e. equality [1.15] is true.

We have the same for the rest $u_i(\overline{x}, t), i = \overline{1, n}$:

$$\frac{\partial}{\partial t} u_i(\overline{x}, t) = -\lambda u_i(\overline{x}, t) + v(\overline{\tau}_0, \nabla) u_0(\overline{x}, t) + \lambda u_{i+1}(\overline{x}, t),$$

where $i + 1 := 0$ for $i = n$.

Similarly, there is a system corresponding to the uniform change directions. In this case:

$$u_0(\overline{x}, t + \triangle t) = Ef\left(\overline{x} + v\int_0^{t+\triangle t} \overline{\tau}_{\xi_0(u)} du\right) = Ef\left(\overline{x} + v\int_0^{\triangle t} \overline{\tau}_{\xi_0(u)} du + \right.$$

$$\left. v\int_{\triangle t}^{t+\triangle t} \overline{\tau}_{\xi_0(u)} du\right) = P(N(\triangle t) = 0) Ef\left(\overline{x} + v\overline{\tau}_0 \triangle t + v\int_{\triangle t}^{t+\triangle t} \overline{\tau}_{\xi_0(u)} du\right) +$$

$$\sum_{i \neq 0} P(N(\triangle t) = 1) P(ndir(0) = i) Ef\left(\overline{x} + O(\triangle t) + v\int_{\triangle t}^{t+\triangle t} \overline{\tau}_{\xi(u)+i} du\right) +$$

$o(\triangle t), \triangle t \to 0$, where $ndir(0)$ is the number of the direction following the 0-th, and $P(ndir(0) = i) = \frac{1}{n}$ $(i \neq 0)$ by constructing a uniform process. Further calculations are similar.

The theorem is proven.

Note that the function $f(x) = \sum_{j=1}^{n} c_j x_j$ satisfies the conditions of the previous theorem, and therefore the functions [1.10] and [1.11] satisfy the systems [1.12] and [1.13], respectively. Let us put $u_{ij} = (\overline{x}, \overline{y}, t) = P_{ij}(\overline{x} + v\int_0^t \overline{\tau}_{\xi(u)} du, \overline{y})$, where $\overline{x}, \overline{y} \in R^n$, $i, j \in S$ – initial (time 0) and the final (time t) state $\xi(u)$. Here, the process starts from a point $\overline{x}$ and at the moment t falls into $\overline{y}$.

THEOREM 1.9.– *If $f(x)$ satisfies the conditions of theorem 1.8, then $u_j(\overline{y}, t) = u_{ij} = (\overline{x}, \overline{y}, t), \overline{x} \in R^n, i \in S$ satisfy the system of forward Kolmogorov differential equations:*

– *with the cyclic change of directions:*

$$\begin{cases} \frac{\partial}{\partial t} u_0(\overline{y}, t) = -\lambda u_0(\overline{y}, t) - v\frac{\partial}{\partial y_1} u_0(\overline{y}, t) + \lambda u_n(\overline{y}, t) \\ \frac{\partial}{\partial t} u_1(\overline{y}, t) = -\lambda u_1(\overline{y}, t) - v(-\frac{1}{n}\frac{\partial}{\partial y_1} + \sqrt{\frac{(n+1)(n-1)}{n^2}}\frac{\partial}{\partial y_2}) u_1(\overline{y}, t) + \\ +\lambda u_0(\overline{y}, t) \\ \dots \\ \frac{\partial}{\partial t} u_n(\overline{y}, t) = -\lambda u_n(\overline{y}, t) - v(-\frac{1}{n}\frac{\partial}{\partial y_1} - \sqrt{\frac{(n+1)(n-1)}{n^2}}\frac{\partial}{\partial y_2} - \dots - \\ -\frac{1}{n}\sqrt{\frac{(n+1)n}{6}}\frac{\partial}{\partial y_{n-1}} - \frac{1}{n}\sqrt{\frac{(n+1)n}{2}}\frac{\partial}{\partial y_n}) u_n(\overline{y}, t) + \lambda u_{n-1}(\overline{y}, t) \end{cases}$$

with the uniform change of directions:

$$\begin{cases} \frac{\partial}{\partial t}u_0(\overline{y},t) = -\lambda u_0(\overline{y},t) - v\frac{\partial}{\partial y_1}u_0(\overline{y},t) + \frac{\lambda}{n}\sum_{i\neq 0}u_i(\overline{y},t) \\ \frac{\partial}{\partial t}u_1(\overline{y},t) = -\lambda u_1(\overline{y},t) - v(-\frac{1}{n}\frac{\partial}{\partial y_1} + \sqrt{\frac{(n+1)(n-1)}{n^2}}\frac{\partial}{\partial y_2})u_1(\overline{y},t) + \\ +\frac{\lambda}{n}\sum_{i\neq 1}u_i(\overline{y},t) \\ \dots \\ \frac{\partial}{\partial t}u_n(\overline{y},t) = -\lambda u_n(\overline{y},t) - v(-\frac{1}{n}\frac{\partial}{\partial y_1} - \sqrt{\frac{(n+1)(n-1)}{n^2}}\frac{\partial}{\partial y_2} - \dots - \\ -\frac{1}{n}\sqrt{\frac{(n+1)n}{6}}\frac{\partial}{\partial y_{n-1}} - \frac{1}{n}\sqrt{\frac{(n+1)n}{2}}\frac{\partial}{\partial y_n})u_n(\overline{y},t) + \frac{\lambda}{n}\sum_{i\neq n}u_i(\overline{y},t) \end{cases}$$

PROOF.– We have

$$u_{i0}(\overline{x},\overline{y},t+\triangle t) = P_{i0}\left(\overline{x} + v\int_0^{t+\triangle t}\tau_{\xi(u)}du,\overline{y}\right) = P_{i0}\left(\overline{x} + v\int_0^t \tau_{\xi(u)}du + v\times\right.$$

$$\left.\int_t^{\triangle t}\tau_{\xi(u)}du,\overline{y}\right) = P(N(\triangle t) = 0)P_{i0}\left(\overline{x} + v\int_0^t \tau_{\xi(u)}du + v\overline{\tau}_0\triangle t,\overline{y}\right) +$$

$$P(N(\triangle t) = 1)P_{in}\left(\overline{x} + v\int_0^t \tau_{\xi(u)}du + O(\triangle t),\overline{y}\right) + o(\triangle t) = (1-\lambda\triangle t)P_{i0}\left(\overline{x} + \right.$$

$$\left. v\int_0^t \tau_{\xi(u)}du,\overline{y} - v\overline{\tau}_0\triangle t\right) + \lambda\triangle t P_{in}\left(\overline{x} + v\int_0^t \tau_{\xi(u)}du,\overline{y} - O(\triangle t)\right) + o(\triangle t).$$

Cyclic evolution is considered here (from state n, the process enters state 0).

$$u_{i0}(\overline{x},\overline{y},t+\triangle t) - u_{i0}(\overline{x},\overline{y},t) = (1-\lambda\triangle t)P_{i0}\left(\overline{x} + v\int_0^t \tau_{\xi(u)}du,\overline{y} - v\overline{\tau}_0\triangle t\right) -$$

$$P_{i0}\left(\overline{x} + v\int_0^t \tau_{\xi(u)}du,\overline{y}\right) + \lambda\triangle t P_{in}\left(\overline{x} + v\int_0^t \tau_{\xi(u)}du,\overline{y} - O(\triangle t)\right) + o(\triangle t).$$

Dividing by $\triangle t$ and directing $\triangle t$ to 0, we receive

$$\frac{\partial}{\partial t}u_{i0}(\overline{x},\overline{y},t) = -\lambda u_{i0}(\overline{x},\overline{y},t) - v(\overline{\tau}_0,\nabla)u_{i0}(\overline{x},\overline{y},t) + \lambda u_{in}(\overline{x},\overline{y},t),$$

where $\nabla = (\frac{\partial}{\partial y_1},\dots,\frac{\partial}{\partial y_n})$. Here $(\overline{\tau}_0,\nabla) = 1\frac{\partial}{\partial y_1} + 0\frac{\partial}{\partial y_2} + \dots + 0\frac{\partial}{\partial y_n} = \frac{\partial}{\partial y_1}$.

Similarly for other directions:

$$\frac{\partial}{\partial t}u_{ij}(\overline{x},\overline{y},t) = -\lambda u_{ij}(\overline{x},\overline{y},t) - v(\overline{\tau}_j,\nabla)u_{ij}(\overline{x},\overline{y},t) + \lambda u_{i(j-1)}(\overline{x},\overline{y},t), j=\overline{1,n},$$

for any $i=\overline{0,n}, \overline{x}\in R^n$.

With the uniform change in the direction of movement, the system is derived similarly.

The theorem is proven.

Comparing the systems obtained in theorems 1.8 and 1.9 shows that these systems are conjugated. This result is consistent with the results described in Doob (1962) and Chung (2012).

1.4. Evolutionary operator and theorem about weak convergence to the measure of the Wiener process

Here, we will prove the theorem concerning the weak convergence of measures generated by the Markov random evolutionary process, which indicates that in the hydrodynamic limit, the latter is a Wiener process.

Consider the Markov random evolutionary process as in Kisinski (1974), i.e. as a couple $(\overline{x}+v\int_0^t \overline{\tau}_{\xi(u)}du, \xi(t))$ defined by $R^n\times S$. This is a Markov process, for which it is possible to define a semigroup.

Let $f(\overline{x},i): R^n\times S\to R$ be some function, define a semigroup:

$$T(t)f(\overline{x},i) = E\left[f(\overline{x}+v\int_0^t \overline{\tau}_{\xi_i(u)}du, \xi_i(t))|\xi(0)=i\right]. \quad [1.16]$$

Let us verify the properties of the semigroup:

1) $T(0)f(\overline{x},i) = Ef(\overline{x},\xi_i(t)) = f(\overline{x},i)$, for any i;

2) $T(t+s)f(\overline{x},i) = Ef(\overline{x}+v\int_0^{t+s}\overline{\tau}_{\xi_i(u)}du, \xi_i(t+s)) = Ef(\overline{x}+$

$$v\int_0^s \overline{\tau}_{\xi_i(u)}du + v\int_s^{t+s}\overline{\tau}_{\xi_i(u)}du, \xi_i(t+s)\Big) = Ef\left(\overline{x}+v\int_0^s \overline{\tau}_{\xi_i(u)}du+\right.$$

$$\left. v\int_0^t \overline{\tau}_{\xi(u)+\xi_i(s)}du, \xi_i(t+s)\right) \quad [1.17]$$

considering the homogeneity of $\xi(t)$. Furthermore, in view of homogeneity of $\xi(t)$ and permutability of integrations

$$T(t)T(s)f(\overline{x},i) = T(t)Ef\left(\overline{x} + v\int_0^s \overline{\tau}_{\xi_i(u)}du, \xi_i(s)\right) = ET(t)f(\overline{x}+$$

$$v\int_0^s \overline{\tau}_{\xi_i(u)}du, \xi_i(s)\Big) = Ef\left(\overline{x} + v\int_0^s \overline{\tau}_{\xi_i(u)}du + v\int_0^t \overline{\tau}_{\xi(u)+\xi_i(s)}du,\right.$$

$$\left.\xi(t) + \xi_i(s)\right) = Ef\left(\overline{x} + v\int_0^s \overline{\tau}_{\xi_i(u)}du + v\int_0^t \overline{\tau}_{\xi(u)+\xi_i(s)}du, \xi_i(t+s)\right). \quad [1.18]$$

Obviously, [1.18] coincides with [1.17], i.e. $T(t)T(s)f(\overline{x},i) = T(t+s)f(\overline{x},i)$. So, [1.16] defines a semigroup, $t \geq 0$.

THEOREM 1.10.– *Infinitesimal operator of the semigroup* [1.16] *has the form:*

– *in the case of the cyclic change of directions:* $A = T_t'|_{t=0} =$

$$\begin{pmatrix} -\lambda + v(\overline{\tau}_0, \nabla) & \lambda & 0 & \dots & 0 \\ 0 & -\lambda + v(\overline{\tau}_1, \nabla) & \lambda & \dots & 0 \\ \dots & \dots & \dots & \dots & \dots \\ 0 & 0 & \dots & -\lambda + v(\overline{\tau}_{n-1}, \nabla) & \lambda \\ \lambda & 0 & 0 & \dots & -\lambda + v(\overline{\tau}_n, \nabla) \end{pmatrix} =$$

$$= A_0 + A_1,$$

– *in the case of the uniform change of directions:* $A = T_t'|_{t=0} =$

$$\begin{pmatrix} -\lambda + v(\overline{\tau}_0, \nabla) & \frac{\lambda}{n} & \frac{\lambda}{n} & \dots & \frac{\lambda}{n} \\ \frac{\lambda}{n} & -\lambda + v(\overline{\tau}_1, \nabla) & \frac{\lambda}{n} & \dots & \frac{\lambda}{n} \\ \dots & \dots & \dots & \dots & \dots \\ \frac{\lambda}{n} & \frac{\lambda}{n} & \dots & -\lambda + v(\overline{\tau}_{n-1}, \nabla) & \frac{\lambda}{n} \\ \frac{\lambda}{n} & \frac{\lambda}{n} & \frac{\lambda}{n} & \dots & -\lambda + v(\overline{\tau}_n, \nabla) \end{pmatrix} =$$

$$= A_0 + A_1,$$

where $A_0 = \begin{pmatrix} v(\overline{\tau}_0, \nabla) & 0 & \dots & 0 \\ 0 & v(\overline{\tau}_1, \nabla) & \dots & 0 \\ \dots & \dots & \dots & \dots \\ 0 & 0 & \dots & v(\overline{\tau}_n, \nabla) \end{pmatrix}$ *is defined on* R^n,

– *in the case of the cyclic change of directions:* $A_1 = \begin{pmatrix} -\lambda & \lambda & 0 & \dots & 0 \\ \dots & \dots & \dots & \dots & \dots \\ 0 & 0 & \dots & -\lambda & \lambda \\ \lambda & 0 & 0 & \dots & -\lambda \end{pmatrix}$

in the case of the uniform change of directions: $A_1 = \begin{pmatrix} -\lambda & \frac{\lambda}{n} & \frac{\lambda}{n} & \dots & \frac{\lambda}{n} \\ \dots & \dots & \dots & \dots & \dots \\ \frac{\lambda}{n} & \frac{\lambda}{n} & \dots & -\lambda & \frac{\lambda}{n} \\ \frac{\lambda}{n} & \frac{\lambda}{n} & \frac{\lambda}{n} & \dots & -\lambda \end{pmatrix}$ *are defined on* S.

PROOF.– $T(t)f(\overline{x}, i) = Ef(\overline{x}+v\int_0^t \overline{\tau}_{\xi_i(u)}du, \xi_i(t)) = P(N(t) = 0)f(\overline{x}+v\overline{\tau}_i t, i)+$ $P(N(t) = 1)f(\overline{x} + O(t), i + 1) + o(t)$ at $t \to 0$ in the case of the cyclic change of directions; meanwhile, in the case of the uniform change of directions, the second term is equal to $P(N(t) = 1)\sum_{j\neq i} P(\xi(t) = j - i)f(\overline{x} + O(t), j)$, where $N(t)$ is the number of Poisson events in the time interval t.

Thus,

$$T(t)f(\overline{x}, i) - f(\overline{x}, i) = f(\overline{x} + v\overline{\tau}_i t, i) - f(\overline{x}, i) - \lambda t f(\overline{x} + v\overline{\tau}_i t, i)+$$
$$\lambda t f(\overline{x} + O(t), i + 1) + o(t), t \to 0$$

Dividing by t and directing t to 0, we obtain under the condition differentiability of f with respect to x:

$$T_t'|_{t=0} f(\overline{x}, i) = -\lambda f(\overline{x}, i) + v(\overline{\tau}_i, \nabla)f(\overline{x}, i) + \lambda f(\overline{x}, i + 1).$$

Having written $Af(\overline{x}, i) = T_t'|_{t=0} f(\overline{x}, i)$, where $f(\overline{x}, i)$ is differentiable with respect to $x_1, \dots, x_n$, in a matrix form, we get: $A =$

$$\begin{pmatrix} -\lambda + v(\overline{\tau}_0, \nabla) & \lambda & 0 & \dots & 0 \\ 0 & -\lambda + v(\overline{\tau}_1, \nabla) & \lambda & \dots & 0 \\ \dots & \dots & \dots & \dots & \dots \\ 0 & 0 & \dots & -\lambda + v(\overline{\tau}_{n-1}, \nabla) & \lambda \\ \lambda & 0 & 0 & \dots & -\lambda + v(\overline{\tau}_n, \nabla) \end{pmatrix} =$$
$$= A_0 + A_1,$$

where A_0 and A_1 are defined in the condition of the theorem.

Similar calculations are carried out in the case of the uniform change of directions.

The theorem is proven.

COROLLARY 1.1.– *Functions* $u_i(\overline{x}, t) = T(t)f(\overline{x}, i), i = \overline{0, n}$ *satisfy a system of backward Kolmogorov differential equations*

$$\frac{\partial}{\partial t}\begin{pmatrix} u_0 \\ \vdots \\ u_n \end{pmatrix} = A\begin{pmatrix} u_0 \\ \vdots \\ u_n \end{pmatrix} = A_0\begin{pmatrix} u_0 \\ \vdots \\ u_n \end{pmatrix} + A_1\begin{pmatrix} u_0 \\ \vdots \\ u_n \end{pmatrix},$$

coinciding with systems [1.12] *and* [1.13].

Let A^* be the operator conjugate to A. Then, from works Doob (1962) and Chung (2012), it follows that the forward system of Kolmogorov differential equations has the form:

– *in the case of the cyclic change of directions:* $A^* =$

$$\begin{pmatrix} -\lambda - v(\overline{\tau}_0, \nabla) & 0 & 0 & \dots & \lambda \\ \lambda & -\lambda - v(\overline{\tau}_1, \nabla) & 0 & \dots & 0 \\ \dots & \dots & \dots & \dots & \dots \\ 0 & \dots & \lambda & -\lambda - v(\overline{\tau}_{n-1}, \nabla) & 0 \\ 0 & 0 & \dots & \lambda & -\lambda - v(\overline{\tau}_n, \nabla) \end{pmatrix}$$

– *in the case of the uniform change of directions:* $A^* =$

$$\begin{pmatrix} -\lambda - v(\overline{\tau}_0, \nabla) & \frac{\lambda}{n} & \frac{\lambda}{n} & \dots & \frac{\lambda}{n} \\ \frac{\lambda}{n} & -\lambda - v(\overline{\tau}_1, \nabla) & \frac{\lambda}{n} & \dots & \frac{\lambda}{n} \\ \dots & \dots & \dots & \dots & \dots \\ \frac{\lambda}{n} & \frac{\lambda}{n} & \dots & -\lambda - v(\overline{\tau}_{n-1}, \nabla) & \frac{\lambda}{n} \\ \frac{\lambda}{n} & \frac{\lambda}{n} & \frac{\lambda}{n} & \dots & -\lambda - v(\overline{\tau}_n, \nabla) \end{pmatrix},$$

and $\frac{\partial}{\partial t}\begin{pmatrix} u_0 \\ \vdots \\ u_n \end{pmatrix} = A^* \begin{pmatrix} u_0 \\ \vdots \\ u_n \end{pmatrix}$, *that coincides with the result of theorem 1.9.*

Results on the central limit theorem for models similar to the Markov random evolutionary process were obtained in works by Korolyuk and Swishchuk (1995a, 1995b). Let us prove a more general result about the convergence of the measures generated by the random evolutionary process to the measure of the Wiener process.

For any $t \geq 0$, we define a probability measure μ_t^c as in Kisinski (1974)

$$\mu_t^c(B) = P\left(\left(v\int_0^t \overline{\tau}_{\xi(u)}du, \overline{\tau}_{\xi(t)}\right) \in B\right)$$

for any Borel set $B \in R^n \times \{\overline{\tau}_0, \dots, \overline{\tau}_n\}$. Here, $c = v, c^2 = \lambda; \frac{v^2}{\lambda} \to 1, c \to \infty$.

The measures μ_t^c have a compact support, namely $supp\ \mu_t^c = \{(\zeta, k) : \zeta \in Tetr(0, vt); k = \overline{\tau}_i, i = \overline{0, n}\}$, where $Tetr(0, vt)$ is an $n+1$-hedron inscribed in a sphere of radius vt.

THEOREM 1.11.– *Measures* $\mu_t^c(B) = P\left(\left(v\int_0^t \overline{\tau}_{\xi(u)}du, \overline{\tau}_{\xi(t)}\right) \in B\right)$ *for* $c \to \infty$ *weakly converge to the measure of an* n*-dimensional Wiener process with a zero transfer vector and a unit diffusion operator.*

PROOF.– To prove the theorem, it is necessary to prove the weak compactness of the set of measures $\{\mu_t^c\}$ and the weak convergence of the process $v\int_0^t \overline{\tau}_{\xi(u)}du$ to the Wiener process.

In Korolyuk and Turbin (1993), it was proved that the distributions of the process $v\int_0^t \overline{\tau}_{\xi(u)}du$ at $v \to \infty, \lambda \to \infty : \frac{v^2}{\lambda} \to 1$ converge to distributions n-dimensional Wiener process with a zero transfer vector and a unit diffusion operator.

It remains to be proven the weak compactness of the set of measures $\{\mu_t^c\}$. Let us use Prokhorov's theorem. It is necessary to prove that for $\forall\varepsilon > 0$, there exists a compact $K : \sup\limits_c\{\mu_t^c(R^n - K)\} < \varepsilon$.

Indeed, $\sup\limits_c P\left(\left(v\int_0^t \overline{\tau}_{\xi(u)}du, \overline{\tau}_{\xi(t)}\right) \in K\right) = 1 > 1 - \varepsilon, \forall\varepsilon > 0$, since with probability 1 for any finite c, the evolutionary process is within the $n+1$-hedron inscribed in the sphere of radius vt which is compact. Thus, the set of measures is weakly compact.

The theorem is proven.

2

Symmetry of Markov Random Evolutionary Processes in R^n

2.1. Symmetrization: definition and properties

Let us introduce into R^n the notion of symmetrization of a random vector, which generalizes the concept of symmetrization of a random variable and has interesting group properties. In the following, the symmetry of the Markov random evolutionary process is proven.

Firstly, we introduce $\overline{x} = \sum_{j=1}^{n} x_j \overline{\tau}_j$: vector of n-dimensional space with a fixed basis $\overline{\tau}_1, \ldots, \overline{\tau}_n$. If $pi_j(\cdot)$ is some permutation, and $\pi_j(\overline{x}) = \sum_{k=1}^{n} x_{j_k} \overline{\tau}_k$, the transformation of the vector $\overline{x}$ obtained from this vector by rearranging its component, then we can write $\pi_j(\overline{x}) = \prod_j^0 \overline{x}$, where $\prod_j^0$ represents permutation $n_j(\cdot)$ in the group of permutated $n \times N$ matrices $P^0 = \prod_0^0, \ldots, \prod_{n!-1}^0$, each of which contains one row and each column unit and $n-1$ zeros, $\prod_0^0 = I$: unit $n \times n$ matrix, ordering is arbitrary but fixed.

Let $\prod_j^0, j = \overline{0, n!-1}$ be one of the matrices in the group P^0. Let us fix $i = \overline{1, n}$ and replace all elements of the i-th column with -1. We denote the resulting matrix by $\prod_j^i$. In this way, we obtain the set $GM_{S_{n+1}}(F_3)$ $(n+1)!$ of Galois matrices on the Galois field F_3.

The following theorem is well known.

THEOREM 2.1.– *The group of matrices $GM_{S_{n+1}}(F_3)$ is isomorphic to the group of permutations S_{n+1} of order $(n+1)!$.*

In R^n with the standard basis $\overline{e_1}, \overline{e_2} \dots \overline{e_n}$, we will write

$$\overline{\tau}_k = \sum_{i=1}^{n} \tau_k^{(i)} \overline{e_i} \qquad [2.1]$$

where

$$\tau_k^{(i)} = \begin{cases} -\frac{1}{n}\sqrt{\frac{n(n+1)}{(n-i+1)(n-i+2)}}, i < k+1, \\ \sqrt{\frac{(n-k)(n+1)}{n(n-k+1)}}, i = k+1, \\ 0, i > k+1. \end{cases} \qquad ; i = \overline{1,n}, k = \overline{0,n}$$

Let $\xi_0, \xi_1, \dots, \xi_n$ be independent identically distributed random variables, having the distribution function $F(x)$.

Consider a random vector

$$\overline{\xi} = \xi_0 \overline{\tau}_0 + \dots + \xi_n \overline{\tau}_n = \left(\sum_{k=0}^{n} \xi_k \tau_1^{(k)} \right) \overline{e}_1 + \dots + \left(\sum_{k=0}^{n} \xi_k \tau_n^{(k)} \right) \overline{e}_n. \qquad [2.2]$$

Components of the vector $\overline{\xi}$ on the basis $\overline{e}_1, \dots, \overline{e}_n$ are dependent and have different distributions. Nevertheless, it turns out that the distribution of $\overline{\xi}$ invariant with respect to the action of the group of proper self-combinations $n+1$-hedron in R^n that is isomorphic to the permutation group S_{n+1}.

Let π_{n+1} be a cyclic permutation of the $n+1$-th order, π_n is a cyclic permutation of the n-th order, and so on, π_2 is a cyclic permutation of the second order in S_{n+1}, and π_0 is an identical substitution. We denote

$$\begin{aligned} & g_0 = \pi_0, g_1 = \pi_{n+1}, g_2 = \pi_{n+1}^2, \dots, g_n = \pi_{n+1}^n, g_{n+1} = \pi_n, \\ & g_{n+2} = \pi_n^2, \dots, g_{2n-1} = \pi_n^{n-1}, \dots, g_{\frac{(n+1)n}{2}} = \pi_2, \\ & g_{\frac{(n+1)n}{2}+1} = \pi_{n+1}\pi_n\pi_{n+1}^n, g_{\frac{(n+1)n}{2}+2} = \pi_{n+1}^2\pi_n\pi_{n+1}^{n-1}, \dots \end{aligned} \qquad [2.3]$$

Then, $S_{n+1} = \{g_0, \dots, g_{(n+1)!-1}\}$.

Consider the set of $(n+1)!$ square matrices of the n-th order

$$GM_{S_{n+1}}(F_3) = \{\Pi_0^0, \dots, \Pi_{n!-1}^0, \Pi_0^1, \dots, \Pi_{n!-1}^1, \dots, \Pi_0^n, \dots, \Pi_{n!-1}^n\},$$

as specified above.

Between matrices from the set $GM_{S_{n+1}}(F_3)$ and representations [2.3], it is possible to establish a mutually unique correspondence by theorem 2.1. Let us redefine the matrices so that the correspondence takes place $L_j \longleftrightarrow g_j, j = \overline{0, (n+1)! - 1}$.

Vectors $\overline{\tau_1}, \dots, \overline{\tau_n}$ in [2.1] are linearly independent and can be chosen as a new affine base. On this basis, for $\overline{\xi}$ in equation [2.2], we have

$$\overline{\xi} = \sum_{i=1}^{n} (\xi_i - \xi_0)\overline{\tau_i}, \qquad [2.4]$$

since $\sum_{k=0}^{n} a_i^{(k)} = 0, i = \overline{1, n}$. It follows from the independence of ξ_i that $\xi_i - \xi_0, i = \overline{1, n}$, are equally distributed and symmetrical.

For the elements L_j of the S_{n+1} representation, we put $L_j = \{l^j_{km}, k, m = \overline{1, n}\}, j = \overline{0, (n+1)! - 1}$. We define the action $g_j\overline{x}$ of the group S_{n+1} in R^n as $(\overline{x} = \sum_{i=1}^{n} x_i\overline{\tau_i})$:

$$g_j\overline{x} := L_j\overline{x} := \sum_{i=1}^{n}(\sum_{k=1}^{n} l^j_{ik}x_k)\overline{\tau_i}.$$

THEOREM 2.2 (ABOUT SYMMETRIZATION IN R^n).– *For any $g \in S_{n+1}$ and $\overline{\xi}$ of the form* [2.2]

$$\overline{\xi} \doteq g\overline{\xi}.$$

The sign $\doteq$ means equality by distribution.

PROOF.– Since the vector $\overline{\xi}$ of the form [2.2] can be written in the form [2.4], and $g_j\overline{\xi} = L_j\overline{\xi}$, then we will exactly consider the following operation: $L_j\overline{\xi} = \sum_{i=1}^{n}(\sum_{k=1}^{n} l^j_{ik}(\xi_k - \xi_0))\overline{\tau_i}$.

In each sum $\sum_{k=1}^{n} l^j_{ik}(\xi_k - \xi_0)$ either one $l^j_{im} = 1$, where $1 \le m \le n$ and the rest are equal to 0, or two l^j_{im}, l^j_{is}, where $1 \le m, s \le n$ are -1 and 1 accordingly, the remainder is 0, so we have two cases:

$$\sum_{k=1}^{n} l^j_{ik}(\xi_k - \xi_0) = \begin{cases} \xi_m - \xi_0, 1 \le m \le n \\ \xi_m - \xi_s, 1 \le m, s \le n \end{cases} \qquad [2.5]$$

Thus, $g_j\overline{\xi}$ is the sum of differences of the form [2.5], multiplied by the vectors $\overline{\tau_i}$. But since all ξ_i are equally distributed, then $g_j\overline{\xi} \doteq \sum_{i=1}^{n}(\xi_i - \xi_0)\overline{\tau_i} = \overline{\xi}$.

The theorem is proven.

REMARK 2.1.– *Since the components in the right-hand side of equation* [2.4] *are symmetric random variables, then*

$$\overline{\xi} \doteq -\overline{\xi},$$

which is not obvious for equation [2.2] *(the result of the strong dependence of components in the original basis* $\overline{e}_1, \ldots, \overline{e}_n$*).*

DEFINITION 2.1.– *A number*

$$\gamma(\overline{x}) = \sum_{j=1}^{n} x_j - (n+1)\min\{0, x_1, \ldots, x_n\}$$

is called the γ*-module of the vector* $\overline{x}$*.*

The γ-module has the following properties:

1) $\gamma(\overline{x}) \geq 0$.

2) $\gamma(\overline{x}) = 0$, if and only if $x_1 = \cdots = x_n = 0$.

3) $\gamma(\alpha\overline{x}) = |\alpha|\gamma(\overline{x})$.

4) $\gamma(\overline{x} + \overline{y}) \leq \gamma(\overline{x}) + \gamma(\overline{y})$.

5) γ-module is invariant with respect to actions of group $GM_{S_{n+1}}(F_3)$: $\gamma(\prod_i^j \overline{x}) = \gamma(\overline{x})$ for any $i = \overline{0, n! - 1}, j = \overline{1, n}$.

REMARK 2.2.– *Since the distributions of functionals from identically distributed random vectors also coincide, and the* γ*-module is itself a functional, the following relation holds true: for any* $g \in S_{n+1}$*:*

$$\gamma(\overline{\xi}) = \sum_{i=1}^{n} \xi_i - n\xi_0 - (n+1) \cdot \min\{0, \xi_1 - \xi_0, \ldots, \xi_n - \xi_0\} \doteq \gamma(g\overline{\xi}).$$

2.2. Examples of symmetric distributions in R^n and distributions on $n+1$-hedra

2.2.1. *Symmetric distributions*

Symmetrical distributions play a significant role in probability theory and mathematical statistics. In particular, we should mention the triangular distribution, the double exponential distribution and the Bessel distribution. Random variables with such distributions are symmetrical due to the fact that they can be written as the difference of two independent identically distributed random variables. Let us study the distributions that arise when applying a more general algebraic structure. Let $\overline{\xi} = \overline{\tau}_0\xi_0 + \cdots + \overline{\tau}_n\xi_n$, where the vectors $\overline{\tau}_0, \ldots, \overline{\tau}_n$ are defined in the previous section, then the distributions $\overline{\xi}$ and $\overline{\eta}$, where $\overline{\eta}$ is obtained from $\overline{\xi}$ by $\overline{\tau}_i$, coincide.

We are dealing not with two, but with n independent identically distributed random variables. Let us consider the distributions that $\overline{\xi}$ can have: multidimensional analogs of symmetric distributions which are of interest for probability theory and mathematical statistics.

1) Generalization of the triangular distribution (Feller 1971).

Symmetrization of the distribution uniform on [0,1] in R^1 leads to triangular distribution. It is defined on a regular rhombohedron inscribed into the unit sphere

$$Rb_n(0,1) = \left\{ \overline{x} = \sum_{i=1}^{n} x_i \overline{\tau_i} \in R^n : x_i \in [0,1], i = \overline{1,n} \right\}.$$

The sets

$$Rb_n^0\left(\frac{t}{2}(\overline{\tau}_1 + \cdots + \overline{\tau}_n), t\right) = \{\overline{x} = x_1\overline{\tau}_1 + \cdots + x_n\overline{\tau}_n \in R^n : x_1, \ldots, x_n \in [0,t]\},$$

$$Rb_n^1\left(-\frac{t}{2}\overline{\tau}_1, t\right) = \{\overline{x} = -x_1\overline{\tau}_1 + (x_2 - x_1)\overline{\tau}_2 + \cdots + (x_n - x_1)\overline{\tau}_n \in R^n :$$

$x_1, \ldots, x_n \in [0,t]\}$,

...

$$Rb_n^n\left(-\frac{t}{2}\overline{\tau}_n, t\right) = \{\overline{x} = (x_1 - x_n)\overline{\tau}_1 + \cdots - x_n\overline{\tau}_n \in R^n : x_1, \ldots, x_n \in [0,t]\}$$

are rhombohedrons with centers in $\frac{t}{2}(\overline{\tau_1} + \cdots + \overline{\tau_n}), -\frac{t}{2}\overline{\tau}_1, \ldots, -\frac{t}{2}\overline{\tau}_n$, respectively, and the length of the side equal to t. Their union gives the rhombohedron $Rb_n(0,t), t \in (0,1]$. Considering the symmetry of $Rb_n(0,t)$ with respect to rotations given by the group C_{n+1}, we have: $P\{\overline{\xi} \in Rb_n^0(\frac{t}{2}(\overline{\tau}_1 + \cdots + \overline{\tau}_n), t\} = P\{\overline{\xi} \in Rb_n^1(-\frac{t}{2}\overline{\tau}_1, t)\} = \cdots = P\{\overline{\xi} \in Rb_n^n(-\frac{t}{2}\overline{\tau}_n, t)\}$;

$$P\left\{\overline{\xi} \in Rb_n^0\left(\frac{t}{2}(\overline{\tau}_1 + \cdots + \overline{\tau}_n)\right), t\right\} = P\{0 \le \xi_1 - \xi_0 \le t, \ldots, 0 \le \xi_n - \xi_0 \le t\} =$$

$$\int_0^1 P\{u \le \xi_1 \le t + u, \ldots, u \le \xi_n \le t + u\} du = \int_0^1 P^n\{u \le \xi_1 \le t + u\} du =$$

$$\int_0^{1-t} t^n du + \int_{1-t}^1 (1-u)^n du = t^n(1-t) - \frac{1}{n+1} t^{n+1} = t^n - \frac{n}{n+1} t^{n+1}.$$

Thus,

$$P\{\overline{\xi} \in Rb_n(0,t)\} = (n+1)t^n - nt^{n+1}.$$

Consider a random variable $\overline{\xi} = \overline{\tau}_0\xi_0 + \cdots + \overline{\tau}_n\xi_n$. In the standard orthonormal basis $\overline{e}_1, \ldots, \overline{e}_n$, the random variable $\overline{\xi}$ has unequally distributed components. Therefore, it is difficult to find a common distribution function for the components. But if we write $\overline{\xi}$ in the form $\overline{\xi} = \overline{\tau}_1(\xi_1 - \xi_0) + \cdots + \overline{\tau}_n(\xi_n - \xi_0)$, where $\overline{\tau}_1, \ldots, \overline{\tau}_n$ are linearly independent and form an affine basis, then in this basis, the joint distribution function is clearly written, which is a consequence of a strong dependence of the components in the basis $\overline{\tau}_1, \ldots, \overline{\tau}_n$.

Let us put $\Phi(t_1, \ldots, t_n) = P(\xi_1 - \xi_0 \leq t_1, \ldots, \xi_n - \xi_0 \leq t_n)$ as the joint distribution function in the affine basis $\overline{\tau_1}, \ldots, \overline{\tau_n}$. Then,

$$\Phi(t_1, \ldots, t_n) = \int_0^1 F(t_1 + u) \cdot \ldots \cdot F(t_n + u)du,$$

where $F(t)$ is the distribution function of a random variable uniformly distributed on [0,1].

2) Generalization of the double exponential distribution (Feller 1971).

Symmetrization of an exponentially distributed random variable gives a double exponential distribution.

Let ξ_j in equation [2.2] be independent exponentially distributed with parameter λ. In the notations of the previous section, we have

$$P\left\{\overline{\xi} \in Rb_n^0\left(\frac{t}{2}(\overline{\tau}_1 + \cdots + \overline{\tau}_n), t\right)\right\} = \lambda \int_0^\infty e^{-\lambda u} P\{u < \xi_1 \leq t + u, \ldots,$$

$$u < \xi_n \leq t + u\}du = \lambda \int_0^\infty e^{-\lambda u}[e^{-\lambda u} - e^{-\lambda(u+t)}]^n du = \frac{1}{n+1}(1 - e^{-\lambda t})^n.$$

Thus,

$$P\{\overline{\xi} \in Rb_n(0, t)\} = (1 - e^{-\lambda t})^n.$$

3) Generalization of the Bessel distribution.

Symmetrization of the Poisson distribution leads to the Bessel distribution (Feller 1971).

Denote

$$\Re_{n+1}(R^n) = \{\overline{x} \in R^n : \overline{x} = m_0\overline{\tau}_0 + \cdots + m_n\overline{\tau}_n, m_j \in Z\},$$

where Z is the ring of integers.

Let ξ_j in equation [2.2] be independent and have Poisson distribution with parameter λ. In the basis $\overline{\tau}_1, \dots, \overline{\tau}_n$, points $\Re_{n+1}(R^n)$ are uniquely written in the form $m_1\overline{\tau}_1 + \dots + m_n\overline{\tau}_n, m_j \in Z$. Thus, ($m_* = \min\{0, m_1, \dots, m_n\}$)

$$P\{\overline{\xi} = \sum_{i=1}^{n} m_i\overline{\tau}_i\} = P\{\xi_1\overline{\tau}_1 + \dots + \xi_n\overline{\tau}_n = (m_1 + \xi_0)\overline{\tau}_1 + \dots + (m_n - \xi_0)\overline{\tau}_n\} =$$

$$e^{-\lambda}\sum_{k=0}^{\infty}\frac{\lambda^k}{k!}P\{\xi_1\overline{\tau}_1 + \dots + \xi_n\overline{\tau_n} = (m_1 + k)\overline{\tau}_1 + \dots + (m_n - k)\overline{\tau}_n\} =$$

$$e^{-\lambda}\sum_{k=-m_*}^{\infty}\frac{\lambda^k}{k!}P\{\xi_1 = (m_1 + k), \dots, \xi_n = m_n + k\} = e^{-\lambda}\sum_{k=-m_*}^{\infty}\frac{\lambda^k}{k!}P\{\xi_1 =$$

$$(m_1 + k)\} \dots P\{\xi_n = m_n + k\} = e^{-(n+1)\lambda}\sum_{k=-m_*}^{\infty}\frac{\lambda^k\lambda^{m_1+k}\cdot\dots\cdot\lambda^{m_n+k}}{k!(m_1 + k)!\cdot\dots\cdot(m_n + k)!} =$$

$$e^{-(n+1)\lambda}\sum_{k=0}^{\infty}\frac{\lambda^{(n+1)k+m_1+\dots+m_n-(n+1)m_*}}{(k - m_*)!(m_1 + k - m_*)!\cdot\dots\cdot(m_n + k - m_*)!}$$

Here, it is taken into account that $m_i - k \geq 0, i = \overline{1, n}$; therefore, $k \geq -m_*$.

This is the Bessel G-function of the multi-index $< m_1, \dots, m_n >$. So, the Bessel G-function has the property

$$P\{\overline{\xi} = m_1\overline{\tau}_1 + \dots + m_n\overline{\tau}_n\} = e^{-(n+1)\lambda}Z_{<m_1,\dots,m_n>}(\lambda).$$

It follows from the last equality that

$$\sum_{m_1\in Z}\dots\sum_{m_n\in Z} Z_{<m_1,\dots,m_n>}(\lambda) = e^{(n+1)\lambda}.$$

2.2.2. *Distributions on* $n + 1$*-hedra*

Let us consider a random variable $\zeta = \gamma(\xi_1, \dots, \xi_n) = \sum_{i=1}^{n}\xi_i - (n + 1)\min\{0, \xi_1, \dots, \xi_n\}$. Since the γ-module is invariant with respect to the action of the group $GM_{S_{n+1}}(F_3)$, the random variable ζ is symmetric with respect to the action of this group.

Since the group $GM_{S_{n+1}}(F_3)$ is isomorphic to the group of self-combinations of $n + 1$-hedron, ζ is defined on $n + 1$-hedra.

1) Bernoulli distribution on $n+1$-hedra.

Let $\xi_i = \{-1, 1\}$ with probability $\frac{1}{2}$ each. Then, for $\zeta = \sum_{i=1}^{n} \xi_i - (n+1)\min\{0, \xi_1, \ldots, \xi_n\}$, the following options are possible:

a) all ξ_i are equal to -1, then $\zeta = -n + (n+1) = 1$. The probability of such an event is $\frac{1}{2^n}$;

b) one of ξ_i is -1, then $\zeta = n - 2 + (n+1) = 2n - 1$. The probability of such an event is $\frac{1}{2^n}n$;

c) two of ξ_i are equal to -1, $\zeta = n - 4 + (n+1) = 2n - 3$. The probability is $\frac{1}{2^n}C_n^2$, and so on;

d) one of ξ_i is equal to 1, $\zeta = n - 4 + (n+1) = 2n - 3$. The probability is equal to $\frac{1}{2^n}C_n^{n-1}$;

e) all ξ_i are equal to 1, $\zeta = n$. The probability is equal to $\frac{1}{2^n}$.

Thus:

$$P(\zeta = 1) = \frac{1}{2^n}C_n^n,$$

$$P(\zeta = n) = \frac{1}{2^n}C_n^1,$$

$$P(\zeta = 2n - (2k-1)) = \frac{1}{2^n}C_n^k, k = \overline{2, n-1}.$$

2) Poisson distribution on $n+1$-hedra.

Let ξ_i have the Bessel distribution $P(\xi_i = k) = e^{-2\lambda}\sum_{j=0}^{\infty} \frac{\lambda^{2j+k-2k_*}}{(j-k_*)!(k+j-k_*)!}$, where $k_* = \min\{0, k\}, k \in Z$. Then, for $\zeta = \xi_1 + \xi_2 - 3\min\{0, \xi_1, \xi_2\}$, we have ($\zeta \geq 0$ by property 1) of the γ-module, so for any $m \in R$, we consider $P(\zeta = |m|)$): $P(\zeta = |m|) = P(\xi_1 = |m| - \xi_2 + 3\min\{0, \xi_1, \xi_2\})$, where $m \neq 0$, since for $m = 0$: trivially, $\xi_1 = \xi_2 = 0$. Let $k < 0$, then $P(\xi_2 = k) = e^{-2\lambda}\sum_{j=0}^{\infty} \frac{\lambda^{2j+k-2k_*}}{(j-k_*)!(k+j-k_*)!}$. Two variants are possible:

1) $\xi_1 \leq k$, then $\xi_1 = |m| - k + 3\xi_1$; $\xi_1 = \frac{k-|m|}{2}$, thus $\frac{k-|m|}{2} \leq k$; $|m| \geq -k$.

2) $\xi_1 > k$, then $\xi_1 = |m| - k + 3k$; $\xi_1 = |m| + 2k$; thus $|m| + 2k > k$; $|m| > -k$.

For $k \geq 0$ $P(\xi_2 = k) = e^{-2\lambda}\sum_{j=0}^{\infty} \frac{\lambda^{2j+k-2k_*}}{(j-k_*)!(k+j-k_*)!}$. Similarly:

1) $\xi_1 \leq 0$, then $\xi_1 = |m| - k + 3\xi_1$; $\xi_1 = \frac{k-|m|}{2}$; hence, $\frac{k-|m|}{2} \leq 0$; $|m| \geq k$.

2) $\xi_1 > 0$, then $\xi_1 = |m| - k$; hence, $|m| - k > 0$; $|m| > 0$.

So, $P(\zeta = |m|) = e^{-2\lambda} \sum_{k=-|m|}^{0} \sum_{j=0}^{\infty} \frac{\lambda^{2j+k-2k_*}}{(j-k_*)!(k+j-k_*)!} \{e^{-2\lambda} \times$

$$\sum_{i=0}^{\infty} \frac{\lambda^{2j+[\frac{k-|m|}{2}]-2[\frac{k-|m|}{2}]_*}}{(j-[\frac{k-|m|}{2}]_*)!(k+j-[\frac{k-|m|}{2}]_*)!} + e^{-2\lambda} \times$$

$$\sum_{i=0}^{\infty} \frac{\lambda^{2j+|m|+2k-2(|m|+2k)_*}}{(j-(|m|+2k)_*)!(k+j-(|m|+2k)_*)!}\},$$

where $[\cdot]$ - is the integer part of a number.

Then, $P(\zeta = |m|) = e^{-4\lambda} \sum_{k=-|m|}^{|m|} \sum_{j=0}^{\infty} \frac{\lambda^{2j+k-2k_*}}{(j-k_*)!(k+j-k_*)!} \{Z_{[\frac{k-|m|}{2}]}(2\lambda) + Z_{|m|-\gamma(0,k)}(2\lambda)\}$, where $k_* = \min\{0, k\}$.

So, we have

$$P(\zeta = |m|) = e^{-4\lambda} \sum_{k=-|m|}^{|m|} I_k(2\lambda)\{Z_{[\frac{k-|m|}{2}]}(2\lambda) + Z_{|m|-\gamma(0,k)}(2\lambda)\},$$

where $I_k(x)$, modified Bessel function, $\gamma(0,k) = k - 2(0 \bigwedge k) = |k|$.

For $\zeta = \xi_1 + \xi_2 + \xi_3 - 4\min\{0, \xi_1, \xi_2, \xi_3\}$ after carrying out similar calculations, we get:

$$P(\zeta = |m|) = e^{-6\lambda} \sum_{k_1=-|m|}^{|m|} \sum_{k_2=[\frac{k_1-|m|}{2}]}^{|m|-\gamma(0,k_1)} I_{<k_1,k_2>}(2\lambda)\{Z_{[\frac{k_1+k_2-|m|}{3}]}(2\lambda)+$$

$Z_{|m|-\gamma(0,k_1,k_2)}(2\lambda)\}$, where $I_{<k_1,k_2>}(2\lambda) = \sum_{j_1,j_2=0}^{\infty} \frac{\lambda^{2(j_1+j_2)+k_1+k_2-3k\ ast}}{j_1!(j_2-k_*)!(j_1+k_1-k_*)!(j_2+k_2-k_*)!}$.

For an arbitrary n, we obtain by induction:

$$P(\xi_1 + \cdots + \xi_n - (n+1)\min\{0, \xi_1, \ldots, \xi_n = |m|\} = e^{-2n\lambda} \sum_{k_1=-|m|}^{|m|} \sum_{k_2=[\frac{k_1-|m|}{2}]}^{|m|-\gamma(0,k)} \cdots$$

$$\cdots \sum_{k_{n-1}=[\frac{k_1+\cdots+k_{n-2}-|m|}{n-1}]}^{|m|-\gamma(0,k_1,\ldots,k_{n-2})} I_{<k_1,\ldots,k_{n-1}>}(2\lambda)\{Z_{[\frac{k_1+\cdots+k_{n-1}-|m|}{n}]}(2\lambda)+$$

$Z_{|m|-\gamma(0,k_1,\ldots,k_{n-1})}(2\lambda)\}$,

where $I_{<k_1,\ldots,k_{n-1}>}(2\lambda) = \sum_{j_1,\ldots,j_{n-1}=0}^{\infty} \frac{\lambda^{2(j_1+\cdots+j_{n-1})+k_1+\cdots+k_{n-1}-nk_*}}{j_1!\ldots j_{n-2}!(j_{n-1}-k_*)!(j_1+k_1-k_*)!\ldots(j_{n-1}+k_{n-1}-k_*)!}$.

3) Distributions of continuous random variables.

Let ξ_i have density $f(x)$ and distribution function $F(x)$. Denoting $\zeta = \xi_1 + \xi_2 - 3\min\{0, \xi_1, \xi_2\}$, we get: $F_\zeta(x) = P(\zeta < x) = 0$ at $x \leq 0$.

For $\xi_2 = y < 0$, we have two options:

1) If $\xi_1 < y$, then $\xi_1 + y - 3\xi_1 < x, \xi_1 > \frac{y-x}{2}$ and $\frac{y-x}{2} < y, y > -x$.

2) If $\xi_1 \geq y$, then $\xi_1 + y - 3y < x, \xi_1 < x + 2y$ and $x + 2y \geq y, y \geq -x$ so that $F_\zeta(x) = \int_{-x}^{0} dF(y)[F(x+2y) - F(\frac{y-x}{2})]$.

For $\xi_2 = y \geq 0$ we get:

1) If $\xi_1 < 0$, then $\xi_1 > \frac{y-x}{2}$ and $y < x$.

2) If $\xi_1 \geq 0$, then $\xi_1 < x - y$ and $y < x$, and thus as a result:

$$F_\zeta(x) = \int_{-x}^{x} dF(y) \left[F(x+2y) - F\left(\frac{y-x}{2}\right)\right],$$

and differentiating with respect to x, we obtain:

$$f_\zeta(x) = \int_{-x}^{x} f(y) \left[f(x+2y) + \frac{1}{2} f\left(\frac{y-x}{2}\right)\right] dy + f(x)\left(F(3x) - F(0)\right).$$

EXAMPLE 2.1.– *If* $f(x) = \frac{\lambda}{2}e^{-\lambda|x|}$, *then*

$$f_\zeta = \begin{cases} \frac{2\lambda}{3}e^{-\frac{\lambda x}{2}} + (\frac{\lambda^2 x}{4} - \frac{\lambda}{4})e^{-\lambda x} - \frac{\lambda}{6}e^{-2\lambda x} - \frac{\lambda}{4}e^{-4\lambda x}, x > 0 \\ 0, x \leq 0 \end{cases}$$

By analogy with the Bessel distribution on $n+1$*-hedra, we derive by induction:*

$$F_\zeta(x) = \int_{-x}^{x} \int_{\frac{y_1 - x}{2}}^{x+\gamma(0,y_1)} \cdots \int_{\frac{y_1+\cdots+y_{n-1}-x}{n-1}}^{x+\gamma(0,y_1,\ldots,y_{n-1})} dF(y_1)\ldots dF(y_{n-1})[F(x-$$

$$\gamma(0, y_1, \ldots, y_{n-1})) - F\left(\frac{y_1 + \cdots + y_n - x}{n}\right)].$$

3

Hyperparabolic Equations, Integral Equation and Distribution for Markov Random Evolutionary Processes

3.1. Hyperparabolic equations and methods of solving Cauchy problems

Equations for processes similar to the Markov random evolutionary process were studied by some authors. However, their models were constructed in such a way that the resulting equation was factorized and its solutions could be found as a linear combination of the solutions of the factorization elements. The resulting equations in our models cannot be factorized, but in the following sections it is possible to find their solutions using methods that have not been used before when studying similar models.

In order to reduce the system of backward Kolmogorov equations [1.12] and [1.13] to the hyperparabolic equation, we use the results of Turbin and Kolesnik (1992), according to which each of the functions $u_i(\overline{x}, t), i = \overline{0, n}$, satisfying the systems [1.12] and [1.13], also satisfies equations

$$det \begin{pmatrix} \frac{\partial}{\partial t} - v(\overline{\tau}_0, \nabla) + \lambda & -\lambda & 0 \ \ldots & 0 \\ 0 & \frac{\partial}{\partial t} - v(\overline{\tau}_1, \nabla) + \lambda & -\lambda \ \ldots & 0 \\ \ldots & \ldots & \ldots \ \ldots & \ldots \\ -\lambda & 0 & \ldots \ 0 & \frac{\partial}{\partial t} - v(\overline{\tau}_n, \nabla) + \lambda \end{pmatrix} \times$$

$$\times u(\overline{x}, t) = 0, \qquad [3.1]$$

$$det \begin{pmatrix} \frac{\partial}{\partial t} - v(\overline{\tau}_0, \nabla) + \lambda & -\frac{\lambda}{n} & -\frac{\lambda}{n} \dots & -\frac{\lambda}{n} \\ -\frac{\lambda}{n} & \frac{\partial}{\partial t} - v(\overline{\tau}_1, \nabla) + \lambda & -\frac{\lambda}{n} \dots & -\frac{\lambda}{n} \\ \dots & \dots & \dots \dots & \dots \\ -\frac{\lambda}{n} & -\frac{\lambda}{n} & \dots -\frac{\lambda}{n} & \frac{\partial}{\partial t} - v(\overline{\tau}_n, \nabla) + \lambda \end{pmatrix} \times$$

$$\times u(\overline{x}, t) = 0 \qquad [3.2]$$

correspondingly. Here, $u(\overline{x}, t)$ – any of the functions $u_i(\overline{x}, t), i = \overline{0, n}$.

Let us first consider equation [3.1]. We have:

$$\left[det \begin{pmatrix} \frac{\partial}{\partial t} - v(\overline{\tau}_0, \nabla) + \lambda & 0 & 0 \dots & 0 \\ 0 & \frac{\partial}{\partial t} - v(\overline{\tau}_1, \nabla) + \lambda & 0 \dots & 0 \\ \dots & \dots & \dots \dots & \dots \\ 0 & 0 & \dots 0 & \frac{\partial}{\partial t} - v(\overline{\tau}_n, \nabla) + \lambda \end{pmatrix} + \right.$$

$$\left. det \begin{pmatrix} 0 & -\lambda & 0 & \dots & 0 \\ 0 & 0 & -\lambda & \dots & 0 \\ \dots & \dots & \dots & \dots & \dots \\ 0 & 0 & \dots & 0 & -\lambda \\ -\lambda & 0 & \dots & 0 & 0 \end{pmatrix} \right] u(\overline{x}, t) = 0,$$

and $\prod_{i=0}^{n} (\frac{\partial}{\partial t} + \lambda - v(\overline{\tau}_i, \nabla)) u(\overline{x}, t) + (-\lambda)(-1)^{n+2}(-\lambda)^n u(\overline{x}, t) = 0$.

Thus,

$$\prod_{i=0}^{n} \left(\frac{\partial}{\partial t} + \lambda - v(\overline{\tau}_i, \nabla) \right) u(\overline{x}, t) = \lambda^{n+1} u(\overline{x}, t). \qquad [3.3]$$

Let us write the Cauchy problem for equation [3.3], the solutions of which will be functions $u_i(\overline{x}, t), i = \overline{0, n}$. To do this, we define the initial conditions for $u(\overline{x}, t) = \sum_{i=0}^{n} r_i u_i(\overline{x}, t)$, where r_i is the probability that the initial direction of movement will be the i-th direction, $\sum_{i=0}^{n} r_i = 1$.

As soon as $u_i(\overline{x}, t) = Ef(\overline{x} + v \int_0^t \overline{\tau}_{\xi_i(u)} du)$, then $u_i(\overline{x}, 0) = Ef(\overline{x}) = f(\overline{x}), i = \overline{0, n}$. So, $u(\overline{x}, 0) = \sum_{i=0}^{n} r_i u_i(\overline{x}, 0) = f(\overline{x})$.

Since the function f is continuously differentiable, it can be differentiated under the sign of mathematical expectation, and then from the system of backward Kolmogorov equations, we have:

$$\frac{\partial}{\partial t} u_0(\overline{x}, t)|_{t=0} = -\lambda u_0(\overline{x}, t)|_{t=0} + v \frac{\partial}{\partial x_1} u_0(\overline{x}, t)|_{t=0} + \lambda u_1(\overline{x}, t)|_{t=0} = -\lambda f(\overline{x}) +$$

$$vE(f(\overline{x}+v\int_0^t \overline{\tau}_{\xi_0(u)}du)'_{x_1})|_{t=0}+\lambda f(\overline{x})=vE(f'_{x_1}(\overline{x}+v\int_0^t \overline{\tau}_{\xi_0(u)}du))|_{t=0}=$$

$$vE(f'_{x_1}(\overline{x}))=v(f'_{x_1}(\overline{x}))=v(\overline{\tau}_0,\nabla)f(\overline{x}).$$

Similarly, $\frac{\partial}{\partial t}u_i(\overline{x},t)|_{t=0}=v(\overline{\tau}_i,\nabla)f(\overline{x})$. Thus,

$$\frac{\partial}{\partial t}u(\overline{x},t)|_{t=0}=\sum_{i=0}^{n} r_i\frac{\partial}{\partial t}u_i(\overline{x},t)|_{t=0}=v\sum_{i=0}^{n} r_i(\overline{\tau}_i,\nabla)f(\overline{x}).$$

Higher derivatives can be found by differentiating the equations of system [1.12] by t. For this, we introduce the operator $D\sum_{i=0}^{n} r_i(\overline{\tau}_i,\nabla)f(\overline{x}) = \lambda\sum_{i=0}^{n} r_i[-(\overline{\tau}_i,\nabla)+(\overline{\tau}_{i+1},\nabla)]f(\overline{x})+v^2\sum_{i=0}^{n} r_i(\overline{\tau}_i,\nabla)^2 f(\overline{x})$.

We have initial conditions:

$$u(\overline{x},0)=f(\overline{x}),$$

$$\frac{\partial}{\partial t}u(\overline{x},t)|_{t=0}=v\sum_{i=0}^{n} r_i(\overline{\tau}_i,\nabla)f(\overline{x}),$$

$$\frac{\partial^2}{\partial t^2}u(\overline{x},t)|_{t=0}=Du'_t(x,t)|_{t=0}=vD\sum_{i=0}^{n} r_i(\overline{\tau}_i,\nabla)f(\overline{x})=$$

$$\lambda v\sum_{i=0}^{n} r_i[-(\overline{\tau}_i,\nabla)+(\overline{\tau}_{i+1},\nabla)]f(\overline{x})+v^2\sum_{i=0}^{n} r_i(\overline{\tau}_i,\nabla)^2 f(\overline{x}),$$

$$\ldots$$

$$\frac{\partial^n}{\partial t^n}u(\overline{x},t)|_{t=0}=D^{n-1}u'_t(x,t)|_{t=0}=vD^{n-1}\sum_{i=0}^{n} r_i(\overline{\tau}_i,\nabla)f(\overline{x}). \qquad [3.4]$$

EXAMPLE 3.1.– *In the case* $f(\overline{x})=\sum_{j=1}^{n} c_j x_j$

$$u_i(\overline{x},t)|_{t=0}=E\left(\sum_{j=1}^{n} c_j x_j\right)=\sum_{j=1}^{n} c_j x_j=f(\overline{x}).$$

From the system [1.12], we have

$$\frac{\partial}{\partial t}u_0(\overline{x},t)|_{t=0}=-\lambda u_0(\overline{x},t)|_{t=0}+v\frac{\partial}{\partial x_1}u_0(\overline{x},t)|_{t=0}+\lambda u_1(\overline{x},t)|_{t=0}=-\lambda f(\overline{x})+$$

$$v(E\left(\sum_{j=1}^{n} c_j x_j\right))'_{x_1}|_{t=0} + \lambda f(\overline{x}) = v\left(\sum_{j=1}^{n} c_j x_j\right)'_{x_1}|_{t=0} = vc_1,$$

thus, $\frac{\partial}{\partial t}u_0(\overline{x},t)|_{t=0} = v(\overline{\tau}_0, \overline{c})$, where $\overline{\tau}_0 = (1, 0, \ldots, 0), \overline{c} = (c_1, \ldots, c_n)$.

Similarly: $\frac{\partial}{\partial t}u_i(\overline{x},t)|_{t=0} = v(\overline{\tau}_i, \overline{c}), i = \overline{1,n}$.

Higher derivatives can be found by differentiating the equations of the system [1.12]. Obviously, these are linear functions from $c_1, \ldots, c_n$.

So,

$$u_i(\overline{x},t)|_{t=0} = f(\overline{x}),$$

$$\frac{\partial}{\partial t}u_i(\overline{x},t)|_{t=0} = v\sum_{i=0}^{n} r_i(\overline{\tau}_i, \overline{c})f(\overline{x}),$$

$$\frac{\partial^2}{\partial t^2}u(\overline{x},t)|_{t=0} = vD\sum_{i=0}^{n} r_i(\overline{\tau}_i, \overline{c})f(\overline{x}) =$$

$$\lambda v\sum_{i=0}^{n} r_i[-(\overline{\tau}_i, \overline{c}) + (\overline{\tau}_{i+1}, \overline{c})]f(\overline{x}) + v^2\sum_{i=0}^{n} r_i(\overline{\tau}_i, \overline{c})^2 f(\overline{x}),$$

$$\ldots$$

$$\frac{\partial^n}{\partial t^n}u(\overline{x},t)|_{t=0} = D^{n-1}u'_t(x,t)|_{t=0} = vD^{n-1}\sum_{i=0}^{n} r_i(\overline{\tau}_i, \overline{c})f(\overline{x}). \quad [3.5]$$

Let $u_i(\overline{x},t), i = \overline{0,n}$ be solutions of equation [3.3]. Then, $w_i(\overline{x},t) = e^{\lambda t}u_i(\overline{x},t)$ are solutions of the equation

$$\prod_{i=0}^{n}\left(\frac{\partial}{\partial t} - v(\overline{\tau}_i, \nabla)\right)w(\overline{x},t) = \lambda^{n+1}w(\overline{x},t). \quad [3.6]$$

Let us replace the variables: $y_0 = \frac{1}{2}(t - \frac{1}{v}x_1), y_1 = \frac{1}{3}\left(t + \frac{n}{v}x_1 - \frac{1}{v\sqrt{\frac{(n+1)(n-1)}{n^2}}}\right)$, $\ldots, y_k = \frac{1}{k+2}\left(t - \sum_{i=1}^{k+1}\frac{x_i}{v\tau_k^{(i)}}\right), k = \overline{0, n-1}, y_n = \frac{1}{n+2}\left(t - \sum_{i=1}^{n}\frac{x_i}{v\tau_n^{(i)}}\right)$.

Then, equation [3.6] will take the form

$$\frac{\partial^{n+1}}{\partial y_0 \ldots \partial y_n}w(y_0, \ldots, y_n) = \lambda^{n+1}w(y_0, \ldots, y_n). \quad [3.7]$$

In the work of Turbin and Plotkin, an equation of this type was studied, and the following was proven (the ideas used in the following and corresponding references could be found in Turbin and Plotkin (1991)). Let us write $z = z(y_0, \dots, y_n) = (y_0 y_1 \dots y_n)^{\frac{1}{n}}$. The solution of equation [3.7] has the property $w(y_0, \dots, y_n) = v(z(y_0, \dots, y_n))$, and the function $v(z)$ satisfies the $n+1$ order Bessel equation:

$$\left(z \frac{d}{dz}\right)^{n+1} v(z) = (\lambda n)^{n+1} v(z). \qquad [3.8]$$

The solution of equation [3.8] is the Bessel function of $n+1$-th order.

Let us replace the variables in the initial conditions in order to obtain the Cauchy problem for equation [3.8]. Let us put $w_i(\overline{x}, t) = e^{\lambda t} u_i(\overline{x}, t)$; thus, from conditions [3.4] we have the initial conditions for equation [3.6]: $(w(\overline{x}, t) = \sum_{i=0}^{n} r_i w_i(\overline{x}, t))$

$$w(\overline{x}, t)|_{t=0} = e^{\lambda t} u(\overline{x}, t)|_{t=0} = f(\overline{x}),$$

$$w'_t(\overline{x}, t)|_{t=0} = \lambda e^{\lambda t} u(\overline{x}, t)|_{t=0} + e^{\lambda t} u'_t(\overline{x}, t)|_{t=0} = \lambda f(\overline{x}) + v \sum_{i=0}^{n} r_i(\overline{\tau}_i, \nabla) f(\overline{x}),$$

...

To find the initial conditions for equation [3.7], note that y_i and t are connected by the relation: $S(\overline{y}) = \frac{2n}{(n+1)} y_0 + \frac{(n-1)3}{n(n+1)} y_1 + \dots + \frac{3(n-1)}{4\dots(n+1)} y_{n-3} + \frac{2n}{3\dots(n+1)} y_{n-2} + \frac{(n+1)}{2\dots(n+1)} y_{n-1} + \frac{(n+1)}{2\dots(n+1)} y_n = t$ (a consequence of the fact that $\sum_{i=0}^{n} \overline{\tau}_i = 0$ by the construction of $n+1$-hedra). Then, for $t = 0$, we have $S(\overline{y}) = 0$; therefore,

$$w(\overline{y})|_{S(\overline{y})=0} = f(\overline{y}),$$

$$w'_t(\overline{y})|_{t=0} = \sum_{j=0}^{n} \frac{\partial w}{\partial y_i} \frac{\partial y_i}{\partial t} |_{S(\overline{y})=0} = \left(\sum_{j=0}^{n-1} \frac{1}{j+2} \frac{\partial w}{\partial y_j} + \frac{1}{n+1} \frac{\partial w}{\partial y_n} \right) |_{S(\overline{y})=0} =$$

$$\lambda f(\overline{x}) + v \sum_{i=0}^{n} r_i(\overline{\tau}_i, \nabla) f(\overline{x}),$$

and so on.

For equation [3.8] $y_k = \frac{z}{n z'_{y_k}}$, from where: $M(z) = \frac{2n}{(n+1)} \frac{z}{n z'_{y_0}} + \frac{(n-1)3}{n(n+1)} \frac{z}{n z'_{y_1}} + \dots + \frac{(n+1)}{2\dots(n+1)} \frac{z}{n z'_{y_n}} = 0$ at $t = 0$, and thus:

$$v(z)|_{M(z)=0} = f(z),$$

$$v_z'(z)|_{t=0} = \sum_{j=0}^{n} \frac{dv}{dz}\frac{\partial z}{\partial y_j}\frac{\partial y_j}{\partial t}|_{M(z)=0} = \left(\sum_{j=0}^{n-1} \frac{1}{j+2}\frac{dv}{dz}\frac{\partial z}{\partial y_j} + \right.$$

$$\left.\frac{1}{n+1}\frac{dv}{dz}\frac{\partial z}{\partial y_n}\right)|_{M(z)=0} = \left(\sum_{j=0}^{n-1} \frac{1}{j+2}\frac{dv}{dz}z'_{y_j} + \frac{1}{n+1}\frac{dv}{dz}z'_{y_n}\right)|_{M(z)=0} =$$

$\lambda f(\overline{x}) + v\sum_{i=0}^{n} r_i(\overline{\tau}_i, \nabla)f(\overline{x})$, and so on.

Therefore,

$$v(z)|_{M(z)=0} = f(z),$$

$$\left(\sum_{j=0}^{n-1} \frac{1}{j+2}\frac{dv}{dz}z'_{y_j} + \frac{1}{n+1}\frac{dv}{dz}z'_{y_n}\right)|_{M(z)=0} = \lambda f(\overline{x}) + v\sum_{i=0}^{n} r_i(\overline{\tau}_i, \nabla)f(\overline{x}),$$

[3.9]

...

We will write down the obtained result in the form of a theorem.

THEOREM 3.1.– *Function $u(\overline{x}, t) = r_0 u_0(\overline{x}, t) + \cdots + r_n u_n(\overline{x}, t)$, where $u_i(\overline{x}, t)$ are defined in equation* [1.9], *in the case of the cyclic change in the direction of motion, satisfies the hyperparabolic equation* [3.3] *with initial conditions* [3.4]. *Equation* [3.3] *and initial conditions* [3.4] *can be reduced to the $n+1$ order Bessel equation* [3.8] *with the initial conditions* [3.9] *by replacing the variables.*

In the case $f(\overline{x}) = \sum_{j=1}^{n} c_j x_j$, it is possible to specify the explicit form of the hyperparabolic equation solutions. The initial conditions can be changed by replacing $c_1, \ldots, c_n$, which distinguishes this case from the general case, where the initial conditions are determined by solutions and cannot be changed.

LEMMA 3.1.– *The function* [1.10] *is a solution of the hyperparabolic equation* [3.3] *with initial conditions* [3.5].

The proof directly follows from example 1.5, example 3.1 and the fact that the function $f(\overline{x}) = \sum_{i=1}^{n} c_i x_i$ satisfies the conditions of theorem 1.8.

Consider equation [3.2]. Let us calculate the determinant, using the well-known ratio: $det \begin{pmatrix} a_1 & x & \ldots & x \\ x & a_2 & \ldots & x \\ \ldots & \ldots & \ldots & \ldots \\ x & x & \ldots & a_n \end{pmatrix} = x(a_1 - x)\ldots(a_n - x)\left(\frac{1}{x} + \frac{1}{a_1 - x} + \cdots + \frac{1}{a_n - x}\right) =$
$(a_1 - x)\ldots(a_n - x) + x(a_2 - x)\ldots(a_n - x) + \cdots + x(a_1 - x)\ldots(a_{n-1} - x)$, so

we have

$$\left[\prod_{i=0}^{n}\left(\frac{\partial}{\partial t}-v(\overline{\tau}_i,\nabla)+\frac{n+1}{n}\lambda\right)-\frac{\lambda}{n}\sum_{i=0}^{n}\prod_{j\neq i}\left(\frac{\partial}{\partial t}-v(\overline{\tau}_j,\nabla)+\frac{n+1}{n}\lambda\right)\right]u(\overline{x},t)=0. \qquad [3.10]$$

From the system of backward Kolmogorov equations, we find the initial conditions, in which the function satisfies $u(\overline{x},t)=r_0u_0(\overline{x},t)+\ldots+r_nu_n(\overline{x},t)$, where r_i are the probabilities of the initial distribution ($\sum_0^n r_i=1$, $D\sum_{i=0}^n r_i(\overline{\tau}_i,\nabla)f(\overline{x})= -\lambda\sum_{i=0}^n r_i(\overline{\tau}_i,\nabla)f(\overline{x})+\frac{1}{3}\lambda\sum_{i=0}^n r_i\sum_{j\neq i}(\overline{\tau}_j,\nabla)f(\overline{x})+v\sum_{i=0}^n r_i(\overline{\tau}_i,\nabla)^2f(\overline{x})$):

$$u(\overline{x},0)=f(\overline{x}),$$

$$u_t'(\overline{x},t)|_{t=0}=v\sum_{i=0}^{n}r_i(\overline{\tau}_i,\nabla)f(\overline{x}),$$

$$u_{tt}''(\overline{x},t)|_{t=0}=Du_t'(\overline{x},t)|_{t=0}=vD\sum_{i=0}^{n}r_i(\overline{\tau}_i,\nabla)f(\overline{x})=v\left[-\lambda\sum_{i=0}^{n}r_i(\overline{\tau}_i,\nabla)f(\overline{x})+\right.$$

$$\left.\frac{1}{3}\lambda\sum_{i=0}^{n}r_i\sum_{j\neq i}(\overline{\tau}_j,\nabla)f(\overline{x})+v\sum_{i=0}^{n}r_i(\overline{\tau}_i,\nabla)^2f(\overline{x})\right]$$

...

$$u_t^{(n)}(\overline{x},t)|_{t=0}=vD^{(n-1)}\sum_{i=0}^{n}r_i(\overline{\tau}_i,\nabla)f(\overline{x}). \qquad [3.11]$$

Thus, the following theorem holds true.

THEOREM 3.2.– *Function* $u(\overline{x},t)=r_0u_0(\overline{x},t)+\cdots+r_nu_n(\overline{x},t)$, *where* $u_i(\overline{x},t)$ *are defined in equation* [1.9], *in the case of uniform changes in the directions of motion, satisfies equation* [3.10] *with initial conditions* [3.11].

Systems of Kolmogorov's forward differential equations from theorem 1.9 are reduced to hyperparabolic equations:

$$\prod_{i=0}^{n}\left(\frac{\partial}{\partial t}+\lambda+v(\overline{\tau}_i,\nabla)\right)u(\overline{x},t)=\lambda^{n+1}u(\overline{x},t),$$

$$\left[\prod_{i=0}^{n}\left(\frac{\partial}{\partial t}+v(\overline{\tau}_i,\nabla)+\frac{n+1}{n}\lambda\right)-\frac{\lambda}{n}\sum_{i=0}^{n}\prod_{j\neq i}\left(\frac{\partial}{\partial t}+v(\overline{\tau}_j,\nabla)+\right.\right.$$

$$\left.\left.\frac{n+1}{n}\lambda\right)\right]u(\overline{x},t)=0$$

in cyclic and uniform cases in accordance.

The initial conditions are as follows:

$$u_{in}(\overline{x}, \overline{y}, 0+) = P_{in}\left(\overline{x} + v\int_0^{0+} \overline{\tau}_{\xi(u)}du, \overline{y}\right) = \delta_{in}\delta(\overline{xy}),$$

where δ is the Dirac delta-function. Initial conditions for derivatives are obtained by differentiating the systems from theorem 1.9.

Note that equations [3.3] and [3.10] in the case of $n = 1$ reduce to the telegraph equation:

$$\frac{\partial^2}{\partial t^2}u(x,t) = v^2\frac{\partial^2}{\partial x^2}u(x,t) - 2\lambda\frac{\partial}{\partial t}u(x,t). \qquad [3.12]$$

Thus, the proposed model is a generalized Goldstein–Kac model for the case of the R^n space. Equation [3.12] with initial conditions $u(x,0) = f(x), u_t'(x,t)|_{t=0} = g(x)$ may be solved by the Riemann method. There have been attempts to extend the Riemann method to the case of the R^n space. There are no other methods of analytically solving hyperparabolic equations. Here, we propose two new methods for solving both the telegraph equation [3.12] and its multivariate analogues: probabilistic solution for real-analytic conditions (section 3.2) and the reduction of the Cauchy problem for hyperparabolic equation to an integral equation with its subsequent solution by the method of successive approximations (section 3.3).

3.2. Analytical solution of a hyperparabolic equation with real-analytic initial conditions

When studying the Goldstein–Kac model, it turns out that the functions from the Markov random evolutionary process satisfy the Cauchy problem for the telegraph equation. When studying a one-dimensional model, a second-order equation arises. This is due to the fact that the equation is obtained from the system of lower-order equations. The Riemann method is used for the mentioned Cauchy problem. However, this method does not allow us to write down the singular and regular part of the solution. In addition, the Riemann method cannot be applied to the hyperparabolic equations obtained in the previous section. Based on these considerations, the application of the following probabilistic solution method to hyperparabolic equations is proposed.

The solution of Cauchy's problem for the telegraph equation

$$\frac{\partial^2}{\partial t^2}u(t,x) + 2\lambda\frac{\partial}{\partial t}u(t,x) = v^2\frac{\partial^2}{\partial x^2}u(t,x)$$

$$u(0,x) = f(x), \frac{\partial}{\partial t}u(t,x)|_{t=0} = g(x). \qquad [3.13]$$

constructed by the Riemann method has the view:

$$u(t,x) = \frac{1}{2}e^{-\lambda t}\left[(f(x+vt)+f(x-vt))+\right.$$

$$v\int_{x-vt}^{x+vt} f(y)\frac{\partial}{\partial t}I_0\left(\sqrt{\frac{\lambda}{v}\left(t^2-v^2(x-y)^2\right)}\right)dy+$$

$$\left. v\int_{x-vt}^{x+vt}\left[f(y)+\lambda g(y)\right]I_0\left(\sqrt{\frac{\lambda}{v}\left(t^2-v^2(x-y)^2\right)}\right)dy\right]. \quad [3.14]$$

We realize our algorithm in the case of real-analytic initial conditions

$$\begin{cases} f(x) = \sum_{k=0}^{\infty} f_k x^k, x \in R; \\ g(x) = \sum_{k=0}^{\infty} g_k x^k, x \in R. \end{cases} \quad [3.15]$$

At the same time, we require both series to converge over the entire space R.

Let us put $\varepsilon^2 = \frac{1}{2\lambda}$ and write the equation [3.13] in the form of

$$\varepsilon^2\frac{\partial^2}{\partial t^2}U(t,x) = \left(\frac{v^2}{2\lambda}\frac{\partial^2}{\partial x^2} - \frac{\partial}{\partial t}\right)U(t,x). \quad [3.16]$$

In the hydrodynamic limit (Korolyuk and Turbin 1993), when $v \to \infty,\ \lambda \to \infty$ so that $\frac{v^2}{\lambda} \to \sigma^2$, equation [3.16] has the form of a singularly perturbed differential equation with a small parameter at the highest derivative with respect to t. In the theory of singularly perturbed evolutionary equations in many cases, it is natural for the solution to have a regular (in ε) component and a singular component containing functions of the form $e^{-\frac{t}{\varepsilon^2}}$, in our case $e^{-2\lambda t} = e^{-\frac{t}{\varepsilon^2}}$ (Korolyuk and Turbin 1993). In the Riemann solution [3.14], singular functions are clearly not contained, which is due to the analytical-geometric approach to constructing [3.13]. In the solutions constructed below, the regular and the singular components are found in an explicit form.

Let us write $b_r^{\lambda,v}(t,x;n) = E\left(x + v\int_0^t(-1)^{\xi_r^{\lambda}(s)}ds\right)^n$. Then, the function $b_r^{\lambda,v}(t,x;n)$ is a solution of the telegraph equation [3.13] with initial conditions

$$\begin{aligned} f(x) &= x^n \\ g(x) &= rvnx^{n-1}. \end{aligned} \quad [3.17]$$

If in equation [3.15] $g(x) = 0$, then the solution $u(t,x)$ of the Cauchy problem [3.13] for the real-analytic function $f(x)$ has the form

$$u_0(t,x) = \sum_{k=0}^{\infty} f_k b_0^{\lambda,v}(t,x;k).$$

If $r \neq 0$, then the function $(m \geq 1)$ $\frac{1}{rvm}\left[b_r^{\lambda,v}(t,x;m) - b_0^{\lambda,v}(t,x;m)\right]$ satisfies the telegraph equation [3.13] and the initial conditions

$$f(x) = 0,\ g(x) = x^m,$$

and then the function

$$u_r(t,x) = \sum_{m=1}^{\infty} \frac{g_m}{rvm}\left[b_r^{\lambda,v}(t,x;m) - b_0^{\lambda,v}(t,x;m)\right]$$

satisfies equation [3.13] and the initial conditions

$$f(x) = 0,\ g(x) = \sum_{m=1}^{\infty} g_m x^m$$

Hence, the function

$$u_0(t,x) + u_r(t,x) = f_0 b_0^{\lambda,v}(t,x;0) + \sum_{k=1}^{\infty}\left[f_k b_0^{\lambda,v}(t,x;k) + \frac{g_k}{rvk}\times \left(b_r^{\lambda,v}(t,x;k) - b_0^{\lambda,v}(t,x;k)\right)\right]$$

is a solution of equation [3.13] with initial conditions $f(x) = \sum_{k=0}^{\infty} f_k x^k,\ g(x) = \sum_{k=1}^{\infty} g_k x^k$. Noting now that the function $\frac{g_0}{2\lambda}\left(1 - e^{-2\lambda t}\right)$ satisfies equation [3.13] with the initial conditions $f(x) = 0,\ g(x) = g_0$, we arrive at the following result.

THEOREM 3.3.– *Let $b_r^{\lambda,v}(t,x;n)$ be the solution* [3.13] *with initial conditions* [3.17]. *Then, the solution $u(x,t)$ of the Cauchy problem* [3.13] *with real-analytic initial conditions* [3.15] *is given by the formula*

$$u(t,x) = f_0 + \frac{g_0}{2\lambda}\left(1 - e^{-2\lambda t}\right) + \sum_{k=1}^{\infty}\left[f_k b_0^{\lambda,v}(t,x;k) + \frac{g_k}{rvk}\times \left(b_r^{\lambda,v}(t,x;k) - b_0^{\lambda,v}(t,x;k)\right)\right].$$

The problem of constructing a solution is thus reduced to the calculation of moments $b_r^{\lambda,v}(t,x;k)$ of a one-dimensional Markov random evolutionary process.

LEMMA 3.2.–

$$\lim_{\substack{\lambda\to\infty \\ v\to\infty \\ \frac{v^2}{\lambda}\to\sigma^2}} b_r^{\lambda,v}(t,x;n) = \sum_{i=0}^{\left[\frac{n}{2}\right]} \binom{n}{2i} x^{n-2i}\theta_{2i}\left(\frac{v^2}{\lambda}t\right)^i \qquad [3.18]$$

where $[p]$ *is an integer part of the number* p,

$$\theta_{2j} = \begin{cases} 1 \cdot 3 \cdot \dots \cdot (2j-1), j = 2k \\ 0, j = 2k+1. \end{cases}$$

PROOF.– By the definition

$$b_{r,x}^{\lambda,v} = E\left(x + v\int_0^t (-1)^{\xi_r^\lambda(s)} ds\right)^n = \sum_{i=0}^{n} \binom{n}{i} x^{n-i} E\left(v\int_0^t (-1)^{\xi_r^\lambda(s)} ds\right)^i.$$

From weak convergence of the process $v\int_0^t (-1)^{\xi_r^\lambda(s)} ds$ at $\lambda \to \infty$, $v \to \infty$, $\frac{v^2}{\lambda} \to \sigma^2$ to the Wiener process $\sigma w(t)$, $Dw(t) = 1$ (Korolyuk and Turbin 1993), it follows that

$$\lim_{\substack{\lambda\to\infty \\ v\to\infty \\ \frac{v^2}{\lambda}\to\sigma^2}} E\left[v\int_0^t (-1)^{\xi_r^\lambda(s)} ds\right]^{2n} = \theta_{2n}\left(\frac{v^2}{\lambda}t\right)^n,$$

which gives equation [3.18].

The lemma is proven.

The lemma allows for finding solutions to equation [3.13] with initial conditions [3.17] in the form of

$$b_r^{\lambda,v}(t,x;n) = x^n + \frac{rvnx^{n-1}}{2\lambda}\left(1 - e^{-2\lambda t}\right) + \sum_{i=1}^{\left[\frac{n}{2}\right]} \binom{n}{2i} x^{n-2i}\theta_{2i}\left(\frac{v^2}{\lambda}t\right)^i +$$

$$a_n(t,x) + c_n(t,x)\left(1 - e^{-2\lambda t}\right), \qquad [3.19]$$

where the functions $a_n(t,x)$ and $c_n(t,x)$ are polynomials in x and t that do not contain powers of t higher than the $n-2$th. Since there must be $b_r^{\lambda,v}(0,x;n) = x^n$, then $a(0,x) = 0$. By differentiating equation [3.19] with respect to t, we find

$$\frac{\partial}{\partial t} b_r^{\lambda,v}(t,x;n) = rvnx^{n-1}e^{-2\lambda t} + \sum_{i=1}^{\left[\frac{n}{2}\right]} \binom{n}{2i} x^{n-2i} i\theta_{2i}\left(\frac{v^2}{\lambda}\right)^i t^{i-1} + \frac{\partial}{\partial t}a(t,x) +$$

$$\left(\frac{\partial}{\partial t}c(t,x)\right)\left(1 - e^{-2\lambda t}\right) - 2\lambda c(t,x)e^{-2\lambda t}.$$

Since $\frac{\partial}{\partial t} b_r^{\lambda,v}(t,x;n)\Big|_{t=0} = rvx^{n-1}$, we get another condition on $a_n(t,x)$ and $c_n(t,x)$:

$$\binom{n}{2} x^{n-2}\theta_2\left(\frac{v^2}{\lambda}\right)^2 + \frac{\partial}{\partial t}a_n(t,x)\Big|_{t=0} = 2\lambda c_n(0,x). \qquad [3.20]$$

THEOREM 3.4.– *Functions $a_n(t,x)$ and $c_n(t,x)$, have the form:*

$$a_n(t,x) = \sum_{j=1}^{\frac{n}{2}-1} \sum_{i=1}^{\frac{n}{2}-j} b_j^{(i)} x^{n-2(i+j)} t^i + \sum_{j=0}^{\frac{n}{2}-2} \sum_{i=1}^{\frac{n}{2}-j-1} d_j^{(i)} x^{n-2(i+j)-1} t^i,$$

$$c_n(t,x) = \sum_{j=0}^{\frac{n}{2}-1} \sum_{i=1}^{\frac{n}{2}-j} e_j^{(i)} x^{n-2(i+j)} t^{i-1} + \sum_{j=1}^{\frac{n}{2}-1} \sum_{i=1}^{\frac{n}{2}-j} f_j^{(i)} x^{n-2(i+j)+1} t^{i-1} + \sum_{i=2}^{\frac{n}{2}} f_0^{(i)} \times$$

$$x^{n-2i+1} t^{i-1},$$

if n is even;

$$a_n(t,x) = \sum_{j=1}^{\left[\frac{n}{2}\right]-1} \sum_{i=1}^{\left[\frac{n}{2}\right]-j} b_j^{(i)} x^{n-2(i+j)} t^i + \sum_{j=0}^{\left[\frac{n}{2}\right]-2} \sum_{i=1}^{\left[\frac{n}{2}\right]-j-1} d_j^{(i)} x^{n-2(i+j)-1} t^i,$$

$$c_n(t,x) = \sum_{j=0}^{\left[\frac{n}{2}\right]-1} \sum_{i=1}^{\left[\frac{n}{2}\right]-j} e_j^{(i)} x^{n-2(i+j)} t^{i-1} + \sum_{j=1}^{\left[\frac{n}{2}\right]} \sum_{i=1}^{\left[\frac{n}{2}\right]-j+1} f_j^{(i)} x^{n-2(i+j)+1} t^{i-1} +$$

$$\sum_{i=2}^{\left[\frac{n}{2}\right]+1} f_0^{(i)} x^{n-2i+1} t^{i-1},$$

if n is odd.

Here,

$$e_j^{(i)} = \frac{b_j^{(1)}}{2\lambda};\ e_j^{(i)} = \frac{1}{2\lambda(i-1)} \Big(e_{j-1}^{(i+1)} i(i-1) -$$

$$-v^2 e_j^{(i-1)} (k - 2(i+j-1))(k - 2(i+j-1) - 1) \Big),\ i \neq 1;$$

$$b_j(i) = \frac{1}{2\lambda i} \Big(2\lambda e_{j-1}^{(i+1)} i - b_{j-1}(i+1)(i+1)i + a_{j-2}^{(i+1)} (i+1)i +$$

$$v^2 b_j^{(i-1)} (k - 2(i+j-1))(k - 2(i+j-1) - 1) - v^2 e_{j-1}^{(i)} (k - 2(i+j-1)) \times$$

$$(k - 2(i+j-1) - 1));$$

$$f_j^{(i)} = \frac{d_{j-1}^{(1)}}{2\lambda};\ f_j^{(i)} = \frac{1}{2\lambda(i-1)} \Big(f_{j-1}^{(i+1)} i(i-1) -$$

$$v^2 f_j^{(i-1)} (k - 2(i+j-1) + 1)(k - 2(i+j-1)) \Big),\ i \neq 1;$$

$$d_j(i) = \frac{1}{2\lambda i} \Big(2\lambda f_j^{(i+1)} i - d_{j-1}(i+1)(i+1)i + f_{j-1}^{(i+2)} (i+1)i$$

$v^2 d_j^{(i-1)}(k-2(i+j-1)-1)(k-2(i+j-1)) - v^2 f_j^{(i)}(k-2(i+j)+1)\times$
$(k-2(i+j)))$.

At the same time, we consider $b_0^{(i)} = \binom{n}{2i}\theta_{2i}\left(\frac{v^2}{\lambda}\right)^i$, $i = 0,\ldots,\left[\frac{n}{2}\right]$, $f_0^{(1)} = -\frac{rvn}{2\lambda}$, *and if* i *and* j *go beyond the specified limits, we consider* $b_j^{(i)} = d_j^{(i)} = e_j^{(i)} = f_j^{(i)} = 0$.

PROOF.– Let us write $\gamma_n(t,x) = \sum_{i=1}^{\left[\frac{n}{2}\right]}\binom{n}{2i}x^{n-2i}\theta_{2i}\left(\frac{v^2}{\lambda}t\right)^i + a_n(t,x)$. Then $b_r^{\lambda,v}(t,x;n) = x^n + \frac{rvnx^{n-1}}{2\lambda}\left(1-e^{-2\lambda t}\right) + \gamma_n(t,x) + c_n(t,x)\left(1-e^{-2\lambda t}\right)$. Substitute this expression into equation [3.13], then group and equate terms at $e^{-2\lambda t}$. We get

$$\frac{\partial^2}{\partial t^2}c_n - 2\lambda\frac{\partial}{\partial t}c_n = v^2\frac{\partial^2}{\partial x^2}c_n - \frac{k(k-1)(k-2)rv^3x^{k-3}}{2\lambda}, \qquad [3.21]$$

$$\frac{\partial^2}{\partial t^2}\gamma_n - \frac{\partial^2}{\partial t^2}c_n + 2\lambda\frac{\partial}{\partial t}\gamma_n - 2\lambda\frac{\partial}{\partial t}c_n = v^2(k-1)kx^{k-2}+$$

$$\frac{k(k-1)(k-2)rv^3x^{k-3}}{2\lambda} + v^2\frac{\partial^2}{\partial x^2}\gamma_n - v^2\frac{\partial^2}{\partial x^2}c_n. \qquad [3.22]$$

Ratio [3.20] can be written in the form of:

$$\left.\frac{\partial}{\partial t}\gamma_n(t,x)\right|_{t=0} = 2\lambda c_n(0,t). \qquad [3.23]$$

The polynomial $\gamma_n(t,x)$ contains the sum $\sum_{i=1}^{\left[\frac{n}{2}\right]}\binom{n}{2i}x^{n-2i}\theta_{2i}\left(\frac{v^2}{\lambda}t\right)^i$, denoting the coefficient at $x^{n-2i}t^i$ due to $b_0^{(i)}$. Since in relations [3.21] and [3.22] connecting polynomials γ_n and c_n, differentiation with respect to x is performed twice, the degree of each subsequent term in x will be 2 less than the previous one, so we denote the coefficient at $x^{n-2(i+j)}t^i$ $b_j^{(i)}$.

It can be seen from equation [3.23] that the polynomial $c_n(t,x)$ contains the term $\frac{b_0^{(1)}}{2\lambda}x^{n-2}$. Let us denote $e_0^1 = \frac{b_0^{(1)}}{2\lambda}$ and, similarly to the previous one, the coefficient at $x^{n-2(i+j)}t^{i-1}$ through $e_j^{(i)}$. Collecting in equation [3.21] coefficients with matching powers of x after differentiation and t, we get:

$$e_{j-1}^{(i+1)}(i-1)i - 2\lambda(i-1)e_j^{(i)} = v^2e_j^{(i-1)}(k-2(i+j-1))(k-2(i+j-1)-1).$$

Coefficients with smaller indices are calculated before coefficients with larger indices. For example, $e_0^{(1)}$ is known, we assume $e_{-1}^{(3)}$ is equal to 0 because j exceeds the specified change limits, and we find $e_0^{(2)}$:

$$e_j^{(i)} = \frac{\left(e_{j-1}^{(i+1)} i(i-1) - v^2 e_j^{(i-1)}(k-2(i+j-1))(k-2(i+j-1)-1)\right)}{2\lambda(i-1)}.$$

Since the power of x during differentiation decreases by 2, the term with x^{k-3} does not yet appear, and therefore the presence of the expression $\frac{k(k-1)(k-2)rv^3x^{k-3}}{2\lambda}$ in equations [3.21] and [3.22] will be taken into account below.

Similarly, collecting the coefficients in equation [3.22], we obtain:

$$b_{j-1}^{(i+1)}(i+1)i - e_{j-2}^{(i+1)}(i+1)i + 2\lambda b_j^{(i)} i - 2\lambda e_{j-1}^{(i+1)} = v^2 b_j^{(i-1)}(k-2(i+j-1))\times$$

$$(k-2(i+j-1)-1) - v^2 e_{j-1}^{(i)}(k-2(i+j-1))(k-2(i+j-1)-1).$$

Since we know the coefficients of smaller indices, for example, b_0^i and e_0^i, then we can write down

$$b_j(i) = \frac{1}{2\lambda i}\left(2\lambda e_{j-1}^{(i+1)} i - b_{j-1}(i+1)(i+1)i + a_{j-2}^{(i+1)}(i+1)i + \right.$$

$$v^2 b_j^{(i-1)}(k-2(i+j-1))(k-2(i+j-1)-1) - v^2 e_{j-1}^{(i)}\times$$

$$\left.(k-2(i+j-1))(k-2(i+j-1)-1)\right).$$

Then, from equation [3.23], we find $e_j^{(1)} = \frac{b_j^{(1)}}{2\lambda}$ and repeat the same procedure. The change limits of i and j can be found for the reasons that polynomials have a degree no higher than $n-2$ and the variables x and t cannot have a degree lower than 0.

However, relations [3.21] and [3.22] contain terms $\frac{k(k-1)(k-2)rv^3x^{k-3}}{2\lambda}$, which contribute to $\gamma_n(t,x)$ and $c_n(t,x)$. Let us denote that $f_0^{(1)} = -\frac{rvn}{2\lambda}$ is the coefficient at $x^{n-1}\left(1-e^{-2\lambda t}\right)$, and in general $f_j^{(i)}$ is the coefficient at $x^{n-2(i+j)+1}t^{i-1}\left(1-e^{-2\lambda t}\right)$, and $d_j^{(i)}$ at $x^{n-2(i+j)-1}t^i$. Applying the procedure described above, we will have the necessary ratios.

Theorem is proven.

Consider equation [3.16] in the form of a singularly perturbed Cauchy problem:

$$\varepsilon^2\frac{\partial^2}{\partial t^2}u(t,x) = \left(\frac{\sigma^2}{2}\frac{\partial^2}{\partial x^2} - \frac{\partial}{\partial t}\right)u(t,x)$$

$$u(0,x) = f(x),\ \frac{\partial}{\partial t}u(t,x)\bigg|_{t=0} = r\frac{\sigma}{\sqrt{2}\varepsilon}f'(x),\ r \in R.$$

Using theorem 3.4, we present the solutions of this Cauchy problem for conditions of independent interest, i.e. for the moments of the Markov random evolutionary process (the regular part of the solution is highlighted in square brackets):

$$f(x) = x\ :\ u(t,x) = \left[x + \frac{r}{\sqrt{2}}\sigma\varepsilon\right] - \frac{r}{\sqrt{2}}\sigma\varepsilon e^{-\frac{t}{\varepsilon^2}};$$

$$f(x) = x^2\ :\ u(t,x) = \left[x^2 + \sigma^2 t + r\sigma\sqrt{2}\varepsilon x - \sigma^2\varepsilon^2\right] + \left(\sigma^2\varepsilon^2 - r\sigma\sqrt{2}\varepsilon\right)\times$$
$$e^{-\frac{t}{\varepsilon^2}};$$

$$f(x) = x^3\ :\ u(t,x) = \left[x^3 + 3x\sigma^2 t - 3x\sigma^2\varepsilon^2 + \frac{3r}{\sqrt{2}}\sigma\varepsilon x^2 - \frac{3r}{\sqrt{2}}\sigma^3\varepsilon^3\right] +$$
$$(3x\sigma^2\varepsilon^2 - \frac{3r}{\sqrt{2}}\sigma\varepsilon x^2 + \frac{3r}{\sqrt{2}}\sigma^3\varepsilon t + \frac{3r}{\sqrt{2}}\sigma^3\varepsilon^3)e^{-\frac{t}{\varepsilon^2}};$$

$$f(x) = x^4\ :\ u(t,x) = [x^4 + 1\cdot 3\cdot(\sigma^2 t)^2 + (6x^2\sigma^2 - 18\sigma^4\varepsilon^2)t - 6x^2\sigma^2\varepsilon^2 +$$
$$6t\sigma^4\varepsilon^2 + +18\sigma^4\varepsilon^4 + 2r\sigma\sqrt{2}\varepsilon x^3 + 6r\sigma^3\sqrt{2}\varepsilon xt - 12r\sigma^3\sqrt{2}\varepsilon^3 x\Big] + \Big(6x^2\sigma^2\varepsilon^2 -$$
$$2r\sigma\sqrt{2}\varepsilon x^3 + 12r\sigma^3\sqrt{2}\varepsilon^3 x + 6r\sigma^3\sqrt{2}\varepsilon xt - 6\sigma^4\varepsilon^2 t - 18\sigma^4\varepsilon^4\Big)\, e^{-\frac{t}{\varepsilon^2}};$$

$$f(x) = x^5\ :\ u(t,x) = [x^5 - 10x^3\sigma^2\varepsilon^2 + 90x\sigma^4\varepsilon^4 + 10x^3 t\sigma^2 +$$
$$15x\left(\sigma^2 t\right)^2 - 60xt\sigma^4\varepsilon^2 + 5\frac{r}{\sqrt{2}}x^4\sigma\varepsilon - 15rx^2 t\sigma^3\sqrt{2}\varepsilon + 15\frac{r}{\sqrt{2}}t^2\sigma^5\varepsilon -$$
$$30rx^2\sigma^3\sqrt{2}\varepsilon^3 + +45rt\sigma^5\sqrt{2}\varepsilon^3 + 120r\sigma^5\sqrt{2}\varepsilon^5\Big] + \Big(10x^3\sigma^2\varepsilon^2 - 90x\sigma^4\varepsilon^4 -$$
$$30xt\sigma^4\varepsilon^2 - \frac{5r}{\sqrt{2}}x^4\sigma\varepsilon - 15rx^2 t\sigma^3\sqrt{2}\varepsilon - 15\frac{r}{\sqrt{2}}t^2\sigma^5\varepsilon + 30rx^2\sigma^3\sqrt{2}\varepsilon^3 -$$
$$45rt\sigma^5\sqrt{2}\varepsilon^3 - 120r\sigma^5\sqrt{2}\varepsilon^5\Big)\, e^{-\frac{t}{\varepsilon^2}};$$

$$f(x) = x^6\ :\ u(t,x) = [x^6 - 15x^4\sigma^2\varepsilon^2 + 270x^2\sigma^4\varepsilon^4 + \left(45x^2\sigma^4 - 135\sigma^6\varepsilon^2\right)t^2 +$$
$$\left(15x^4\sigma^2 - 180x^2\sigma^4\varepsilon^2 + 540\sigma^6\varepsilon^4\right)t - 900\sigma^6\varepsilon^6 + 3rx^5\sigma\sqrt{2}\varepsilon -$$
$$60x^3\sigma^3\sqrt{2}\varepsilon^3 + 180x\sigma^5\sqrt{2}\varepsilon^5 + 30rx^3 t\sigma^3\sqrt{2}\varepsilon + 90rxt\sigma^5\sqrt{2}\varepsilon^3 +$$

$$45rxt^2\sigma^5\sqrt{2}\varepsilon\Big] + \left(15x^4\sigma^2\varepsilon^2 - 270x^2\sigma^4\varepsilon^4 - 90x^2t\sigma^4\varepsilon^2 + \right.$$

$$45t^2\sigma^6\varepsilon^2 + 360t\sigma^6\varepsilon^4 + 900\sigma^6\varepsilon^6 - 3rx^5\sigma\sqrt{2}\varepsilon + 60x^3\sigma^3\sqrt{2}\varepsilon^3 -$$

$$\left. 180x\sigma^5\sqrt{2}\varepsilon^5 + 30rx^3t\sigma^3\sqrt{2}\varepsilon - 270rxt\sigma^5\sqrt{2}\varepsilon^3 - 45rxt^2\sigma^5\sqrt{2}\varepsilon\right) e^{-\frac{t}{\varepsilon^2}}.$$

The question arises about the convergence of the series which represents the solution in the case of real-analytic initial conditions

$$\begin{cases} f(x) = \sum_{k=0}^{\infty} f_k x^k, x \in R; \\ g(x) = rvf'(x), x \in R. \end{cases}$$

But since the initial conditions are represented by series which are convergent on the entire R, the series which will represent the solution will also converge on the entire R. This is due to the fact that the solution is limited since its argument is determined by evolution and not extended beyond the evolution front, which is a regular triangle which vertices lie at a distance vt from its center.

For high-order hyperparabolic equations [3.10], we apply a similar method. In the case of a linear function $f(x) = x_1 + \cdots + x_n$ using relation [1.7], we have:

$$u(\overline{x}, t) = r_0 E\left(x_1 + \cdots + x_n + v\left[\int_0^t \tau^{(1)}_{\xi_0(u)} du + \cdots + \int_0^t \tau^{(n)}_{\xi_0(u)} du\right]\right) + \cdots +$$

$$r_n E\left(x_1 + \cdots + x_n + v\left[\int_0^t \tau^{(1)}_{\xi_n(u)} du + \cdots + \int_0^t \tau^{(n)}_{\xi_n(u)} du\right]\right) = x_1 + \cdots + x_n -$$

$$\frac{n}{n+1}\frac{v}{\lambda}(e^{-\frac{n+1}{n}\lambda t} - 1)[r_0(\overline{\tau}_0, \overline{e}) + \cdots + r_n(\overline{\tau}_n, \overline{e})], \overline{e} = (1, \ldots, 1). \quad [3.24]$$

For an arbitrary Cauchy problem with analytic $f(\overline{x})$, we look for a solution in the form $u(\overline{x}, t) = \gamma(\overline{x}, t) + (e^{-\frac{n+1}{n}\lambda t} - 1)\delta(\overline{x}, t)$.

For unknown functions $\gamma(\overline{x}, t)$ and $\delta(\overline{x}, t)$, we write the ratio from the equation and initial conditions for $f(\overline{x}) = x_1^{k_1} \ldots x_n^{k_n}$. From these ratios, we find the unknown $\gamma(\overline{x}, t)$ and $\delta(\overline{x}, t)$. For example, in the case of $n = 2$, the equation has the form:

$$\left[\frac{\partial^3}{\partial t^3} + 3\lambda\frac{\partial^2}{\partial t^2} + \frac{9\lambda^2}{4}\frac{\partial}{\partial t} - \frac{3v^2}{4}\left(\frac{\partial^3}{\partial x_1^2\partial t} + \frac{\partial^3}{\partial x_2^2\partial t}\right) - \frac{3\lambda v^2}{4}\left(\frac{\partial^2}{\partial x_1^2} + \frac{\partial^2}{\partial x_2^2}\right) - \right.$$

$$\left.\frac{v^3}{4}\frac{\partial^3}{\partial x_1^3} + \frac{3v^3}{4}\frac{\partial^3}{\partial x_1\partial x_2^2}\right] u(x_1, x_2, t) = 0, \quad [3.25]$$

and initial conditions

$$u(x_1, x_2, 0) = f(x_1, x_2),$$

$$u'_t(x_1, x_2, t)|_{t=0} = v\left[(r_0 - \frac{1}{2}r_1 - \frac{1}{2}r_2)f'_{x_1} + \left(\frac{\sqrt{3}}{2}r_1 - \frac{\sqrt{3}}{2}r_2\right)f'_{x_2}\right],$$

$$u''_{tt}(x_1, x_2, t)|_{t=0} = -\frac{3}{2}\lambda v\left[(r_0 - \frac{1}{2}r_1 - \frac{1}{2}r_2)f'_{x_1} + \left(\frac{\sqrt{3}}{2}r_1 - \frac{\sqrt{3}}{2}r_2\right)f'_{x_2}\right] +$$

$$v^2\left[\left(r_0 + \frac{1}{4}r_1 + \frac{1}{4}r_2\right)f''_{x_1x_1} + \left(-\frac{\sqrt{3}}{2}r_1 + \frac{\sqrt{3}}{2}r_2\right)f''_{x_1x_2} + \left(\frac{3}{4}r_1 - \frac{3}{4}r_2\right)f''_{x_2x_2}\right].$$

Let $f(x_1, x_2) = x_1^{k_1}x_2^{k_2}$. We look for a solution in the form:

$$u(x_1, x_2, t) = \gamma(x_1, x_2, t) + (e^{-\frac{3}{2}\lambda t} - 1)\delta(x_1, x_2, t).$$

For a linear function, we have from equation [3.24]:

$$u(x_1, x_2, t) = x_1 + x_2 - \frac{2v}{3\lambda}(e^{-\frac{3}{2}\lambda t} - 1)\left[r_0 + \left(-\frac{1}{2} + \frac{\sqrt{3}}{2}\right)r_1 + \left(-\frac{1}{2} - \frac{\sqrt{3}}{2}\right)r_2\right]. \quad [3.26]$$

From here, we find $v\int_0^t E\tau^{(1)}_{\xi(u)}du = \frac{2v}{3\lambda}(1 - e^{-\frac{3}{2}\lambda t})[r_0 - \frac{1}{2}r_1 - \frac{1}{2}r_2]$ and $v\int_0^t E\tau^{(2)}_{\xi(u)}du = \frac{2v}{3\lambda}(1 - e^{-\frac{3}{2}\lambda t})[\frac{\sqrt{3}}{2}r_1 - \frac{\sqrt{3}}{2}r_2]$.

For $f(x_1, x_2) = x_1x_2$, we have: $u(x_1, x_2, t) = E\left[x_1x_2 + x_1v\int_0^t \tau^{(2)}_{\xi(u)}du + x_2v\int_0^t \tau^{(1)}_{\xi(u)}du + v^2\int_0^t\int_0^t \tau^{(1)}_{\xi(u_1)}\tau^{(2)}_{\xi(u_2)}du_1du_2\right]$. All terms of the sum, except the last one, are known, so we look for a solution in the form $u(x_1, x_2, t) = [x_1x_2 - \frac{2v}{3\lambda}(e^{-\frac{3}{2}\lambda t} - 1)[(r_0 - \frac{1}{2}r_1 - \frac{1}{2}r_2)x_1 + (\frac{\sqrt{3}}{2}r_1 - \frac{\sqrt{3}}{2})r_2)x_2] + \gamma(t) + (e^{-\frac{3}{2}\lambda t} - 1)\delta(t)]$, where γ and δ depend only on t.

From equation [3.25] and the initial conditions, we have:

$$\frac{\partial^3}{\partial t^3}\gamma(t) + 3\lambda\frac{\partial^2}{\partial t^2}\gamma(t) + \frac{9\lambda^2}{4}\frac{\partial}{\partial t}\gamma(t) - \frac{\partial^3}{\partial t^3}\delta(t) - 3\lambda\frac{\partial^2}{\partial t^2}\delta(t) -$$

$$\frac{9\lambda^2}{4}\frac{\partial}{\partial t}\delta(t) + \frac{\partial^3}{\partial t^3}\gamma(t)e^{-\frac{3}{2}\lambda t} - \frac{3\lambda}{2}\frac{\partial^2}{\partial t^2}\delta(t)e^{-\frac{3}{2}\lambda t} = 0,$$

$$v\left[\left(r_0 - \frac{1}{2}r_1 - \frac{1}{2}r_2\right)x_2 + \left(\frac{\sqrt{3}}{2}r_1 - \frac{\sqrt{3}}{2}r_2\right)x_1\right] + \frac{\partial}{\partial t}\gamma(t)|_{t=0} - \frac{3\lambda}{2}\frac{\partial}{\partial t}\delta(t)|_{t=0} =$$

$$v\left[\left(r_0-\frac{1}{2}r_1-\frac{1}{2}r_2\right)x_2+\left(\frac{\sqrt{3}}{2}r_1-\frac{\sqrt{3}}{2}r_2\right)x_1\right],$$

$$-\frac{3}{2}\lambda v\left[\left(r_0-\frac{1}{2}r_1-\frac{1}{2}r_2\right)x_2+\left(\frac{\sqrt{3}}{2}r_1-\frac{\sqrt{3}}{2}r_2\right)x_1\right]+\frac{\partial^2}{\partial t^2}\gamma(t)|_{t=0}-$$

$$3\lambda\frac{\partial}{\partial t}\delta(t)|_{t=0}+\frac{9\lambda^2}{4}\delta(0)=-\frac{3}{2}\lambda v\left[\left(r_0-\frac{1}{2}r_1-\frac{1}{2}r_2\right)x_2+\left(\frac{\sqrt{3}}{2}r_1-\right.\right.$$

$$\left.\left.\frac{\sqrt{3}}{2}r_2\right)x_1\right]+v^2\left(-\frac{\sqrt{3}}{2}r_1+\frac{\sqrt{3}}{2}r_2\right).$$

Collecting terms at $e^{-\frac{3}{2}\lambda t}$ and free terms, and taking into account that $\gamma(t)$ and $\delta(t)$ do not depend on x_1, x_2, and therefore the terms containing them can be discarded, we get four ratios:

$$\frac{\partial^3}{\partial t^3}\gamma(t)+3\lambda\frac{\partial^2}{\partial t^2}\gamma(t)+\frac{9\lambda^2}{4}\frac{\partial}{\partial t}\gamma(t)-\frac{\partial^3}{\partial t^3}\delta(t)-3\lambda\frac{\partial^2}{\partial t^2}\delta(t)-\frac{9\lambda^2}{4}\frac{\partial}{\partial t}\delta(t)=0,$$

$$\frac{\partial^3}{\partial t^3}\gamma(t)-\frac{3\lambda}{2}\frac{\partial^2}{\partial t^2}\delta(t)=0,$$

$$\frac{\partial}{\partial t}\gamma(t)|_{t=0}=\frac{3\lambda}{2}\frac{\partial}{\partial t}\delta(t)|_{t=0},$$

$$\frac{\partial^2}{\partial t^2}\gamma(t)|_{t=0}=3\lambda\frac{\partial}{\partial t}\delta(t)|_{t=0}-\frac{9\lambda^2}{4}\delta(0)+v^2\left(-\frac{\sqrt{3}}{2}r_1+\frac{\sqrt{3}}{2}r_2\right).$$

When solving the equation, it should be taken into account that $\gamma(t)$ and $\delta(t)$ have in t a degree no higher than k_1+k_2-1, i.e. in this case no higher than 1, so $\frac{\partial^3}{\partial t^3}\gamma(t)$, $\frac{\partial^2}{\partial t^2}\gamma(t)$, $\frac{\partial^3}{\partial t^3}\delta(t)$, $\frac{\partial^2}{\partial t^2}\gamma(t)$ are equal to 0. Therefore, it is necessary to solve the system

$$\begin{cases}\frac{\partial}{\partial t}\gamma(t)=\frac{\partial}{\partial t}\delta(t),\\ \frac{\partial}{\partial t}\gamma(t)|_{t=0}=\frac{3\lambda}{2}\frac{\partial}{\partial t}\delta(t)|_{t=0},\\ 3\lambda\frac{\partial}{\partial t}\delta(t)|_{t=0}=\frac{9\lambda^2}{4}\delta(0)-v^2(-\frac{\sqrt{3}}{2}r_1+\frac{\sqrt{3}}{2}r_2).\end{cases}$$

By substituting the value of the derivative of $\gamma(t)$ from the first to the second equality, we get:

$$\begin{cases}-\frac{3\lambda}{2}\lambda\frac{\partial}{\partial t}\delta(t)|_{t=0}=-\frac{9\lambda^2}{4}\delta(0),\\ 3\lambda\frac{\partial}{\partial t}\delta(t)|_{t=0}=\frac{9\lambda^2}{4}\delta(0)-v^2(-\frac{\sqrt{3}}{2}r_1+\frac{\sqrt{3}}{2}r_2).\end{cases}$$

and $\frac{3\lambda}{2}\lambda\frac{\partial}{\partial t}\delta(t)|_{t=0} = -v^2(-\frac{\sqrt{3}}{2}r_1 + \frac{\sqrt{3}}{2}r_2)$. Thus, $\delta(t) = -\frac{2v^2}{3\lambda}t(-\frac{\sqrt{3}}{2}r_1 + \frac{\sqrt{3}}{2}r_2) + \dots$

From the third equation, we get $\frac{9\lambda^2}{4}\delta(0) = -v^2(-\frac{\sqrt{3}}{2}r_1 + \frac{\sqrt{3}}{2}r_2)$, and finally $\delta(t) = -\frac{2v^2}{3\lambda}t(\frac{\sqrt{3}}{2}r_2 - \frac{\sqrt{3}}{2}r_1) - \frac{4v^2}{9\lambda^2}(\frac{\sqrt{3}}{2}r_2 - \frac{\sqrt{3}}{2}r_1)$.

From the first equation, we have: $\gamma(t) = -\frac{2v^2}{3\lambda}t(\frac{\sqrt{3}}{2}r_2 - \frac{\sqrt{3}}{2}r_1)$

Thus, for $f(x_1, x_2) = x_1x_2$:

$$u(x_1, x_2, t) = x_1x_2 - \frac{2v^2}{3\lambda}t\left(\frac{\sqrt{3}}{2}r_2 - \frac{\sqrt{3}}{2}r_1\right) - (e^{-\frac{3}{2}\lambda t} - 1)\left(\frac{2v}{3\lambda}\left(\left(r_0 - \frac{1}{2}r_1 - \frac{1}{2}r_2\right)x_1 + \left(\frac{\sqrt{3}}{2}r_1 - \frac{\sqrt{3}}{2}\right)r_2\right)x_2 + \frac{2v^2}{3\lambda}t\left(\frac{\sqrt{3}}{2}r_2 - \frac{\sqrt{3}}{2}r_1\right) + \frac{4v^2}{9\lambda^2}\times\left(\frac{\sqrt{3}}{2}r_2 - \frac{\sqrt{3}}{2}r_1\right)\right). \quad [3.27]$$

From here, we find $v^2\int_0^t\int_0^t \tau^{(1)}_{\xi(u_1)}\tau^{(2)}_{\xi(u_2)}du_1du_2 = e^{-\frac{3}{2}\lambda t}\frac{2v^2}{3\lambda}t(\frac{\sqrt{3}}{2}r_1 - \frac{\sqrt{3}}{2}r_2) - (e^{-\frac{3}{2}\lambda t} - 1)\frac{4v^2}{9\lambda^2}(\frac{\sqrt{3}}{2}r_2 - \frac{\sqrt{3}}{2}r_1)$.

Obviously, in the case of multidimensional hyperparabolic equations, the described method faces difficulties: the solution of any order cannot be found directly: to do this, firstly it is necessary to find solutions of lower degrees. In this regard, it should be noted that the solutions are written using moments of Markov random evolutionary processes, found in section 1.2. For the telegraph equation, we have formulas [2.5]. Similarly, solutions are written using relations [1.5]. In the case of $n = 2$, they coincide with moments [3.26] and [3.27] and higher moments.

In addition, by applying moments [1.8], we can solve equation [3.3] – the case of a cyclic change in the direction of motion – with real-analytic initial conditions.

Questions about the convergence of solutions in the multidimensional case are solved in the same way as in the case of the space R^1, i.e. the solution, as well as the series specifying the initial conditions, coincides in the entire space R^n.

3.3. Integral representation of the hyperparabolic equation

In the Goldstein–Kac model, functions of the form $u(x,t) = Ef\left(x + v\int_0^t(-1)^{\xi(u)}du\right)$ are considered, which satisfy the Cauchy problem:

$$\frac{\partial^2}{\partial t^2}u(x,t) = -2\lambda\frac{\partial}{\partial t}u(x,t) + v^2\frac{\partial^2}{\partial x^2}u(x,t), u(x,0) = f(x), \qquad [3.28]$$

$\frac{\partial}{\partial t}u(x,t)|_{t=0} = v\frac{d}{dx}f(x)$ in the case of start in the positive direction,

$\frac{\partial}{\partial t}u(x,t)|_{t=0} = -v\frac{d}{dx}f(x)$ in the case of start in the negative direction.

Let us write the integral equation for $u_+(x,t)$: the function of the evolutionary process starting in the positive direction over the first jump of the process, which we will call Kolmogorov's integral equation ($N(t)$: the number of Poisson events in the time interval t):

$$u_+(x,t) = P(N(t)=0)Ef(x+vt) + \int_0^t P(N(s)=1)Ef(x+vs+$$

$$v\int_s^t (-1)^{\xi_1(u)}du)ds = e^{-\lambda t}f(x+vt) + \lambda\int_0^t e^{-\lambda s}u_-(x+vs,t-s)ds, \qquad [3.29]$$

where $u_-(x,t)$ is a function from the evolution starting in the negative direction, for which we similarly have

$$u_-(x,t) = e^{-\lambda t}f(x-vt) + \lambda\int_0^t e^{-\lambda s}u_+(x-vs,t-s)ds.$$

Substituting the last expression in equation [3.29], we get

$$u_+(x,t) = e^{-\lambda t}f(x+vt) + \lambda e^{-\lambda t}\int_0^t f(x-v(t-2s))ds+$$

$$\lambda^2\int_0^t\int_0^{t-s} e^{-\lambda(l+s)}u_+(x+v(s-l),t-(l+s))dlds \qquad [3.30]$$

Similarly, for $u_-(x,t)$:

$$u_-(x,t) = e^{-\lambda t}f(x-vt) + \lambda e^{-\lambda t}\int_0^t f(x+v(t-2s))ds+$$

$$\lambda^2\int_0^t\int_0^{t-s} e^{-\lambda(l+s)}u_-(x-v(s-l),t-(l+s))dlds. \qquad [3.31]$$

To reduce equation [3.30] to the Cauchy problem [3.28], let us replace the variables:

$$u_+(x,t) = e^{-\lambda t}f(x+vt) + \lambda e^{-\lambda t}\int_0^t f(x-v(t-2s))ds + \lambda^2\int_0^t\int_s^t e^{-\lambda m}u_+(x+$$

$$v(2s-m),t-m)dmds = e^{-\lambda t}f(x+vt) + \lambda e^{-\lambda t}\int_0^t f(x-v(t-2s))ds +$$

$$\lambda^2 \int_0^t \int_0^m e^{-\lambda m}u_+(x+v(2s-m),t-m)dsdm = e^{-\lambda t}f(x+vt) + \lambda e^{-\lambda t}\times$$

$$\int_0^t f(x-v(t+2s))ds + \lambda^2 e^{-\lambda t}\int_0^t \int_0^{t-k} e^{\lambda k}u_+(x+v(2s+k-t),k)dsdk.$$

By differentiating the last expression with respect to x and t, we get

$$\frac{\partial^2}{\partial x^2}u_+(x,t) = e^{-\lambda t}\frac{d^2}{dx^2}f(x+vt) + \lambda e^{-\lambda t}\int_0^t \frac{d^2}{dx^2}f(x-v(t+2s))ds +$$

$$\lambda^2 e^{-\lambda t}\int_0^t \int_0^{t-k} e^{\lambda k}\frac{\partial^2}{\partial x^2}u_+(x+v(2s+k-t),k)dsdk, \quad [3.32]$$

$$\frac{\partial}{\partial t}u_+(x,t) = -\lambda\left[e^{-\lambda t}f(x+vt) + \lambda e^{-\lambda t}\int_0^t f(x-v(t-2s))ds - \right.$$

$$\left.\lambda^2 e^{-\lambda t}\int_0^t \int_0^{t-k} e^{\lambda k}u_+(x+v(2s+k-t),k)dsdk\right] + \left[ve^{-\lambda t}\frac{d}{dx}f(x+vt) - \right.$$

$$\lambda v e^{-\lambda t}\int_0^t \frac{d}{dx}f(x-v(t-2s))ds + \lambda^2 v e^{-\lambda t}\int_0^t \int_0^{t-k} e^{\lambda k}\times$$

$$\left.\frac{\partial}{\partial x}u_+(x+v(2s+k-t),k)dsdk\right] + \lambda e^{-\lambda t}f(x+vt) + \lambda^2 e^{-\lambda t}\int_0^t e^{\lambda k}\times$$

$$u_+(x+vt-vk,k)dk = -\lambda u_+(x,t) + \left[ve^{-\lambda t}\frac{d}{dx}f(x+vt) - \right.$$

$$\lambda v e^{-\lambda t}\int_0^t \frac{d}{dx}f(x-v(t-2s))ds + \lambda^2 v e^{-\lambda t}\int_0^t \int_0^{t-k} e^{\lambda k}\times$$

$$\left.\frac{\partial}{\partial x}u_+(x+v(2s+k-t),k)dsdk\right] + \lambda e^{-\lambda t}f(x+vt) +$$

$$\lambda^2 e^{-\lambda t}\int_0^t e^{\lambda k}u_+(x+vt-vk,k)dk, \quad [3.33]$$

$$\frac{\partial^2}{\partial t^2}u_+(x,t) = -\lambda\frac{\partial}{\partial t}u_+(x,t) - \lambda\left[ve^{-\lambda t}\frac{d}{dx}f(x+vt) - \lambda ve^{-\lambda t}\times\right.$$

$$\int_0^t \frac{d}{dx}f(x-v(t-2s))ds + \lambda^2 ve^{-\lambda t}\int_0^t\int_0^{t-k} e^{\lambda k}\frac{\partial}{\partial x}u_+(x+v(2s+$$

$$\left.k-t),k)dsdk + \lambda e^{-\lambda t}f(x+vt) - \lambda^2 e^{-\lambda t}\int_0^t e^{\lambda k}u_+(x+vt-vk,k)dk\right]+$$

$$v^2\left[e^{-\lambda t}\frac{d^2}{dx^2}f(x+vt) + \lambda e^{-\lambda t}\int_0^t \frac{d^2}{dx^2}f(x-v(t-2s))ds+\right.$$

$$\left.\lambda^2 e^{-\lambda t}\int_0^t\int_0^{t-k} e^{\lambda k}\frac{\partial^2}{\partial x^2}u_+(x+v(2s+k-t),k)dsdk\right] - \lambda ve^{-\lambda t}\frac{d}{dx}f(x+$$

$$vt) + \lambda^2 ve^{-\lambda t}\int_0^t e^{\lambda k}\frac{d}{dx}u_+(x+vt-vk,k)dk + \lambda ve^{-\lambda t}\frac{d}{dx}f(x+$$

$$vt) + \lambda^2 ve^{-\lambda t}\int_0^t e^{\lambda k}\frac{d}{dx}u_+(x+vt-vk,k)dk + \lambda^2 e^{-\lambda t}e^{\lambda t}u_+(x,t). \qquad [3.34]$$

Combining equations [3.32], [3.33] and [3.34], we get

$$\frac{\partial^2}{\partial t^2}u_+(x,t) = -\lambda\frac{\partial}{\partial t}u_+(x,t) - \lambda\left[\frac{\partial}{\partial t}u_+(x,t) + \lambda u_+(x,t)\right] + v^2\frac{\partial^2}{\partial x^2}u_+(x,t)+$$

$$\lambda^2 u_+(x,t) = -2\lambda\frac{\partial}{\partial t}u_+(x,t) + v^2\frac{\partial^2}{\partial x^2}u_+(x,t).$$

The initial conditions are obviously as follows: $u(x,0) = f(x)$, $\frac{\partial}{\partial t}u(x,t)|_{t=0} = v\frac{d}{dx}f(x)$.

Analogous calculations give the telegraph equation for the function $u_-(x,t)$ with initial conditions: $u(x,0) = f(x)$, $\frac{\partial}{\partial t}u(x,t)|_{t=0} = -v\frac{d}{dx}f(x)$.

Thus, the following theorem is true.

THEOREM 3.5.– *Functions* $u_+(x,t), u_-(x,t)$ – *solutions of the Cauchy problem* [3.28], *under the condition of differentiability* $f(\overline{x})$ *in definition* [1.9] – *satisfy equations* [3.30] *and* [3.31], *respectively. The solutions of the equations satisfy the equations and initial conditions* [3.28].

In other words, the Cauchy problem [3.28] and equations [3.30] and [3.31] are equivalent.

Let us now consider the general Cauchy problem

$$\frac{\partial^2}{\partial t^2}u(x,t) = -2\lambda\frac{\partial}{\partial t}u(x,t) + v^2\frac{\partial^2}{\partial x^2}u(x,t)$$

$$u(x,0) = f(x), \frac{\partial}{\partial t}u(x,t)|_{t=0} = g(x) \qquad [3.35]$$

We derive the corresponding integral equation by solving Cauchy problems with initial conditions

1) $u(x,0) = f(x)$, $\frac{\partial}{\partial t}u(x,t)|_{t=0} = rvf'(x)$ $(r = p - q, p + q = 1)$.

The solution is the function $u(x,t) = pu_+(x,t) + qu_-(x,t)$, which satisfies equation

$$u(x,t) = e^{-\lambda t}\{pf(x+vt) + qf(x-vt)\} + \lambda e^{-\lambda t}\int_0^t \{pf(x - v(t-2s)) + qf(x+$$

$$v(t-2s))\}ds + \lambda^2 \int_0^t \int_0^{t-s} e^{-\lambda(l+s)}u(x + v(s-l), t-(l+s))dlds.$$

Indeed, $\int_0^t \int_0^{t-s} e^{-\lambda(l+s)}u(x+v(s-l), t-(l+s))dlds = \int_0^t \int_0^{t-s} e^{-\lambda(l+s)}u(x - v(l-s), t-(l+s))dlds = \int_0^t \int_0^{t-l} e^{-\lambda(l+s)}u(x - v(l-s), t-(l+s))dsdl$, and $p + q = 1$.

2) $u(x,0) = f(x)$, $\frac{\partial}{\partial t}u(x,t)|_{t=0} = 0$, at $p = q = \frac{1}{2}$.

The corresponding integral equation:

$$u(x,t) = \frac{1}{2}e^{-\lambda t}\{f(x+vt) + f(x-vt)\} + \frac{1}{2}\lambda e^{-\lambda t}\int_0^t \{f(x - v(t-2s)) + f(x+$$

$$v(t-2s))\}ds + \lambda^2 \int_0^t \int_0^{t-s} e^{-\lambda(l+s)}u(x + v(s-l), t-(l+s))dlds.$$

3) $u(x,0) = 0$, $\frac{\partial}{\partial t}u(x,t)|_{t=0} = rvf'(x)$.

The corresponding equation:

$$u(x,t) = e^{-\lambda t}\left\{\left(p - \frac{1}{2}\right)f(x+vt) + \left(q - \frac{1}{2}\right)f(x-vt)\right\} +$$

$$\lambda e^{-\lambda t}\int_0^t\left\{\left(p-\frac{1}{2}\right)f(x-v(t-2s))+\left(q-\frac{1}{2}\right)f(x+v(t-2s))\right\}ds+$$

$$\lambda^2\int_0^t\int_0^{t-s}e^{-\lambda(l+s)}u(x+v(s-l),t-(l+s))dlds.$$

4) $u(x,0)=0, \frac{\partial}{\partial t}u(x,t)|_{t=0}=g(x)$, where $g(x)$ is integrable and $g(x)=rvf'(x)$, so $f(x)=\frac{1}{rv}\int g(x)dx=\frac{1}{rv}G(x)$.

The corresponding equation:

$$u(x,t)=\frac{1}{rv}e^{-\lambda t}\left\{\left(p-\frac{1}{2}\right)G(x+vt)+\left(q-\frac{1}{2}\right)G(x-vt)\right\}+\frac{1}{rv}\lambda e^{-\lambda t}\times$$

$$\int_0^t\left\{\left(p-\frac{1}{2}\right)G(x-v(t-2s))+\left(q-\frac{1}{2}\right)G(x+v(t-2s))\right\}ds+\lambda^2\times$$

$$\int_0^t\int_0^{t-s}e^{-\lambda(l+s)}u(x+v(s-l),t-(l+s))dlds=e^{-\lambda t}\left\{\frac{1}{2v}G(x+vt)-\frac{1}{2v}G(x-\right.$$

$$\left.vt)\right\}+\lambda e^{-\lambda t}\int_0^t\left\{\frac{1}{2v}G(x-v(t-2s))-\frac{1}{2v}G(x+v(t-2s))\right\}ds+\lambda^2\times$$

$$\int_0^t\int_0^{t-s}e^{-\lambda(l+s)}u(x+v(s-l),t-(l+s))dlds,$$

as soon as $\frac{p-\frac{1}{2}}{p-q}=\frac{1}{2}, \frac{q-\frac{1}{2}}{p-q}=-\frac{1}{2}$.

5) $u(x,0)=f(x), \frac{\partial}{\partial t}u(x,t)|_{t=0}=g(x)$.

Finally,

$$u(x,t)=e^{-\lambda t}\left\{\frac{1}{2v}G(x+vt)-\frac{1}{2v}G(x-vt)+\frac{1}{2}f(x+vt)+\frac{1}{2}f(x-vt)\right\}+$$

$$\lambda e^{-\lambda t}\int_0^t\left\{\frac{1}{2v}G(x-v(t-2s))-\frac{1}{2v}G(x+v(t-2s))+\frac{1}{2}f(x-v(t-2s))+\right.$$

$$\left.\frac{1}{2}f(x+v(t-2s))\right\}ds+\lambda^2\int_0^t\int_0^{t-s}e^{-\lambda(l+s)}u(x+v(s-l),t-(l+s))dlds.$$

[3.36]

Thus, the following theorem is proven.

THEOREM 3.6.– *Under the condition of integrability of $f(x)$ and $g(x)$, the function $u(x,t)$ – the solution of the Cauchy problem* [3.35] *– satisfies equation* [3.36]. *The function $u(x,t)$ satisfying equation* [3.36] *under the condition of differentiability $f(\overline{x})$ in definition* [1.9] *satisfies the equation and initial conditions* [3.35].

Let us write the integral equation for the evolution in the R^n space. We have $n+1$ functions, each corresponds to one of $n+1$ initial directions of movement. In the case of a cyclic change of the direction of movement application of the procedure described above gives the general form of the equation $i = \overline{0,n}$:

$$u_i(\overline{x},t) = e^{-\lambda t} f(\overline{x} + \overline{\tau}_i vt) + \lambda e^{-\lambda t} \int_0^t f(\overline{x} + \overline{\tau}_i vs_1 + \overline{\tau}_{i+1} v(t - s_1))ds_1 +$$

$$\lambda^2 e^{-\lambda t} \int_0^t \int_0^{t-s_1} f(\overline{x} + \overline{\tau}_i vs_1 + \overline{\tau}_{i+1} vs_2 + \overline{\tau}_{i+2} v(t - s_1 - s_2)ds_2 ds_1 + \cdots +$$

$$\lambda^n e^{-\lambda t} \int_0^t \int_0^{t-s_1} \cdots \int_0^{t-s_1-\cdots-s_{n-1}} f(\overline{x} + \overline{\tau}_i vs_1 + \overline{\tau}_{i+1} vs_2 + \ldots + \overline{\tau}_{i+n} v(t - s_1 - s_2 -$$

$$\cdots - s_n))ds_n \ldots ds_2 ds_1 + \lambda^{n+1} \int_0^t \int_0^{t-s_1} \cdots \int_0^{t-s_n-\cdots-s_1} e^{-\lambda(s_{n+1}+\cdots+s_2+s_1)} u_i(\overline{x} +$$

$$\overline{\tau}_i vs_1 + \overline{\tau}_{i+1} vs_2 + \cdots + \overline{\tau}_{i+n} vs_{n+1}, t - s_1 - s_2 - \cdots - s_{n+1})ds_{n+1} \ldots ds_2 ds_1. \quad [3.37]$$

Carrying out the described substitution of variables and differentiation, we arrive at Cauchy problems [3.3], [3.4].

EXAMPLE 3.2.– *$n = 2$, the change of movement directions is cyclical. Then, $S(t) = \overline{x} + v \int_0^t \overline{\tau}_{\xi(u)} du$, where $\xi(u) \in \{0,1,2\}$.*

We have $u_0(\overline{x},t) = Ef\left(\overline{x} + v\int_0^t \overline{\tau}_{\xi(u)+0} du\right) = e^{-\lambda t} f(\overline{x} + \overline{\tau}_0 vt) + \lambda \int_0^t e^{-\lambda s} \times u_1(\overline{x} + \overline{\tau}_0 vs, t - s)ds$,

$u_1(\overline{x},t) = Ef\left(\overline{x} + v\int_0^t \overline{\tau}_{\xi(u)+1} du\right) = e^{-\lambda t} f(\overline{x} + \overline{\tau}_1 vt) + \lambda \int_0^t e^{-\lambda s} u_2(\overline{x} + \overline{\tau}_1 vs, t - s)ds$,

$u_2(\overline{x},t) = Ef\left(\overline{x} + v\int_0^t \overline{\tau}_{\xi(u)+2} du\right) = e^{-\lambda t} f(\overline{x} + \overline{\tau}_2 vt) + \lambda \int_0^t e^{-\lambda s} u_0(\overline{x} + \overline{\tau}_2 vs, t - s)ds$.

Substituting expressions for $u_1(\overline{x}, t)$ and $u_2(\overline{x}, t)$ in the first ratio, we obtain

$$u_0(\overline{x}, t) = e^{-\lambda t} f(\overline{x} + \overline{\tau}_0 vt) + \lambda e^{-\lambda t} \int_0^t f(\overline{x} + \overline{\tau}_0 vs + \overline{\tau}_1 v(t-s))ds + \lambda^2 e^{-\lambda t} \times$$

$$\int_0^t \int_0^{t-s} f(\overline{x} + \overline{\tau}_0 vs + \overline{\tau}_1 vl + \overline{\tau}_2 v(t-l-s))dlds + \lambda^3 \int_0^t \int_0^{t-s} \int_0^{t-l-s} e^{-\lambda(m+l+s)} \times$$

$$u_0(\overline{x} + \overline{\tau}_0 vs + \overline{\tau}_1 vl + \overline{\tau}_2 vm, t-l-s-m)dmdlds = e^{-\lambda t} f(\overline{x} + \overline{\tau}_0 vt) + \lambda e^{-\lambda t} \int_0^t f(\overline{x}+$$

$$\overline{\tau}_0 vs + \overline{\tau}_1 v(t-s))ds + \lambda^2 e^{-\lambda t} \int_0^t \int_0^{t-s} f(\overline{x} + \overline{\tau}_0 vs + \overline{\tau}_1 vl + \overline{\tau}_2 v(t-l-s))dlds+$$

$$\lambda^3 e^{-\lambda t} \int_0^t \int_0^t \int_0^{t-k-s} e^{\lambda k} u_0(\overline{x} + \overline{\tau}_0 vs + \overline{\tau}_1 vl + \overline{\tau}_2 v(t-k-l-s), k)dldsdk.$$

Differentiating the last expression, we arrive at the Cauchy problem [3.25].

Equations [3.3], [3.4] are Volterra equations of the second kind. Therefore, according to the well-known results, the following theorem is true.

THEOREM 3.7.– *For $f(x)$ from the space L_p, $1 \leq p \leq \infty$ equations* [3.3] *and* [3.4] *have a unique solution in the space L_p.*

EXAMPLE 3.3.– *For equation* [3.3] *in the case $f(x) = x$, we put $u_0(x, t) = 0$, and then, successively substituting the functions $u_i(x, t)$ in equation* [3.3], *we get*

$$u_1(x, t) = e^{-\lambda t}(x + xt + vt), \ldots,$$

$$u_n(x, t) = e^{-\lambda t} \left(x \sum_{k=0}^{2n-1} \frac{t^k}{k!} \lambda^k + \frac{v}{\lambda} \sum_{k=0}^{[\frac{2n-1}{2}]} \frac{(\lambda t)^{2k}}{(2k)!} \right),$$

$$\lim_{n \to \infty} u_n(x, t) = x + \frac{v}{2\lambda}(1 - e^{-2\lambda t}),$$

which coincides with the first moment of the Markov random evolutionary process calculated in equation [1.5] *in R^1 at $r = 1$.*

Note that the method of successive approximations also solves equation [3.37], which is satisfied by functions from evolutionary processes in the space R^n. Thus, in contrast to Riemann's method, which can be applied only to the telegraph equation, the method proposed in section 3.3 is also applicable to hyperparabolic equations: multidimensional analogues of the telegraph equation.

Application of integral equations to the study of random evolutionary processes has advantages over the application of differential equations. For example, in the case of fading random evolutionary process described in Chapter 4, it is impossible to write a differential equation for a function from the evolution; instead, the integral equation is written out.

In addition, when the evolutionary process is not governed by a Poisson process, but by an arbitrary one, which has the distribution density $g(t)$, it is not always possible to construct a differential equation. Consider the evolution in space R^1:

$$u_+(x,t) = P(N(t)=0)Ef(x+vt) + \int_0^t P(N(s)=1)Ef\left(x+vs+ v\int_s^t (-1)^{\xi_1(u)}du\right)ds = \left[1-\int_0^t g(y)dy\right]f(x+vt) + \int_0^t g(s)u_-(x+vs,t-s)ds$$

$$u_-(x,t) = \left[1-\int_0^t g(y)dy\right]f(x-vt) + \int_0^t g(s)u_+(x-vs,t-s)ds.$$

As a consequence,

$$u_+(x,t) = \left[1-\int_0^t g(y)dy\right]f(x+vt) + \int_0^t g(s)\left[1-\int_0^{t-s} g(y)dy\right]f(x-v(t- 2s))ds + \int_0^t\int_0^{t-s} g(s)g(l)\left[1-\int_0^{t-s} g(y)dy\right]u_+(x+v(s-l),t-(l+s))dlds.$$

Let $g(t)$ be the density of the gamma distribution: $g(t) = \begin{cases} \frac{\beta^\alpha}{\Gamma(\alpha)}t^{\alpha-1}e^{-\beta t}, t>0, \\ 0, t<0. \end{cases}$

Then,

$$u_+(x,t) = \left[1-\int_0^t \frac{\beta^\alpha}{\Gamma(\alpha)}y^{\alpha-1}e^{-\beta y}dy\right]f(x+vt) + \int_0^t \frac{\beta^\alpha}{\Gamma(\alpha)}s^{\alpha-1}e^{-\beta s}\left[1- \int_0^{t-s}\frac{\beta^\alpha}{\Gamma(\alpha)}y^{\alpha-1}e^{-\beta y}dy\right]f(x-v(t-2s))ds + \int_0^t\int_0^{t-s}\frac{\beta^{2\alpha}}{(\Gamma(\alpha))^2}(sl)^{\alpha-1}e^{-\beta(l+s)}\left[1- \int_0^{t-s}\frac{\beta^\alpha}{\Gamma(\alpha)}y^{\alpha-1}e^{-\beta y}dy\right]u_+(x+v(s-l),t-(l+s))dlds = \left[1-\int_0^t\frac{\beta^\alpha}{\Gamma(\alpha)}(t- z)^{\alpha-1}e^{-\beta(t-z)}dz\right]f(x+vt) + \int_0^t\frac{\beta^\alpha}{\Gamma(\alpha)}(t-k)^{\alpha-1}e^{-\beta(t-k)}\left[1-\int_0^{t-k}\frac{\beta^\alpha}{\Gamma(\alpha)}(t-\right.$$

$$z)^{\alpha-1}e^{-\beta(t-z)}dz\Big] f(x-v(t-2s))dk + \int_0^t \int_0^{t-k} \frac{\beta^{2\alpha}}{(\Gamma(\alpha))^2}(t-k)^{\alpha-1}(t-l)^{\alpha-1}$$

$$e^{-\beta(2t-k-l)}\left[1-\int_0^{t-k}\frac{\beta^{\alpha}}{\Gamma(\alpha)}(t-z)^{\alpha-1}e^{-\beta(t-z)}dz\right]u_+(x+v(s-l),t-(l+s))dlds.$$

If α is not an integer, then the integral equation contains Riemann–Liouville integrals (Hille 1948). For integers α, we have the integral equation for which it is possible to write the corresponding partial differential equations.

EXAMPLE 3.4.– *Let $\alpha = 2, \beta = \lambda$, i.e. a process changes direction when two Poisson events occur after the last change. We have the integral equation:*

$$u_+(x,t) = e^{-\alpha t}[1+\alpha t]f(x+vt) + \frac{\alpha^2}{1!}e^{-\alpha t}\int_0^t s(1+(t-s)\alpha)f(x-v(t-2s))ds +$$

$$\frac{\alpha^4}{(1!)^2}\int_0^t\int_0^{t-s}(sl)^{\alpha-1}u_+(x+v(s-l),t-(l+s))dlds.$$

To write down the corresponding differential equations, let us expand the phase space to four states: the evolution can move in a positive or negative direction $(+,-)$, while waiting for the first or second Poisson event $(1,2)$. The corresponding system of differential equations has the form:

$$\begin{cases} \frac{\partial}{\partial t}u_{+1}(x,t) = -\lambda u_{+1}(x,t) + v\frac{\partial}{\partial x}u_{+1}(x,t) + \lambda u_{+2}(x,t) \\ \frac{\partial}{\partial t}u_{+2}(x,t) = -\lambda u_{+2}(x,t) + v\frac{\partial}{\partial x}u_{+2}(x,t) + \lambda u_{-1}(x,t) \\ \frac{\partial}{\partial t}u_{-1}(x,t) = -\lambda u_{-1}(x,t) - v\frac{\partial}{\partial x}u_{-1}(x,t) + \lambda u_{-2}(x,t) \\ \frac{\partial}{\partial t}u_{-2}(x,t) = -\lambda u_{-2}(x,t) - v\frac{\partial}{\partial x}u_{-2}(x,t) + \lambda u_{+1}(x,t) \end{cases}.$$

As above, we find the equation in partial derivatives:

$$\left[\left(\frac{\partial}{\partial t}+\lambda-v\frac{\partial}{\partial x}\right)^2\left(\frac{\partial}{\partial t}+\lambda+v\frac{\partial}{\partial x}\right)^2-\lambda^4\right]u(x,t)=0,$$

$$\left[\left(\left(\frac{\partial}{\partial t}+\lambda\right)^2-v^2\frac{\partial^2}{\partial x^2}\right)^2-\lambda^4\right]u(x,t)=0,$$

$$\left[\frac{\partial^2}{\partial t^2}+2\lambda\frac{\partial}{\partial t}-v^2\frac{\partial^2}{\partial x^2}\right]\left[\frac{\partial^2}{\partial t^2}+2\lambda\frac{\partial}{\partial t}-v^2\frac{\partial^2}{\partial x^2}+2\lambda^2\right]u(x,t)=0. \qquad [3.38]$$

Note that the first component of the factored equation is the telegraph operator. Also, a similar equation with two factorization components, which are operators of the telegraph type, were obtained by Orsingher and Kolesnik (1994) when studying evolution on a plane.

Initial conditions for the function $u(x,t) = pu_{+1}(x,t) + qu_{-1}(x,t)$ *have the form:*

$$u(x,0) = f(x),$$

$$\frac{\partial}{\partial t}u(x,t)|_{t=0} = rvf'(x),$$

$$\frac{\partial^2}{\partial t^2}u(x,t)|_{t=0} = v^2 f''(x),$$

$$\frac{\partial^3}{\partial t^3}u(x,t)|_{t=0} = -2\lambda^2 rf'(x) + rv^3 f'''(x).$$

Moments of this process ($\tilde{\xi}(t)$ *is a process that acquires the values* $\{0, 1, \ldots\}$*, and spends time in each state that has the Erlang distribution with parameters* $\lambda, 2$*):*

$$E[(-1)^{\tilde{\xi}(t)}] = re^{-\lambda t}[\cos\lambda t + \sin\lambda t],$$

$$E[(-1)^{\tilde{\xi}(u)}(-1)^{\tilde{\xi}(t)}] = e^{-\lambda(t-u)}[\cos\lambda(t-u) + \sin\lambda(t-u)],$$

$$E\left(v\int_0^t (-1)^{\tilde{\xi}(u)}du\right) = \frac{vr}{\lambda}[1 - \cos\lambda te^{-\alpha t}],$$

$$E\left(v\int_0^t (-1)^{\tilde{\xi}(u)}du\right)^2 = \frac{v^2}{\lambda}t - \frac{v^2}{2\lambda^2}[1 - \cos\lambda te^{-\alpha t} + \sin\lambda te^{-\alpha t}].$$

Note that in the hydrodynamic limit for moments of the evolutionary process, we will have moments of the Wiener process.

3.4. Distribution function of evolutionary process

In the works Orsingher (2002) and Orsingher and Sommella (2004), the authors managed to receive the obvious view for the distribution functions of random evolutions in R^2 and R^3 with a cyclic change in directions. In Orsingher and Sommella (2004), they also made a conjuncture about the view of the distribution function of the random evolution in R^n.

The following is the generalization of their results on R^n and proof of the corresponding conjuncture. This method may be applied only in the case of a cyclic change in directions as soon as the structure of equations in the case of a uniform change of directions is complicated.

One of the most important characteristics of the random evolutionary process which differs it from the Wiener process is that this process with probability 1 moves into a regular $n+1$-hedra

$$T_{vt} \equiv \Bigg\{ x_1, \ldots, x_n : -\frac{vt}{n} < x_1 < vt, \frac{1}{n-k+1} \left[\sqrt{\frac{(n-1)\ldots(n-k+1)}{(n+1)\ldots(n-k+3)}} x_1 + \right.$$

$$\left. \ldots + \sqrt{\frac{(n-k+1)}{(n-k+3)}} x_{k-1} - vt \sqrt{\frac{(n-1)\ldots(n-k+1)}{(n+1)\ldots(n-k+3)}} \right] < x_k <$$

$$< - \left[\sqrt{\frac{(n-1)\ldots(n-k+1)}{(n+1)\ldots(n-k+3)}} x_1 + \ldots + \sqrt{\frac{(n-k+1)}{(n-k+3)}} x_{k-1} - \right.$$

$$\left. vt \sqrt{\frac{(n-1)\ldots(n-k+1)}{(n+1)\ldots(n-k+3)}}, k = \overline{2, n} \right\}. \qquad [3.39]$$

The probability that evolution is on the edge ∂T_{vt} of $n+1$-hedra is equal to:

$$P\{\overline{S}(t) \in \partial T_{vt}\} = e^{-\lambda t} + \lambda t e^{-\lambda t} + \ldots + \frac{(\lambda t)^{n-1}}{(n-1)!} e^{-\lambda t}.$$

Here, $e^{-\lambda t}$ is the probability of being at time t on the vertices of T_{vt}, $\frac{(\lambda t)^{k-1}}{(k-1)!} e^{-\lambda t}, k = \overline{1, n-1}$ is the probability of being on the k-dimensional edge of T_{vt}.

So, the continuous part of the distribution we are to find has the property:

$$\int \cdots \int_{T_{vt}} f(x_1, \ldots, x_n; t) dx_1 \ldots dx_n = 1 - e^{-\lambda t} - \lambda t e^{-\lambda t} - \ldots - \frac{(\lambda t)^{n-1}}{(n-1)!} e^{-\lambda t}. \qquad [3.40]$$

In other words, we have to find a non-negative continuous function that satisfies system [1.12] and condition [3.40].

Making exponential transformation $u_j = e^{-\lambda t} g_j, j = \overline{0, n}$, we receive from equation [1.12]:

$$\begin{cases} \frac{\partial}{\partial t} g_0(\overline{x}, t) = -v(\overline{\tau}_0, \nabla) g_0(\overline{x}, t) + \lambda g_n(\overline{x}, t) \\ \frac{\partial}{\partial t} g_1(\overline{x}, t) = -v(\overline{\tau}_1, \nabla) g_1(\overline{x}, t) + \lambda g_0(\overline{x}, t) \\ \ldots \\ \frac{\partial}{\partial t} g_n(\overline{x}, t) = -v(\overline{\tau}_n, \nabla) g_n(\overline{x}, t) + \lambda g_{n-1}(\overline{x}, t) \end{cases} \qquad [3.41]$$

THEOREM 3.8.– *The functions $g_j, j = \overline{0,n}$ are solutions of the equation*

$$\frac{\partial g}{\partial y_1 \ldots \partial y_{n+1}} = \left(\frac{\lambda}{v}\right)^{n+1} \left(\frac{\sqrt{n}}{\sqrt{n+1}}\right)^{n+1} \left(\frac{1}{\sqrt[2n+2]{2n+2}}\right)^{n+1} g, \qquad [3.42]$$

where

$$y_1 = \frac{vt}{n} + x_1,$$

$$y_k = \frac{1}{n-k+1}\left[\sqrt{\frac{(n-1)\ldots(n-k+1)}{(n+1)\ldots(n-k+3)}}vt - \sqrt{\frac{(n-1)\ldots(n-k+1)}{(n+1)\ldots(n-k+3)}}x_1 - \right.$$

$$\left. \ldots - \sqrt{\frac{n-k+1}{n-k+3}}x_{k-1}\right] + x_k, k = \overline{2,n},$$

$$y_{n+1} = \sqrt{\frac{(n-1)\ldots 1}{(n+1)\ldots 3}}vt - \sqrt{\frac{(n-1)\ldots 1}{(n+1)\ldots 3}}x_1 - \ldots - \sqrt{\frac{1}{3}}x_{n-1} - x_n. \qquad [3.43]$$

PROOF.– By applying the substitution [3.43] to the system [3.41], we receive:

$$\begin{cases} \frac{n+1}{n} v \frac{\partial g_0}{\partial y_1} = \lambda g_n \\ \frac{\sqrt{(n+1)(n-k+1)}}{\sqrt{n(n-k)}} v \frac{\partial g_k}{\partial y_{k+1}} = \lambda g_{k-1}, k = \overline{1, n-1} \\ \frac{\sqrt{2(n+1)}}{\sqrt{n}} v \frac{\partial g_n}{\partial y_{n+1}} = \lambda g_{n-1}. \end{cases}$$

By differentiation, we easily obtain equation [3.42].

Theorem is proven.

THEOREM 3.9.– *The substitution $z = \sqrt[n+1]{y_1 \ldots y_{n+1}}$converts the equation [3.42] into then + 1-dimensional Bessel equation:*

$$\left(z\frac{\partial}{\partial z}\right)^{n+1} g = \left(\frac{\lambda}{v}\right)^{n+1} \left(\sqrt{n(n+1)}\right)^{n+1} \left(\frac{1}{\sqrt[2n+2]{2n+2}}\right)^{n+1} z^{n+1} g, \qquad [3.44]$$

where g is any of the functions $g_j, j = \overline{0,n}$.

PROOF.– We have not shown the proof since plain calculations are involved.

The solutions of equation [3.44] were found in Turbin and Plotkin (1991). Here, we use one of the functions which is the solution of equation [3.44]:

$$I_{0,n}\left(\frac{\lambda}{v}\frac{\sqrt{n(n+1)}}{\sqrt[2n+2]{2n+2}}z\right)=\sum_{k=0}^{\infty}\left(\frac{\lambda}{v}\frac{\sqrt{n(n+1)}}{\sqrt[2n+2]{2n+2}}\frac{1}{n+1}z\right)^{(n+1)k}\frac{1}{(k!)^{n+1}}. \quad [3.45]$$

REMARK 3.1.– *The proofs demonstrating that this function is the solution of equation* [3.44] *in the case of* $n = 2, 3$ *may also be found in Orsingher (2002) and Orsingher and Sommella (2004).*

Making the backward change of variables in equation [3.45] and exponential substitution, we receive the solution of system [1.12].

Now, we are ready to formulate the main result of this section.

THEOREM 3.10.– *The absolutely continuous component of the distribution of the Markovian random evolutionary process in* R^n *with a cyclic change in directions is:*

$$f(x_1,\ldots,x_n;t)=\frac{(\sqrt{n})^n e^{-\lambda t}}{(\sqrt{n+1})^{n+1}v^n}\left[\lambda^n+\lambda^{n-1}\frac{\partial}{\partial t}+\ldots+\right.$$

$$\left.\frac{\partial^n}{\partial t^n}\right]I_{0,n}\left(\frac{\lambda}{v}\frac{\sqrt{n(n+1)}}{\sqrt[2n+2]{2n+2}}\sqrt[n+1]{y_1\cdots y_{n+1}}\right), \quad [3.46]$$

here and later $y_i, i=\overline{1,n+1}$ *are the linear combinations of* $t, x_i, i=\overline{1,n}$ *pointed in equation* [3.43].

PROOF.– The fact that equation [3.46] is a non-negative function may be easily seen from the view of the series [3.45].

The function [3.46] satisfies equation [3.3]. Really, $I_{0,n}\left(\frac{\lambda}{v}\frac{\sqrt{n(n+1)}}{\sqrt[2n+2]{2n+2}}\times\right.$ $\left.\times\sqrt[n+1]{y_1\cdots y_{n+1}}\right)$, where $y_i, i=\overline{1,n+1}$ are pointed in equation [3.43], satisfies equation [3.42]. Any linear combination of derivatives of the last function with the coefficient $\frac{(\sqrt{n})^n}{(\sqrt{n+1})^{n+1}v^n}$ also satisfies equation [3.42]. So, if we make backward exponential substitution, we receive a solution of equation [3.3].

The last problem is to prove the condition [3.40] for the function $f(x_1,\ldots,x_n;t)$.

We first note that

$$\int\cdots\int_{T_{vt}} I_{0,n}\left(\frac{\lambda}{v}\frac{\sqrt{n(n+1)}}{\sqrt[2n+2]{2n+2}}\sqrt[n+1]{y_1\cdots y_{n+1}}\right)dx_1\ldots dx_n=$$

$$= \sum_{k=0}^{\infty} \left(\frac{\lambda}{(n+1)v} \right)^{(n+1)k} \frac{(\sqrt{n(n+1)})^{(n+1)k}}{(\sqrt[2n+2]{2n+2})^{(n+1)k}} \frac{1}{(k!)^{n+1}} \int_{-\frac{vt}{n}}^{vt} \frac{1}{n^k} [vt+nx_1]^k dx_1 \ldots$$

$$\int_{\frac{1}{2}\left[\sqrt{\frac{(n-1)\ldots 2}{(n+1)\ldots 4}}x_1+\ldots+\sqrt{\frac{2}{4}}x_{n-2}-\sqrt{\frac{(n-1)\ldots 2}{(n+1)\ldots 4}}vt\right]}^{-\left[\sqrt{\frac{(n-1)\ldots 2}{(n+1)\ldots 4}}x_1+\ldots+\sqrt{\frac{2}{4}}x_{n-2}-\sqrt{\frac{(n-1)\ldots 2}{(n+1)\ldots 4}}vt\right]} \frac{1}{2^k} \left[-\sqrt{\frac{(n-1)\ldots 2}{(n+1)\ldots 4}} x_1 - \ldots - \right.$$

$$\left. \sqrt{\frac{2}{4}} x_{n-2} + \sqrt{\frac{(n-1)\ldots 2}{(n+1)\ldots 4}} vt + 2x_{n-1} \right]^k dx_{n-1} \times$$

$$\int_{\left[\sqrt{\frac{(n-1)\ldots 1}{(n+1)\ldots 3}}x_1+\ldots+\sqrt{\frac{1}{3}}x_{n-1}-\sqrt{\frac{(n-1)\ldots 1}{(n+1)\ldots 3}}vt\right]}^{-\left[\sqrt{\frac{(n-1)\ldots 1}{(n+1)\ldots 3}}x_1+\ldots+\sqrt{\frac{1}{3}}x_{n-1}-\sqrt{\frac{(n-1)\ldots 1}{(n+1)\ldots 3}}vt\right]} \left[\left(-\sqrt{\frac{(n-1)\ldots 1}{(n+1)\ldots 3}} x_1 - \right. \right.$$

$$\left. \left. \ldots - \sqrt{\frac{1}{3}} x_{n-1} + \sqrt{\frac{(n-1)\ldots 1}{(n+1)\ldots 3}} vt \right)^2 - x_n^2 \right]^k dx_n. \qquad [3.47]$$

The inner, first, integral could be found by replacing the variables $x_n = \left(-\sqrt{\frac{(n-1)\ldots 1}{(n+1)\ldots 3}} x_1 - \ldots - \sqrt{\frac{1}{3}} x_{n-1} + \sqrt{\frac{(n-1)\ldots 1}{(n+1)\ldots 3}} vt \right) z$. We have:

$$\int_{\left[\sqrt{\frac{(n-1)\ldots 1}{(n+1)\ldots 3}}x_1+\ldots+\sqrt{\frac{1}{3}}x_{n-1}-\sqrt{\frac{(n-1)\ldots 1}{(n+1)\ldots 3}}vt\right]}^{-\left[\sqrt{\frac{(n-1)\ldots 1}{(n+1)\ldots 3}}x_1+\ldots+\sqrt{\frac{1}{3}}x_{n-1}-\sqrt{\frac{(n-1)\ldots 1}{(n+1)\ldots 3}}vt\right]} \left[\left(-\sqrt{\frac{(n-1)\ldots 1}{(n+1)\ldots 3}} x_1 - \ldots - \sqrt{\frac{1}{3}} x_{n-1} + \right. \right.$$

$$\left. \left. \sqrt{\frac{(n-1)\ldots 1}{(n+1)\ldots 3}} vt \right)^2 - x_n^2 \right] dx_n = \left(-\sqrt{\frac{(n-1)\ldots 1}{(n+1)\ldots 3}} x_1 - \ldots - \sqrt{\frac{1}{3}} x_{n-1} + \right.$$

$$\left. \sqrt{\frac{(n-1)\ldots 1}{(n+1)\ldots 3}} vt \right)^{2k+1} \int_{-1}^{1} (1-z^2)^k dz = \left(-\sqrt{\frac{(n-1)\ldots 1}{(n+1)\ldots 3}} x_1 - \ldots - \right.$$

$$\left. \sqrt{\frac{1}{3}} x_{n-1} + \sqrt{\frac{1}{3}} x_{n-1} + \sqrt{\frac{(n-1)\ldots 1}{(n+1)\ldots 3}} vt \right)^{2k+1} \frac{2^{2k+1}(k!)^2}{(2k+1)!}.$$

In the following, second, integral

$$\int_{\frac{1}{2}\left[\sqrt{\frac{(n-1)\ldots 2}{(n+1)\ldots 4}}x_1+\ldots+\sqrt{\frac{2}{4}}x_{n-2}-\sqrt{\frac{(n-1)\ldots 2}{(n+1)\ldots 4}}vt\right]}^{-\left[\sqrt{\frac{(n-1)\ldots 2}{(n+1)\ldots 4}}x_1+\ldots+\sqrt{\frac{2}{4}}x_{n-2}-\sqrt{\frac{(n-1)\ldots 2}{(n+1)\ldots 4}}vt\right]} \frac{1}{2^k} \left[-\sqrt{\frac{(n-1)\ldots 2}{(n+1)\ldots 4}} x_1 - \ldots - \sqrt{\frac{2}{4}} x_{n-2} + \right.$$

$$\sqrt{\frac{(n-1)\ldots 2}{(n+1)\ldots 4}}vt + 2x_{n-1}\Bigg]^k \Bigg[-\sqrt{\frac{(n-1)\ldots 1}{(n+1)\ldots 3}}x_1 - \ldots - \sqrt{\frac{1}{3}}x_{n-1}+$$

$$\sqrt{\frac{(n-1)\ldots 1}{(n+1)\ldots 3}}vt\Bigg]^{2k+1} dx_{n-1} = \int_{\frac{1}{2}\left[\sqrt{\frac{(n-1)\ldots 2}{(n+1)\ldots 4}}x_1+\ldots+\sqrt{\frac{2}{4}}x_{n-2}-\sqrt{\frac{(n-1)\ldots 2}{(n+1)\ldots 4}}vt\right]}^{-\left[\sqrt{\frac{(n-1)\ldots 2}{(n+1)\ldots 4}}x_1+\ldots+\sqrt{\frac{2}{4}}x_{n-2}-\sqrt{\frac{(n-1)\ldots 2}{(n+1)\ldots 4}}vt\right]} \frac{1}{2^k\sqrt{3}^{2k+1}} \times$$

$$\Bigg[-\sqrt{\frac{(n-1)\ldots 2}{(n+1)\ldots 4}}x_1 - \ldots - \sqrt{\frac{2}{4}}x_{n-2} + \sqrt{\frac{(n-1)\ldots 2}{(n+1)\ldots 4}}vt+$$

$$2x_{n-1}\Big]^k \Bigg[-\sqrt{\frac{(n-1)\ldots 2}{(n+1)\ldots 4}}x_1 - \ldots - \sqrt{\frac{2}{4}}x_{n-2} + \sqrt{\frac{(n-1)\ldots 2}{(n+1)\ldots 4}}vt-$$

$$x_{n-1}\Big]^{2k+1} dx_{n-1} = \frac{1}{2^k\sqrt{3}^{2k+1}} \Bigg(-\sqrt{\frac{(n-1)\ldots 2}{(n+1)\ldots 4}}x_1 - \ldots - \sqrt{\frac{2}{4}}x_{n-2}+$$

$$\sqrt{\frac{(n-1)\ldots 2}{(n+1)\ldots 4}}vt\Bigg)^{3k+1} \int_{\frac{1}{2}\left[\sqrt{\frac{(n-1)\ldots 2}{(n+1)\ldots 4}}x_1+\ldots+\sqrt{\frac{2}{4}}x_{n-2}-\sqrt{\frac{(n-1)\ldots 2}{(n+1)\ldots 4}}vt\right]}^{-\left[\sqrt{\frac{(n-1)\ldots 2}{(n+1)\ldots 4}}x_1+\ldots+\sqrt{\frac{2}{4}}x_{n-2}-\sqrt{\frac{(n-1)\ldots 2}{(n+1)\ldots 4}}vt\right]} (1+$$

$$2\frac{x_{n-1}}{\left(-\sqrt{\frac{(n-1)\ldots 2}{(n+1)\ldots 4}}x_1 - \ldots - \sqrt{\frac{2}{4}}x_{n-2} + \sqrt{\frac{(n-1)\ldots 2}{(n+1)\ldots 4}}vt\right)}\Bigg)^k \times$$

$$\left(1 - \frac{x_{n-1}}{\left(-\sqrt{\frac{(n-1)\ldots 2}{(n+1)\ldots 4}}x_1 - \ldots - \sqrt{\frac{2}{4}}x_{n-2} + \sqrt{\frac{(n-1)\ldots 2}{(n+1)\ldots 4}}vt\right)}\right)^{2k+1} dx_{n-1} =$$

$$\frac{3^{3k+1}}{2^{3k+1}\sqrt{3}^{2k+1}} \left(-\sqrt{\frac{(n-1)\ldots 2}{(n+1)\ldots 4}}x_1 - \ldots - \sqrt{\frac{2}{4}}x_{n-2} + \sqrt{\frac{(n-1)\ldots 2}{(n+1)\ldots 4}}vt\right)^{3k+1} \times$$

$$\int_{\frac{1}{2}\left[\sqrt{\frac{(n-1)\ldots 2}{(n+1)\ldots 4}}x_1+\ldots+\sqrt{\frac{2}{4}}x_{n-2}-\sqrt{\frac{(n-1)\ldots 2}{(n+1)\ldots 4}}vt\right]}^{-\left[\sqrt{\frac{(n-1)\ldots 2}{(n+1)\ldots 4}}x_1+\ldots+\sqrt{\frac{2}{4}}x_{n-2}-\sqrt{\frac{(n-1)\ldots 2}{(n+1)\ldots 4}}vt\right]} \left(\frac{1}{3} + \frac{2}{3}\times\right.$$

$$\left.\frac{x_{n-1}}{\left(-\sqrt{\frac{(n-1)\dots 2}{(n+1)\dots 4}}x_1 - \dots - \sqrt{\frac{2}{4}}x_{n-2} + \sqrt{\frac{(n-1)\dots 2}{(n+1)\dots 4}}vt\right)}\right)^k \times$$

$$\left(\frac{2}{3} - \frac{2}{3}\frac{x_{n-1}}{\left(-\sqrt{\frac{(n-1)\dots 2}{(n+1)\dots 4}}x_1 - \dots - \sqrt{\frac{2}{4}}x_{n-2} + \sqrt{\frac{(n-1)\dots 2}{(n+1)\dots 4}}vt\right)}\right)^{2k+1} dx_{n-1}$$

we make the replacement of variables $z = \frac{1}{3} + \frac{2}{3}\frac{x_{n-1}}{\left(-\sqrt{\frac{(n-1)\dots 2}{(n+1)\dots 4}}x_1 - \dots - \sqrt{\frac{2}{4}}x_{n-2} + \sqrt{\frac{(n-1)\dots 2}{(n+1)\dots 4}}vt\right)}$

and so we have

$$\frac{3^{3k+2}}{2^{3k+2}\sqrt{3}^{2k+1}}\left(-\sqrt{\frac{(n-1)\dots 2}{(n+1)\dots 4}}x_1 - \dots - \sqrt{\frac{2}{4}}x_{n-2} + \sqrt{\frac{(n-1)\dots 2}{(n+1)\dots 4}}vt\right)^{3k+2} \times$$

$$\int_0^1 z^k(1-z)^{2k+1}dz = \frac{3^{3k+2}}{2^{3k+2}\sqrt{3}^{2k+1}}\left(-\sqrt{\frac{(n-1)\dots 2}{(n+1)\dots 4}}x_1 - \dots - \sqrt{\frac{2}{4}}x_{n-2} +\right.$$

$$\left.\sqrt{\frac{(n-1)\dots 2}{(n+1)\dots 4}}vt\right)^{3k+2} \frac{\Gamma(k+1)\Gamma(2k+2)}{\Gamma(3k+3)}.$$

The following integrals could be found in the same way. For the m-th integral, we have:

$$\left(\sqrt{\frac{m-1}{m+1}}\right)^{m(k+1)-1}\left(\frac{m+1}{m}\right)^{(m+1)(k+1)-1}\frac{\Gamma(m(k+1))\Gamma(k+1)}{\Gamma((m+1)(k+1))}\times$$

$$\left(-\sqrt{\frac{(n-1)\dots m}{(n+1)\dots(m+2)}}x_1 - \dots - \sqrt{\frac{m}{m+2}}x_{n-m} +\right.$$

$$\left.\sqrt{\frac{(n-1)\dots m}{(n+1)\dots(m+2)}}vt\right)^{(m+1)(k+1)-1}.$$

Substituting the integrals found in equation [3.47] and performing simple calculations, we receive:

$$\int\dots\int_{T_{vt}} I_{0,n}\left(\frac{\lambda}{v}\frac{\sqrt{n(n+1)}}{\sqrt[2n+2]{2n+2}}\sqrt[n+1]{y_1\dots y_{n+1}}\right) = \left(\frac{v}{\lambda}\right)^n\frac{(\sqrt{n+1})^{n+1}}{(\sqrt{n})^n}\times$$

$$\sum_{k=0}^{\infty}\frac{(\lambda t)^{(n+1)(k+1)-1}}{((n+1)(k+1)-1)!}.$$

But to prove equation [3.40], we have to find the following integrals:

$$\int \cdots \int_{T_{vt}} \frac{\partial^m}{\partial t^m} I_{0,n}\left(\frac{\lambda}{v}\frac{\sqrt{n(n+1)}}{\sqrt[2n+2]{2n+2}}\sqrt[n+1]{y_1\dots y_{n+1}}\right)dx_1\dots dx_n, m=\overline{1,n}.$$

To do this, let us find

$$\frac{\partial}{\partial t}\int \cdots \int_{T_{vt}} I_{0,n}\left(\frac{\lambda}{v}\frac{\sqrt{n(n+1)}}{\sqrt[2n+2]{2n+2}}\sqrt[n+1]{y_1\dots y_{n+1}}\right)dx_1\dots dx_n = \frac{\partial}{\partial t}\int_{-\frac{vt}{n}}^{vt}\cdots$$

$$\int_{\frac{1}{2}\left[\sqrt{\frac{(n-1)\dots 2}{(n+1)\dots 4}}x_1+\dots+\sqrt{\frac{2}{4}}x_{n-2}-\sqrt{\frac{(n-1)\dots 2}{(n+1)\dots 4}}vt\right]}^{-\left[\sqrt{\frac{(n-1)\dots 2}{(n+1)\dots 4}}x_1+\dots+\sqrt{\frac{2}{4}}x_{n-2}-\sqrt{\frac{(n-1)\dots 2}{(n+1)\dots 4}}vt\right]}$$

$$\int_{\left[\sqrt{\frac{(n-1)\dots 1}{(n+1)\dots 3}}x_1+\dots+\sqrt{\frac{1}{3}}x_{n-1}-\sqrt{\frac{(n-1)\dots 1}{(n+1)\dots 3}}vt\right]}^{-\left[\sqrt{\frac{(n-1)\dots 1}{(n+1)\dots 3}}x_1+\dots+\sqrt{\frac{1}{3}}x_{n-1}-\sqrt{\frac{(n-1)\dots 1}{(n+1)\dots 3}}vt\right]} I_{0,n}\left(\frac{\lambda}{v}\times\right.$$

$$\left.\times\frac{\sqrt{n(n+1)}}{\sqrt[2n+2]{2n+2}}\sqrt[n+1]{y_1\dots y_{n+1}}\right)dx_1\dots dx_{n-1}dx_n.$$

The main rule for such integrals is: we find the derivative of the above limit and multiply it on the integral in which we substitute the upper limit instead of x_1, then we subtract the derivative of the lower limit multiplied on the integral in which we substitute the down limit instead of x_1, and so on for every integral.

But in our case when we substitute the above limit into the next integral, it becomes equal to 0. This may be easily seen using equation [3.39]. Otherwise, when we substitute the down limit, the argument of the Bessel function becomes equal to 0. This may be seen from equations [3.39] and [3.43]. But it is clear that $I_{0,n}(0)=1$, so the integrand will be always be equal to 1.

In other words, we have the following equality:

$$\frac{\partial}{\partial t}\int \cdots \int_{T_{vt}} I_{0,n}\left(\frac{\lambda}{v}\frac{\sqrt{n(n+1)}}{\sqrt[2n+2]{2n+2}}\sqrt[n+1]{y_1\dots y_{n+1}}\right)dx_1\dots dx_n =$$

$$\frac{\partial}{\partial t}\int \cdots \int_{T_{vt}} 1 dx_1\dots dx_n + \int \cdots \int_{T_{vt}} \frac{\partial}{\partial t} I_{0,n}\left(\frac{\lambda}{v}\frac{\sqrt{n(n+1)}}{\sqrt[2n+2]{2n+2}}\sqrt[n+1]{y_1\dots y_{n+1}}\right)dx_1\dots dx_n.$$

But the first integral is the derivative of $VolT_{vt}$. We may easily find that $VolT_{vt} = \frac{(\sqrt{n+1})^{n+1}}{(\sqrt{n})^n n!}(vt)^n$.

So,

$$\frac{\partial}{\partial t}\int\cdots\int_{T_{vt}} I_{0,n}\left(\frac{\lambda}{v}\frac{\sqrt{n(n+1)}}{\sqrt[2n+2]{2n+2}}\sqrt[n+1]{y_1\cdots y_{n+1}}\right)dx_1\ldots dx_n =$$

$$\frac{(\sqrt{n+1})^{n+1}}{(\sqrt{n})^n(n-1)!}v^n t^{n-1}+\int\cdots\int_{T_{vt}}\frac{\partial}{\partial t}I_{0,n}\left(\frac{\lambda}{v}\frac{\sqrt{n(n+1)}}{\sqrt[2n+2]{2n+2}}\sqrt[n+1]{y_1\cdots y_{n+1}}\right)dx_1\ldots dx_n.$$

For the next derivative, we have:

$$\frac{\partial^2}{\partial t^2}\int\cdots\int_{T_{vt}} I_{0,n}\left(\frac{\lambda}{v}\frac{\sqrt{n(n+1)}}{\sqrt[2n+2]{2n+2}}\sqrt[n+1]{y_1\cdots y_{n+1}}\right)dx_1\ldots dx_n =$$

$$\frac{(\sqrt{n+1})^{n+1}}{(\sqrt{n})^n(n-2)!}v^n t^{n-2}+\frac{\partial}{\partial t}\int\cdots\int_{T_{vt}}\frac{\partial}{\partial t}I_{0,n}\left(\frac{\lambda}{v}\frac{\sqrt{n(n+1)}}{\sqrt[2n+2]{2n+2}}\sqrt[n+1]{y_1\cdots y_{n+1}}\right)dx_1\ldots dx_n.$$

We will find the last integral by the rule we mentioned above, but here the above limit makes the following integral equal to 0, and when we substitute the down limit into the integrand, we have $\frac{\partial}{\partial t}I_{0,n}(0)=0$. So,

$$\frac{\partial^2}{\partial t^2}\int\cdots\int_{T_{vt}} I_{0,n}\left(\frac{\lambda}{v}\frac{\sqrt{n(n+1)}}{\sqrt[2n+2]{2n+2}}\sqrt[n+1]{y_1\cdots y_{n+1}}\right)dx_1\ldots dx_n =$$

$$\frac{(\sqrt{n+1})^{n+1}}{(\sqrt{n})^n(n-2)!}v^n t^{n-2}+\int\cdots\int_{T_{vt}}\frac{\partial^2}{\partial t^2}I_{0,n}\left(\frac{\lambda}{v}\frac{\sqrt{n(n+1)}}{\sqrt[2n+2]{2n+2}}\sqrt[n+1]{y_1\cdots y_{n+1}}\right)dx_1\ldots dx_n.$$

By analogy, for the k-th derivative, we have ($k=\overline{3,n}$):

$$\frac{\partial^k}{\partial t^k}\int\cdots\int_{T_{vt}} I_{0,n}\left(\frac{\lambda}{v}\frac{\sqrt{n(n+1)}}{\sqrt[2n+2]{2n+2}}\sqrt[n+1]{y_1\cdots y_{n+1}}\right)dx_1\ldots dx_n =$$

$$\frac{(\sqrt{n+1})^{n+1}}{(\sqrt{n})^n(n-k)!}v^n t^{n-k}+\int\cdots\int_{T_{vt}}\frac{\partial^k}{\partial t^k}I_{0,n}\left(\frac{\lambda}{v}\frac{\sqrt{n(n+1)}}{\sqrt[2n+2]{2n+2}}\sqrt[n+1]{y_1\cdots y_{n+1}}\right)dx_1\ldots dx_n.$$

Using the formulas found, we receive:

$$\int\cdots\int_{T_{vt}}\left[\lambda^n+\lambda^{n-1}\frac{\partial}{\partial t}+\ldots+\frac{\partial^n}{\partial t^n}\right]I_{0,n}\left(\frac{\lambda}{v}\frac{\sqrt{n(n+1)}}{\sqrt[2n+2]{2n+2}}\sqrt[n+1]{y_1\cdots y_{n+1}}\right)dx_1\ldots dx_n =$$

$$v^n\frac{(\sqrt{n+1})^{n+1}}{(\sqrt{n})^n}\left[e^{-\lambda t}-1-\lambda t-\ldots-\frac{(\lambda t)^{n-1}}{(n-1)!}\right].$$

And finally,

$$\frac{(\sqrt{n})^n}{(\sqrt{n+1})^{n+1}v^n}e^{-\lambda t}\int\cdots\int_{T_{vt}}\left[\lambda^n+\lambda^{n-1}\frac{\partial}{\partial t}+\ldots+\frac{\partial^n}{\partial t^n}\right]I_{0,n}\left(\frac{\lambda}{v}\times\right.$$

$$\left.\frac{\sqrt{n(n+1)}}{\sqrt[2n+2]{2n+2}}\sqrt[n+1]{y_1\ldots y_{n+1}}\right)dx_1\ldots dx_n=1-e^{-\lambda t}-\ldots-\frac{(\lambda t)^{n-1}}{(n-1)!}e^{-\lambda t}.$$

Theorem is proven.

REMARK 3.2.– *In the work (Orsingher and Sommella 2004), Orsingher and Sommella conjectured that the normalizing constant in equation* [3.46] *should be equal to* $\frac{(\sqrt{n})^n}{(\sqrt{n+1})^{n+1}v^n}=\frac{t^n}{n!VolT_{vt}}$. *As we have seen, it is not surprising because this constant appears when we find the integral* $\int\ldots\int_{T_{vt}}1dx_1\ldots dx_n=VolT_{vt}$.

4

Fading Markov Random Evolutionary Process

4.1. Definition of fading Markov random evolutionary process, its moments and limit distribution

The Goldstein–Kac model describes the evolution of a particle on a straight line. At the same time, no external forces act on the particle, and it is impossible to determine the limiting (at $t \to \infty$) distribution of its coordinates.

In the proposed model of the fading evolutionary process, the particle moves in a straight line, being under the influence of an external force, when the speed of movement decreases over time. As a result, the particle is "carried away" to some point where it "freezes" at $t \to \infty$. In contrast to the Goldstein–Kac model, in the case of the fading evolutionary process, it is possible to determine the limit distribution of process coordinates.

DEFINITION 4.1.– *We call a fading telegraphic process in the space R^1 the process $\eta_t = (-a)^{\xi(t)}, 0 < a < 1, \xi(t) \in \{0, 1, \dots\}$ is a Poisson process with parameter λ.*

A fading Markov stochastic evolutionary process corresponding to the fading telegraphic process will be called the process $S(t) = v \int_0^t (-a)^{\xi(u)} du$, where v has the meaning of speed.

A fading multidimensional homogeneous alternating process in the R^n space is called the process $\eta_t = a^{\xi(t)} \overline{\tau}_{\xi(t) \mod (n+1)}, 0 < a < 1, \xi(t) \in \{0, 1, \dots\}$, where $\overline{\tau}_i$ are vectors, specified in section 1.1.

By a fading Markov random evolutionary process in R^n with cyclic (uniform) change in the direction of movement is called a process, subject to the following conditions:

1) The process starts at the point $\overline{x} = (x_1, \ldots, x_n)$.

2) Initial direction of movement $\overline{\tau}_i, i = \overline{0, n}$.

3) If θ *is the time during which the process moves in some direction, then* $P(\theta > t) = e^{-\lambda t}$.

4) k*-th direction is followed by* $k + 1$*-th,* n*-th by* 0*-th (*k*-th is followed by any of the others with probability* $\frac{1}{n}$*).*

5) The speed of movement changes and at the moment t *equals* va^k*, if* k *is the number of changes in the direction of movement until the moment of time* t.

A fading Markov random evolutionary process in R^n can be written using the formula $S(t) = v \int_0^t a^{\xi(u)} \overline{\tau}_{\xi(u) \mod (n+1)} du$, where the change in directions may be cyclic or uniform.

Let us consider some physical characteristics of the fading telegraph process in R^1 and compare them with well-known analogues for the telegraphic process.

Let the parameter of the switching Poisson process change with time. Then, the probability of k Poisson events in the time interval (t_1, t_2) is equal to: $p_k(t_1, t_2) = \frac{(\Lambda(t_1,t_2))^k}{k!} e^{-\Lambda(t_1,t_2)}, k = 0, 1, \ldots,$ where $\Lambda(t_1, t_2) = \int_{t_1}^{t_2} \lambda(t)dt, t_2 > t_1$ ($\lambda(t)$: parameter of the Poisson distribution) and we have an expression for the correlation function $B(t_1, t_2) = m(\eta_{t_1}\eta_{t_2}) = e^{-\Lambda(0,t_2)} - ae^{-\Lambda(0,t_1)} \times \frac{\Lambda(t_1,t_2)}{1!} e^{-\Lambda(t_1,t_2)} + ae^{-\Lambda(0,t_1)} \frac{\Lambda(0,t_1)}{1!} e^{-\Lambda(t_1,t_2)} + ae^{-\Lambda(0,t_1)} \frac{(\Lambda(t_1,t_2))^2}{2!} e^{-\Lambda(t_1,t_2)} - a^3 e^{-\Lambda(0,t_1)} \times \frac{\Lambda(0,t_1)}{1!} e^{-\Lambda(t_1,t_2)} \times \frac{\Lambda(0,t_1)}{1!} + a^4 e^{-\Lambda(0,t_1)} \frac{(\Lambda(0,t_1))^2}{2!} e^{-\Lambda(t_1,t_2)} + \ldots,$ and, using the relation $e^{-\Lambda(0,t_2)} = e^{-\Lambda(0,t_1)} e^{-\Lambda(t_1,t_2)}$, we obtain

$$B(t_1, t_2) = e^{-\Lambda(0,t_2)} \sum_{n=0}^{\infty} \sum_{k=0}^{n} (-a)^n (-a)^{n-k} \frac{(\Lambda(t_1, t_2))^k}{k!} \frac{(\Lambda(0, t_1))^{n-k}}{(n-k)!} =$$

$$v^2 e^{-\Lambda(0,t_2)} \sum_{n=0}^{\infty} \sum_{k=0}^{n} \frac{(-a\Lambda(t_1, t_2))^k}{k!} \frac{\left(a^2 \Lambda(0, t_1))\right)^{n-k}}{(n-k)!} = e^{-\Lambda(0,t_2)} \sum_{k=0}^{\infty}$$

$$\sum_{n=k}^{\infty} \frac{(-a\Lambda(t_1, t_2))^k}{k!} \frac{\left(a^2 \Lambda(0, t_1))\right)^{n-k}}{(n-k)!} = e^{-\Lambda(0,t_2)} e^{-a\Lambda(t_1,t_2)} e^{a^2 \Lambda(0,t_1)} =$$

$$v^2 e^{-(1+a)\Lambda(0,t_2)} e^{(a+a^2)\Lambda(0,t_1)} = e^{-(1+a)(\Lambda(0,t_2) - a\Lambda(0,t_1))}.$$

Obviously, at $a = 1$ $B(t_1, t_2) = e^{-2\Lambda(t_1,t_2)}$, this coincides with the correlation function of the telegraphic process in radiophysics.

If $\lambda(t) = \lambda$, then $\Lambda(t_1, t_2) = \Lambda(t_2 - t_1)$ and $B(t_1, t_2) = e^{-(1+a)[\lambda t_2 - a\lambda t_1]}$, which coincides with $e^{-2\lambda\tau} (\tau = t_2 - t_1)$ at $a = 1$.

Let us find the instantaneous energy spectrum using the formula

$$\Phi(t,\omega) = 4\int_0^\infty B(t,t+\tau)cos\omega td\tau = 4\int_0^\infty e^{-(1+a)[\Lambda(0,t+\tau)-a\Lambda(0,t)]}\times$$

$$cos\omega\tau d\tau = 4e^{-(1-a^2)\Lambda(0,t)}\int_0^\infty e^{-(1+a)\Lambda(t,t+\tau)}cos\omega\tau d\tau.$$

If $\Lambda(t_1,t_2) = \lambda(t_2-t_1)$, then $\Phi(t,\omega) = 4e^{-(1-a^2)\lambda t}\int_0^\infty e^{-(1+a)\lambda\tau}\times cos\omega\tau d\tau = 4e^{(a^2-1)\lambda t}\frac{(1+a)\lambda}{((1+a)\lambda)^2+\omega^2}$.

Note that for $a = 1$ $\Phi(t,\omega) = \frac{8\lambda}{4\lambda^2+\omega^2}$, i.e. the instantaneous energy spectrum is analogous to the spectrum of the telegraphic process.

Thus, the following theorem is true.

THEOREM 4.1.– *The fading telegraphic process has a correlation function*

$$B(t_1,t_2) = e^{-(1+a)(\Lambda(0,t_2)-a\Lambda(0,t_1))}$$

and an instantaneous energy spectrum

$$\Phi(t,\omega) = 4e^{-(1-a^2)\Lambda(0,t)}\int_0^\infty e^{-(1+a)\Lambda(t,t+\tau)}cos\omega\tau d\tau.$$

Consider the moments of the fading telegraphic process in space R^1.

THEOREM 4.2.– *If* $P(\xi(0) = 0) = p$, $P(\xi(0) = 1) = q, p+q = 1, p-q = r$, *then the moments of the fading telegraphic process are given by the formula*

$$E[(-1)^{\xi(u_1)}\dots(-1)^{\xi(u_k)}] =$$

$$\begin{cases} re^{-\lambda[(1-(-a))(u_k-u_{k-1})+(1-(-a)^2)(u_{k-1}-u_{k-2})+\dots+(1-(-a)^k)u_1]}, k = 2n+1 \\ e^{-\lambda[(1-(-a))(u_k-u_{k-1})+(1-(-a)^2)(u_{k-1}-u_{k-2})+\dots+(1-(-a)^k)u_1]}, k = 2n, \end{cases}$$

where $u_1 < \dots < u_k$.

PROOF.– We have

$$E[(-a)^{\xi(u_1)}\dots(-a)^{\xi(u_k)}] = p\sum_{n_1=0}^\infty(-a)^{n_1}P(\xi(u_1) = n_1)\sum_{n_2=n_1}^\infty(-a)^{n_2}P(\xi(u_2-$$

$$u_1) = n_2-n_1)\cdots\sum_{n_{k-1}=n_{k-2}}^\infty(-a)^{n_{k-1}}P(\xi(u_{k-1}-u_{k-2}) = n_{k-1}-n_{k-2})\times$$

$$\sum_{n_k=n_{k-1}}^\infty(-a)^{n_k}P(\xi(u_k-u_{k-1}) = n_k-n_{k-1}) + q\sum_{n_1=0}^\infty(-1)(-a)^{n_1}P(\xi(u_1) = n_1)\times$$

$$\sum_{n_2=n_1}^{\infty}(-1)(-a)^{n_2}P(\xi(u_2-u_1)=n_2-n_1)\cdots\sum_{n_{k-1}=n_{k-2}}^{\infty}(-1)(-a)^{n_{k-1}}P(\xi(u_{k-1}-$$

$$u_{k-2})=n_{k-1}-n_{k-2})\sum_{n_k=n_{k-1}}^{\infty}(-1)(-a)^{n_k}P(\xi(u_k-u_{k-1})=n_k-n_{k-1})=$$

$$p\sum_{n_1=0}^{\infty}(-a)^{n_1}P(\xi(u_1)=n_1)\sum_{n_2=n_1}^{\infty}(-a)^{n_2}P(\xi(u_2-u_1)=n_2-n_1)\cdots\times$$

$$\sum_{n_{k-1}=n_{k-2}}^{\infty}(-a)^{n_{k-1}}P(\xi(u_{k-1}-u_{k-2})=n_{k-1}-n_{k-2})(-a)^{n_{k-1}}e^{-\lambda(1-(-a))(u_k-u_{k-1})}+$$

$$(-1)^k q\sum_{n_1=0}^{\infty}(-a)^{n_1}P(\xi(u_1)=n_1)\sum_{n_2=n_1}^{\infty}(-a)^{n_2}P(\xi(u_2-u_1)=n_2-n_1)\ldots$$

$$\sum_{n_{k-1}=n_{k-2}}^{\infty}(-a)^{n_{k-1}}P(\xi(u_{k-1}-u_{k-2})=n_{k-1}-n_{k-2})(-a)^{n_{k-1}}\times$$

$$e^{-\lambda(1-(-a))(u_k-u_{k-1})}=pe^{-\lambda(1-(-a))(u_k-u_{k-1})}\sum_{n_1=0}^{\infty}(-a)^{n_1}P(\xi(u_1)=n_1)\times$$

$$\sum_{n_2=n_1}^{\infty}(-a)^{n_2}P(\xi(u_2-u_1)=n_2-n_1)\cdots\sum_{n_{k-1}=n_{k-2}}^{\infty}(-a)^{2n_{k-1}}P(\xi(u_{k-1}-u_{k-2})=$$

$$n_{k-1}-n_{k-2})+(-1)^k qe^{-\lambda(1-(-a))(u_k-u_{k-1})}\sum_{n_1=0}^{\infty}(-a)^{n_1}P(\xi(u_1)=n_1)\times$$

$$\sum_{n_2=n_1}^{\infty}(-a)^{n_2}P(\xi(u_2-u_1)=n_2-n_1)\cdots\sum_{n_{k-1}=n_{k-2}}^{\infty}(-a)^{2n_{k-1}}P(\xi(u_{k-1}-u_{k-2})=$$

$$n_{k-1}-n_{k-2})=\cdots=pe^{-\lambda[(1-(-a))(u_k-u_{k-1})+(1-(-a)^2)(u_{k-1}-u_{k-2})+\cdots+(1-(-a)^k)u_1]}+$$

$$(-1)^k qe^{-\lambda[(1-(-a))(u_k-u_{k-1})+(1-(-a)^2)(u_{k-1}-u_{k-2})+\cdots+(1-(-a)^k)u_1]}=$$

$$\begin{cases} re^{-\lambda[(1-(-a))(u_k-u_{k-1})+(1-(-a)^2)(u_{k-1}-u_{k-2})+\cdots+(1-(-a)^k)u_1]}, k=2n+1\\ e^{-\lambda[(1-(-a))(u_k-u_{k-1})+(1-(-a)^2)(u_{k-1}-u_{k-2})+\cdots+(1-(-a)^k)u_1]}, k=2n.\end{cases}$$

Theorem is proven.

EXAMPLE 4.1.– *For the first moment, we have:* $E[(-a)^{\xi(t)}]=re^{-\lambda t}e^{-a\lambda t}$ $(r=p-q)$*, which coincides with the first moment of the telegraphic process at* $a=1$.

For the second moment, we have $(u < t)$*:*

$$E[(-a)^{\xi(u)}(-a)^{\xi(t)}] = p\left[1\frac{(\lambda u)^0}{0!}e^{-\lambda u}(e^{-\lambda(t-u)}e^{-a\lambda(t-u)}) + (-a)\times\right.$$

$$\frac{(\lambda u)^1}{1!}e^{-\lambda u}((-a)\frac{(\lambda(t-u))^0}{0!}e^{-\lambda(t-u)} + (-a)^2\frac{(\lambda(t-u))^1}{1!}e^{-\lambda(t-u)}+$$

$$\ldots) + \ldots] + q\left[-1\frac{(\lambda u)^0}{0!}e^{-\lambda u}(-e^{-\lambda(t-u)}e^{-a\lambda(t-u)}) - (-a)\frac{(\lambda u)^1}{1!}\times\right.$$

$$e^{-\lambda u}(-(-a)\frac{(\lambda(t-u))^0}{0!}e^{-\lambda(t-u)} - (-a)^2\frac{(\lambda(t-u))^1}{1!}e^{-\lambda(t-u)}-$$

$$\ldots) - \ldots] = pe^{-(1+a)\lambda(t-u)}\left(\frac{(\lambda u)^0}{0!}e^{-\lambda u} + (-a)^2\frac{(\lambda u)^1}{1!}e^{-\lambda u}+\right.$$

$$\ldots) + qe^{-(1+a)\lambda(t-u)}\left(\frac{(\lambda u)^0}{0!}e^{-\lambda u} + (-a)^2\frac{(\lambda u)^1}{1!}e^{-\lambda u} + \ldots\right) =$$

$$e^{-(1+a)\lambda(t-u)}e^{-\lambda u}e^{a^2\lambda u} = e^{-\lambda[(1+a)(t-u)+(1-a^2)u]},$$

as soon as $p + q = 1$.

The second moment at $a = 1$ *coincides with the second moment in Example 1.1.*

For the moments of a fading Markov random evolutionary process, we have: $E(v\int_0^t(-a)^{\xi(u)}du) = v\int_0^t E[(-a)^{\xi(u)}]du = rv\int_0^t e^{-(1+a)\lambda t}du = \frac{rv}{(1+a)\lambda}[1 - e^{-(1+a)\lambda t}]$.

THEOREM 4.3.– *The moments of the fading Markov random evolutionary process in* R^1 *satisfy the recurrent correlation:*

$$m_{2k}(v,\lambda,t) = E(v\int_0^t(-1)^{\xi(u)}du)^{2k} = 2kv\int_0^t\frac{e^{-\lambda(1-(-a))u_{2k}}m_{2k-1}(v,a\lambda,u_{2k})}{r}du_{2k},$$

$$m_{2k+1}(v,\lambda,t) = E(v\int_0^t(-1)^{\xi(u)}du)^{2k+1} = (2k+1)rv\int_0^t e^{-\lambda(1-(-a))u_{2k+1}}\times$$

$m_{2k}(v,a\lambda,u_{2k+1})du_{2k+1}$, *where* $m_0(v,\lambda,t) = 1$.

PROOF.– Using the method by Kac (1957) and the relations found in theorem 4.2, we find

$$E\left(v\int_0^t(-1)^{\xi(u)}du\right)^k = k!v^k\int_0^t\cdots\int_0^{u_2}E[(-1)^{\xi(u_1)}\ldots(-1)^{\xi(u_k)}]du_1\ldots du_k =$$

$$\begin{cases} k!v^k \int_0^t \cdots \int_0^{u_2} re^{-\lambda[(1-(-a))(u_k-u_{k-1})+\cdots+(1-(-a)^k)u_1]}du_1 \ldots du_k, k = 2n+1 \\ k!v^k \int_0^t \cdots \int_0^{u_2} e^{-\lambda[(1-(-a))(u_k-u_{k-1})+\cdots+(1-(-a)^k)u_1]}du_1 \ldots du_k, k = 2n, \end{cases} =$$

$$\begin{cases} (2n+1)!v^{2n+1} \int_0^t \cdots \int_0^{u_2} re^{-\lambda[(1-(-a))(u_{2n+1}-u_{2n})+\cdots+(1-(-a)^{2n+1})u_1]}du_1 \ldots du_{2n+1} \\ (2n)!v^{2n} \int_0^t \cdots \int_0^{u_2} e^{-\lambda[(1-(-a))(u_{2n}-u_{2n-1})+\cdots+(1-(-a)^{2n})u_1]}du_1 \ldots du_{2n} \end{cases} =$$

$$\begin{cases} m_{2n+1}(v, \lambda, t) \\ m_{2n}(v, \lambda, t) \end{cases}$$

Obviously,

$$m_{2n+1}(v, \lambda, t) = (2n+1)!v^{2n+1} \int_0^t \cdots \int_0^{u_2} re^{-\lambda[(1-(-a))(u_{2n+1}-u_{2n})+\cdots+(1-(-a)^{2n+1})u_1]}$$

$$du_1 \ldots du_{2n+1} = (2n+1)!rv^{2n+1} \int_0^t e^{-\lambda(1-(-a))u_{2n+1}} \int_0^{u_{2n+1}} \cdots$$

$$\int_0^{u_2} e^{-\lambda[(1-(-a))(-u_{2n})+\cdots+(1-(-a)^{2n+1})u_1]}du_1du_2 \ldots du_{2n+1} = (2n+1)!rv^{2n+1} \times$$

$$\int_0^t e^{-\lambda(1-(-a))u_{2n+1}} \int_0^{u_{2n+1}} \cdots \int_0^{u_2} e^{-\lambda[((-a)-(-a)^2)u_{2n}+\cdots+((-a)^{2n}-(-a)^{2n+1})u_1]}$$

$$du_1du_2 \ldots du_{2n+1} = (2n+1)!rv^{2n+1} \int_0^t e^{-\lambda(1-(-a))u_{2n+1}} \int_0^{u_{2n+1}} \cdots$$

$$\int_0^{u_2} e^{a\lambda(1-(-a))u_{2n}} e^{((-a)-(-a)^2)u_{2n-1})} \cdots e^{((-a)^{2n-1}-(-a)^{2n})u_1} du_1du_2 \ldots du_{2n+1} =$$

$$(2n+1)!rv^{2n+1} \int_0^t e^{-\lambda(1-(-a))u_{2n+1}} \int_0^{u_{2n+1}} \cdots$$

$$\int_0^{u_2} e^{a\lambda[(1-(-a))(u_{2n}-u_{2n-1})+(1-(-a)^2)(u_{2n-1}-u_{2n-2})+\cdots+(1-(-a)^{2n})u_1]}du_1du_2 \ldots du_{2n+1} =$$

$$(2n+1)rv \int_0^t e^{-2\lambda u_{2n+1}} m_{2n}(v, a\lambda, u_{2n+1})du_{2n+1},$$

at the same time $m_1(v, \lambda, t) = E\left(v \int_0^t (-a)^{\xi(u_1)}du_1\right) = rv \int_0^t e^{-(1-(-a))\lambda u}du$, and we put $m_0(v, \lambda, t) = 1$.

Similarly, we have:

$$m_{2n}(v, \lambda, t) = (2n)!v^{2n} \int_0^t \cdots \int_0^{u_2} e^{-\lambda[(1-(-a))(u_{2n}-u_{2n-1})+\cdots+(1-(-a)^{2n})u_1]}du_1 \ldots$$

$$du_{2n} = (2n)!v^{2n} \int_0^t e^{-(1-(-a))\lambda u_{2n}} \int_0^{u_{2n}} \cdots \int_0^{u_2} e^{-\lambda[(1-(-a))(-u_{2n-1})+\cdots+(1-(-a)^{2n})u_1]}$$

$$du_1du_2 \ldots du_{2n} = (2n)!v^{2n} \int_0^t e^{-(1-(-a))\lambda u_{2n}} \int_0^{u_{2n}} \cdots \int_0^{u_2} e^{-\lambda(1-(-a))(u_{2n-1}-u_{2n-2})} \cdots$$

$$e^{(1-(-a)^{2n-1})u_1} du_1du_2 \ldots du_{2n} = 2nv \int_0^t e^{-2\lambda u_{2n}} \frac{m_{2n-1}(v, a\lambda, u_{2n})}{r} du_{2n}.$$

Theorem is proven.

Note that for $a = 1$ we have the moments found in theorem 1.6.

As in the non-fading case, consider the moments of a multidimensional fading homogeneous alternating process which, in the case of a uniform change in the direction of motion, have the form ($i = \overline{1, n}$):

$$m_0^{(i)}(u_1) = E[\tau_{\xi_0(u_1)}^{(i)} a^{\xi_0(u_1)}] = \tau_0^{(i)} \frac{(\lambda u_1)^0}{0!} e^{-\lambda u_1} + \frac{a}{n}(\tau_1^{(i)} + \cdots + \tau_n^{(i)}) \frac{(\lambda u_1)^1}{1!} e^{-\lambda u_1} +$$
$$\frac{a^2}{n^2}[(\tau_0^{(i)} + \tau_2^{(i)} \cdots + \tau_n^{(i)}) + (\tau_0^{(i)} + \tau_1^{(i)} + \tau_3^{(i)} + \cdots + \tau_n^{(i)}) + \cdots + (\tau_0^{(i)} + \cdots + \tau_{n-1}^{(i)})] \times$$
$$\frac{(\lambda u_1)^2}{2!} e^{-\lambda u_1} + \cdots = \tau_0^{(i)} \frac{(\lambda u_1)^0}{0!} e^{-\lambda u_1} + \tau_0^{(i)} \frac{(-\frac{a}{n}\lambda u_1)^1}{1!} e^{-\lambda u_1} + \tau_0^{(i)} \frac{(-\frac{a}{n}\lambda u_1)^2}{2!} e^{-\lambda u_1} +$$
$$\cdots = \tau_0^{(i)} e^{-\lambda u_1 \frac{n+a}{a}}, \text{ as soon as for any } i = \overline{0, n} : \tau_0^{(i)} + \cdots + \tau_n^{(i)} = 0.$$

In the case when the initial direction of movement is i-th with probability r_i, $(\sum_{i=0}^n r_i = 1)$, $E[\tau_{\xi(u_1)}^{(i)} a^{\xi(u_1)}] = \sum_{j=0}^n r_j \tau_j^{(i)} e^{-\lambda u_1 \frac{n+a}{a}} = \sum_{j=0}^n r_j m_j^{(i)}(u_1)$, which coincides with the corresponding moment at $a = 1$.

For the mixed moment, we have:

$$E[\tau_{\xi(u_1)}^{(i_1)} a^{\xi(u_1)} \tau_{\xi(u_2)}^{(i_2)} a^{\xi(u_2)}] = r_0 \sum_{n_1=0}^{\infty} \tau_{n_1}^{(i_1)} a^{n_1} P(\xi(u_1) = n_1) \sum_{n_2=n_1}^{\infty} \tau_{n_2}^{(i_2)} a^{n_2} P(\xi(u_2-$$
$$u_1) = n_2 - n_1) + \cdots + r_n \sum_{n_1=n}^{\infty} \tau_{n_1}^{(i_1)} a^{n_1} P(\xi(u_1) = n_1) \sum_{n_2=n_1}^{\infty} \tau_{n_2}^{(i_2)} a^{n_2} P(\xi(u_2-$$
$$u_1) = n_2 - n_1) = r_0 \sum_{n_1=0}^{\infty} \tau_{n_1}^{(i_1)} a^{2n_1} P(\xi(u_1) = n_1) m_{n_1}^{(i_2)}(u_2 - u_1) + \cdots + r_n \sum_{n_1=n}^{\infty} \tau_{n_1}^{(i_1)} \times$$
$$a^{2n_1} P(\xi(u_1) = n_1) m_{n_1}^{(i_2)}(u_2 - u_1) = \sum_{j=0}^{n} r_j m^{(i_1, i_2)} 2_j(u_1, u_2 - u_1).$$

By induction, we show that

$$E[\tau_{\xi(u_1)}^{(i_1)} a^{\xi(u_1)} \cdots \tau_{\xi(u_k)}^{(i_k)} a^{\xi(u_k)}] = \sum_{j=0}^{n} r_j m_j^{(i_1, \ldots, i_k)}(u_1, u_2 - u_1, \ldots, u_k - u_{k-1}) =$$
$$\sum_{j=0}^{n} r_j \sum_{n_1=j}^{\infty} \tau_{n_1}^{(i_1)} a^{n_1} P(\xi(u_1) = n_1) m_{n_1}^{(i_2, \ldots, i_k)}(u_2 - u_1, \ldots, u_k - u_{k-1}).$$

With a cyclic change ($i = \overline{1, n}$):

$$m_0^{(i)}(u_1) = E[\tau_{\xi_0(u_1)}^{(i)} a^{\xi(u_1)}] = \tau_0^{(i)} \frac{(\lambda u_1)^0}{0!} e^{-\lambda u_1} + a\tau_1^{(i)} \frac{(\lambda u_1)^1}{1!} e^{-\lambda u_1} + \cdots + a^n \tau_n^{(i)} \times$$

$$\frac{(\lambda u_1)^n}{n!} e^{-\lambda u_1} + a^{n+1}\tau_0^{(i)} \frac{(\lambda u_1)^{n+1}}{(n+1)!} e^{-\lambda u_1} + \cdots = e^{-\lambda u_1}[\tau_0^{(i)} ch_{n+1,0}(a\lambda u_1) + \tau_1^{(i)} \times$$

$$ch_{n+1,n}(a\lambda u_1) + \cdots + \tau_n^{(i)} ch_{n+1,1}(a\lambda u_1)].$$

In the case when the initial direction of movement is i-th with probability $r_i, (\sum_{i=0}^n r_i = 1)$,

$$E[\tau_{\xi(u_1)}^{(i)} a^{\xi(u_1)}] = [\tau_0^{(i)}(r_0 e^{-\lambda u_1} ch_{n+1,0}(a\lambda u_1) + \cdots + r_n e^{-\lambda u_1} ch_{n+1,n}(a\lambda u_1)] + \cdots +$$

$$[\tau_n^{(i)}(r_0 e^{-\lambda u_1} ch_{n+1,1}(a\lambda u_1) + \cdots + r_n e^{-\lambda u_1} ch_{n+1,0}(a\lambda u_1)] = [\tau_0^{(i)} \frac{e^{-\lambda u_1}}{n+1}(r_0 \times$$

$$\{e^{a\lambda u_1} + e^{\omega_{n+1} a\lambda u_1} + \cdots + e^{\omega_{n+1}^n a\lambda u_1}\} + \cdots + r_n\{a^n\lambda^n e^{a\lambda u_1} + \cdots + a^n\lambda^n \omega_{n+1}^{n^2} e^{\omega_{n+1}^n a\lambda u_1}\}) +$$

$$\cdots + \tau_n^{(i)} \frac{e^{-\lambda u_1}}{n+1}(r_0\{a\lambda e^{a\lambda u_1} + \cdots + a\lambda\omega_{n+1}^n e^{a\omega_{n+1}^n \lambda u_1}\} + \cdots + r_n\{e^{a\lambda u_1} + \cdots +$$

$$e^{\omega_{n+1}^n a\lambda u_1}\})] = \frac{1}{n+1}[\tau_0^{(i)}(r_0\{1 + e^{(a\omega_{n+1}-1)\lambda u_1} + \cdots + e^{(a\omega_{n+1}^n - 1)\lambda u_1}\} + \cdots + r_n\{a^n\lambda^n +$$

$$\cdots + a^n\lambda^n\omega_{n+1}^{n^2} e^{(a\omega_{n+1}^n - 1)\lambda u_1}\}) + \cdots + \tau_n^{(i)}(r_0\{a\lambda + \cdots + a\lambda\omega_{n+1}^n e^{(a\omega_{n+1}^n - 1)\lambda u_1}\} +$$

$$\cdots + r_n\{1 + \cdots + e^{(a\omega_{n+1}^n - 1)\lambda u_1}\})] = \frac{1}{n+1}[\{1 + e^{(a\omega_{n+1}-1)\lambda u_1} + \cdots +$$

$$e^{(a\omega_{n+1}^n - 1)\lambda u_1}\}(r_0\tau_0^{(i)} + r_1\tau_1^{(i)} + \cdots + r_n\tau_n^{(i)}) + \{a\lambda + a\lambda\omega_{n+1} e^{(a\omega_{n+1}-1)\lambda u_1} + \cdots +$$

$$a\lambda\omega_{n+1}^n e^{(a\omega_{n+1}^n - 1)\lambda u_1}\}(r_0\tau_n^{(i)} + r_1\tau_0^{(i)} + \cdots + r_n\tau_{n-1}^{(i)}) + \cdots + \{a^n\lambda^n + a^n\lambda^n\omega_{n+1}^n \times$$

$$e^{(a\omega_{n+1}-1)\lambda u_1} + \cdots + a^n\lambda^n\omega_{n+1}^{n^2} e^{(a\omega_{n+1}^n - 1)\lambda u_1}\}(r_0\tau_1^{(i)} + r_1\tau_2^{(i)} + \cdots + r_n\tau_0^{(i)})] =$$

$\sum_{j=0}^n r_j m_j^{(i)}(u_1)$, which coincides with the corresponding moment at $a = 1$.

Similarly to the previous one, we have:

$$E[\tau_{\xi(u_1)}^{(i_1)} a^{\xi(u_1)} \cdots \tau_{\xi(u_k)}^{(i_k)} a^{\xi(u_k)}] = \sum_{j=0}^n r_j m_j^{(i_1,\ldots,i_k)}(u_1, u_2 - u_1, \ldots, u_k - u_{k-1}) =$$

$$\sum_{j=0}^n r_j \sum_{n_1=j}^\infty \tau_{n_1}^{(i_1)} a^{n_1} P(\xi(u_1) = n_1) m_{n_1}^{(i_2,\ldots,i_k)}(u_2 - u_1, \ldots, u_k - u_{k-1}).$$

As in the one-dimensional case, using the results in the work by Kac (1957) and moments of the fading alternating process, we find moments of the fading Markov random evolutionary process in R^n.

THEOREM 4.4.– *The moments of the fading Markov random evolutionary process in R^n have the form:*

With the uniform change of direction of movement

$$E\left(v\int_0^t a^{\xi(u)}\tau^{(i)}_{\xi(u)}du\right) = -v\left[\frac{n}{n+a}\frac{1}{\lambda}\right](\tau_0^{(i)}r_0+\cdots+\tau_n^{(i)}r_n)(e^{-\frac{n+a}{n}\lambda t}-1),$$

$$E\left(v\int_0^t a^{\xi(u_1)}\tau^{(1)}_{\xi(u_1)}du_1\right)^{k_1}\cdots\left(v\int_0^t a^{\xi(u_n)}\tau^{(n)}_{\xi(u_n)}du_n\right)^{k_n} = \sum\int_0^t\int_0^{\theta_2}\cdots$$

$$\int_0^{\theta_{k_1+\cdots+k_n}} E\left[a^{\xi(\theta_1)}\tau^{(1)}_{\xi(\theta_1)}\cdots a^{\xi(\theta_{k_1+\cdots+k_n})}\tau^{(n)}_{\xi(\theta_{k_1+\cdots+k_n})}\right]d\theta_1\ldots d\theta_{k_1+\cdots+k_n},$$

$$0\le\theta_1<\cdots<\theta_{k_1+\cdots+k_n}\le t,$$

where all possible permutations $\tau_j^{(i)}$ are summed up (there are $(k_1+\cdots+k_n)!$).

With the cyclic change of direction of movement

$$E\left(v\int_0^t a^{\xi(u)}\tau^{(i)}_{\xi(u)}du\right) = \frac{v}{n+1}\left[\left\{t+\frac{1}{(a\omega_{n+1}-1)\lambda}(e^{(a\omega_{n+1}-1)\lambda t}-1)+\cdots+\right.\right.$$

$$\left.\frac{1}{(a\omega^n_{n+1}-1)\lambda}(e^{a(\omega^n_{n+1}-1)\lambda t}-1)\right\}(r_0\tau_0^{(i)}+r_1\tau_1^{(i)}+\cdots+r_n\tau_n^{(i)})+\{a\lambda t+$$

$$\left.\frac{a\lambda\omega_{n+1}}{(a\omega_{n+1}-1)\lambda}(e^{(a\omega_{n+1}-1)\lambda t}-1)+\cdots+\frac{a\lambda\omega^n_{n+1}}{(a\omega^n_{n+1}-1)\lambda}(e^{(a\omega^n_{n+1}-1)\lambda t}-1)\right\}(r_0\tau_n^{(i)}+$$

$$r_1\tau_0^{(i)}+\cdots+r_n\tau_{n-1}^{(i)})+\cdots+\left\{a^n\lambda^n t+\frac{a^n\lambda^n\omega^n_{n+1}}{(a\omega_{n+1}-1)\lambda}(e^{(a\omega_{n+1}-1)\lambda t}-1)+\cdots+\right.$$

$$\left.\left.\frac{a^n\lambda^n\omega^{n^2}_{n+1}}{(a\omega^n_{n+1}-1)\lambda}(e^{(a\omega^n_{n+1}-1)\lambda t}-1)\right\}(r_0\tau_1^{(i)}+r_1\tau_2^{(i)}+\cdots+r_n\tau_0^{(i)})\right],$$

$$E\left(v\int_0^t a^{\xi(u_1)}\tau^{(1)}_{\xi(u_1)}du_1\right)^{k_1}\cdots\left(v\int_0^t a^{\xi(u_n)}\tau^{(n)}_{\xi(u_n)}du_n\right)^{k_n} = \sum\int_0^t\int_0^{\theta_2}\cdots$$

$$\int_0^{\theta_{k_1+\cdots+k_n}} E\left[a^{\xi(\theta_1)}\tau^{(1)}_{\xi(\theta_1)}\cdots a^{\xi(\theta_{k_1+\cdots+k_n})}\tau^{(n)}_{\xi(\theta_{k_1+\cdots+k_n})}\right]d\theta_1\ldots d\theta_{k_1+\cdots+k_n},$$

$$0\le\theta_1<\cdots<\theta_{k_1+\cdots+k_n}\le t,$$

where all possible permutations $\tau_j^{(i)}$ are summed up (there are $(k_1+\cdots+k_n)!$).

Let us study the limit distribution of the coordinate of the fading Markov random evolutionary process for $t\to\infty$.

Consider the series $S(\infty)=\int_0^\infty(-a)^{\xi(u)}du = u_1-au_2+a^2u_3-\ldots$. Here, u_i are the random exponentially distributed values. The series is convergent by the three series theorem. Let us find the distribution of $S(\infty)$.

THEOREM 4.5.– $F_{S(\infty)}(x) = P\{S(\infty) < x\} = \int_0^\infty dF(y)[1 - F(\frac{(y-x)}{a})]$, *where* $F(x) = 1 - s^{-1}[e^{-\lambda x} - \frac{a^2}{1-a^2}e^{-\frac{\lambda x}{a^2}} + \frac{a^6}{(1-a^2)(1-a^4)}e^{-\frac{\lambda x}{a^4}} - \dots], x \geq 0,$

$$s = 1 + \sum_{n=1}^{\infty}(-1)^n \prod_{k=1}^{2n} \frac{a^k}{1-a^k}. \quad [4.1]$$

REMARK 4.1.– $s = 1 + \sum_{n=1}^{\infty}(-1)^n \prod_{k=1}^{2n} \frac{a^k}{1-a^k} =$

$$1 - \frac{1}{c^2-1} + \frac{1}{(c^2-1)(c^4-1)} - \dots, \quad [4.2]$$

where $c = \frac{1}{a} > 1$. *Then,* $s = \sum_0^\infty (-1)^n \frac{(0)_{c^2,n}}{(c^2)_{c^2,n}} = {}_1\Phi_0(0; -1; c^2)$, *where* $(c)_{q,n} = (1-c)(1-cq)\dots(1-cq^n)$; ${}_r\Phi_s(\begin{smallmatrix}\alpha_1,\dots,\alpha_r;z\\ \beta_1,\dots,\beta_s;q\end{smallmatrix})$*: basic hypergeometric series (Bateman and Erdelyi 1953a, 1953b, 1955).*

Obviously, the sum of the series [4.1] is positive, since $0 < a < 1$; therefore, $F(x) \leq 1$; the series [4.2] is convergent because it changes sign and the limit of the n-th term converges to zero.

PROOF OF THEOREM 4.5.– $S(\infty) = u_1 - au_2 + a^2u_3 - \dots = [u_1 + au_3 + \dots] - a[u_2 + au_4 + \dots], 0 < a < 1$. Since u_i are equally distributed with the parameter λ, we will find the distribution function for $\zeta = u_1 + a^2u_3 + \dots$: $F(x) = P\{\zeta < x\} = P\{u_1 + a^2\zeta' < x\} = \lambda\int_0^\infty e^{-\lambda u}P\{u + a^2\zeta' < x\}du = \lambda\int_0^x e^{-\lambda u}P\{\zeta' < \frac{x-u}{a^2}\}du$. Thus,

$$F(x) = \lambda \int_0^x e^{-\lambda u} F\left(\frac{x-u}{a^2}\right) du. \quad [4.3]$$

Obviously, $F(0) = 0$. We are looking for $F(x)$ in the form:

$$F(x) = 1 + a_1e^{-\lambda x} + a_2e^{-\frac{\lambda x}{a^2}} + a_3e^{-\frac{\lambda x}{a^4}} + \dots + a_ne^{-\frac{\lambda x}{a^{2n-1}}} + \dots$$

Substituting this expression into the right-hand side of equation [4.3], we get

$$F(x) = \lambda \int_0^x e^{-\lambda u}[1 + a_1e^{-\frac{\lambda(x-u)}{a^2}} + a_2e^{-\frac{\lambda(x-u)}{a^4}} + \dots + a_ne^{-\frac{\lambda x}{a^{2n-1}}} + \dots]du =$$

$$1 - e^{-\lambda x} + \frac{a_1a^2e^{-\frac{\lambda x}{a^2}}}{1-a^2}(e^{\frac{(1-a^2)\lambda x}{a^2}} - 1) + \frac{a_2a^4e^{-\frac{\lambda x}{a^4}}}{1-a^4}(e^{\frac{(1-a^4)\lambda x}{a^4}} - 1) + \dots +$$

$$\frac{a_na^{2^{n-1}}e^{-\frac{\lambda x}{a^{2n-1}}}}{1-a^{2n-1}}(e^{\frac{(1-a^{2^{n-1}})\lambda x}{a^{2n-1}}} - 1) + \dots$$

Let us replace $F(x)$ in the left part of its expression [4.3] and equate the coefficients:

at $e^{-\lambda x}$: $a_1 = -1 + \frac{a_1 a^2}{1-a^2} + \frac{a_2 a^4}{1-a^4} + \ldots,$

at $e^{-\frac{\lambda x}{a^2}}$: $a_2 = -\frac{a_1 a^2}{1-a^2},$

at $e^{-\frac{\lambda x}{a^4}}$: $a_3 = -\frac{a_2 a^4}{1-a^4} \ldots,$

at $e^{-\frac{\lambda x}{a^{2n-1}}}$: $a_n = -\frac{a_{n-1} a^{2^{n-1}}}{1-a^{2^{n-1}}}.$

From the first two equalities, we get $a_1 = -1 + \frac{a_1 a^2}{1-a^2} - \frac{a_1 a^6}{(1-a^2)(1-a^4)} + \ldots,$ where $a_1[1 - \frac{a^2}{1-a^2} + \frac{a^6}{(1-a^2)(1-a^4)} - \ldots] = -1$. We denote the sum of the series in square brackets, which is convergent according to remark 4.1, by s. Then, $a_1 = -\frac{1}{s}; a_2 = \frac{a^2}{s(1-a^2)}; a_3 = -\frac{a^6}{s(1-a^2)(1-a^4)}; \ldots; a_n = -\frac{a^{(n-1)(1+2^{n-2})}}{s(1-a^2)(1-a^4)\ldots(1-a^{2^{n-1}})}$. Thus, the distribution function of $\zeta = u_1 + a^2 u_3 + \ldots$ is given by the formula $F(x) = 1 - s^{-1}[e^{-\lambda x} - \frac{a^2}{1-a^2} e^{-\frac{\lambda x}{a^2}} + \frac{a^6}{(1-a^2)(1-a^4)} e^{-\frac{\lambda x}{a^4}} - \ldots], x \geq 0$.

Now, for $S(\infty) = [u_1 + a^2 u_3 + \ldots] - a[u_2 + a^2 u_4 + \ldots]$, we have $F_{S(\infty)}(x) = P\{S(\infty) < x\} = P\{-a[u_2 + a^2 u_4 + \ldots] < x - [u_1 + a^2 u_3 + \ldots]\} = P\{[u_2 + a^2 u_4 + \ldots] > \frac{[u_1 + a^2 u_3 + \ldots] - x}{a}\} = \int_0^\infty dF(y)[1 - F(\frac{y-x}{a})]$.

The theorem is proven.

A similar result holds for cyclic evolution in R^n.

THEOREM 4.6.– $F_{S(\infty)}(x) = \int_0^\infty \cdots \int_0^\infty dF(y_1) \ldots dF(y_n) \left[1 - F\left(\frac{(y_1 \tau_0^{(i)} + a y_2 \tau_1^{(i)} + \cdots + a^{n-1} y_n \tau_{n-1}^{(i)} - x)}{a^n \tau_n^{(i)}}\right)\right]$, *where* $F(x) = 1 - [{}_1\Phi_0(0; -1; c^{n+1})]^{-1} \times [e^{-\lambda x} - \frac{a^{n+1}}{1-a^{n+1}} e^{-\frac{\lambda x}{a^{n+1}}} + \frac{a^{n+1+(n+1)^2}}{(1-a^{n+1})(1-a^{(n+1)^2})} e^{-\frac{\lambda x}{a^{(n+1)^2}}} - \ldots], x \geq 0$, $c = \frac{1}{a} > 1$, $\tau_j^{(i)}$: *the i-th component of the vector* $\overline{\tau}_j$, $i = \overline{1, n}, j = \overline{0, n}$.

PROOF.– We write $S(\infty) = \tau_0^{(i)} u_1 + a \tau_1^{(i)} u_2 + a^2 \tau_2^{(i)} u_3 + \cdots = \tau_0^{(i)} [u_1 + a^{n+1} u_{n+1} + \ldots] + a \tau_1^{(i)} [u_2 + a^{n+2} u_{n+2} + \ldots] + \cdots + a^n \tau_n^{(i)} [u_{n+1} + a^{n+1} u_{2n+1} + \ldots], 0 < a < 1$. Since u_i are equally distributed with the parameter λ, then it is enough to find the distribution function of $\zeta = u_1 + a^{n+1} u_{n+1} + \ldots$ We have $F(x) = P\{\zeta < x\} = P\{u_1 + a^{n+1} \zeta' < x\} = \lambda \int_0^\infty e^{-\lambda u} P\{u + a^{n+1} \zeta' < x\} du = \lambda \int_0^x e^{-\lambda u} P\{\zeta' < \frac{x-u}{a^{n+1}}\} du$. Therefore,

$$F(x) = \lambda \int_0^x e^{-\lambda u} F\left(\frac{x-u}{a^{n+1}}\right) du. \qquad [4.4]$$

Obviously, $F(0) = 0$. We are looking for $F(x)$ in the form:

$$F(x) = 1 + a_1 e^{-\lambda x} + a_2 e^{-\frac{\lambda x}{a^{n+1}}} + a_3 e^{-\frac{\lambda x}{a^{(n+1)^2}}} + \cdots + a_n e^{-\frac{\lambda x}{a^{(n+1)^{n-1}}}} + \ldots$$

By substituting this expression into the right-hand side of equation [4.4], we get

$$F(x) = \lambda \int_0^x e^{-\lambda u}[1 + a_1 e^{-\frac{\lambda(x-u)}{a^{n+1}}} + a_2 e^{-\frac{\lambda(x-u)}{a^{(n+1)^2}}} + \cdots + a_n e^{-\frac{\lambda x}{a^{(n+1)^{n-1}}}} + \ldots]du =$$

$$1 - e^{-\lambda x} + \frac{a_1 a^{n+1} e^{-\frac{\lambda x}{a^{n+1}}}}{1 - a^{n+1}}(e^{\frac{(1-a^{n+1})\lambda x}{a^{n+1}}} - 1) + \frac{a_2 a^{(n+1)^2} e^{-\frac{\lambda x}{a^{(n+1)^2}}}}{1 - a^{(n+1)^2}}(e^{\frac{(1-a^{(n+1)^2})\lambda x}{a^{(n+1)^2}}} -$$

$$1) + \cdots + \frac{a_n a^{(n+1)^{n-1}} e^{-\frac{\lambda x}{a^{(n+1)^{n-1}}}}}{1 - a^{(n+1)^{n-1}}}(e^{\frac{(1-a^{(n+1)^{n-1}})\lambda x}{a^{(n+1)^{n-1}}}} - 1) + \ldots$$

Let us replace $F(x)$ in the left part with its expression [4.4] and equate the coefficients:

at $e^{-\lambda x}$: $a_1 = -1 + \frac{a_1 a^2}{1-a^{n+1}} + \frac{a_2 a^{(n+1)^2}}{1-a^{(n+1)^2}} + \ldots,$

at $e^{-\frac{\lambda x}{a^{n+1}}}$: $a_2 = -\frac{a_1 a^{n+1}}{1-a^{n+1}},$

at $e^{-\frac{\lambda x}{a^{(n+1)^2}}}$: $a_3 = -\frac{a_2 a^{(n+1)^2}}{1-a^{(n+1)^2}}, \ldots,$

at $e^{-\frac{\lambda x}{a^{(n+1)^{n-1}}}}$: $a_n = -\frac{a_{n-1} a^{(n+1)^{n-1}}}{1-a^{(n+1)^{n-1}}}.$

From the first two equalities, we get

$$a_1 = -1 + \frac{a_1 a^{n+1}}{1 - a^{n+1}} - \frac{a_1 a^{n+1+(n+1)^2}}{(1 - a^{n+1})(1 - a^{(n+1)^2})} + \ldots,$$

from where

$$a_1[1 - \frac{a^{n+1}}{1 - a^{n+1}} + \frac{a^{n+1+(n+1)^2}}{(1 - a^{n+1})(1 - a^{(n+1)^2})} - \ldots] = -1.$$

We denote the sum of the convergent series in square brackets by s. Then,

$$a_1 = -\frac{1}{s};$$

$$a_2 = \frac{a^{n+1}}{s(1 - a^{n+1})};$$

$$a_3 = -\frac{a^{n+1+(n+1)^2}}{s(1 - a^{n+1})(1 - a^{(n+1)^2})};$$

$\dots;$

$$a_n = -\frac{a^{(n-1)(1+(n+1)^{n-2})}}{s(1-a^{n+1})(1-a^{(n+1)^2})\dots(1-a^{(n+1)^{n-1}})}.$$

Thus, the distribution function of $\zeta = u_1 + a^{n+1}u_3 + \dots$ is given by the formula

$$F(x) = 1 - s^{-1}[e^{-\lambda x} - \frac{a^{n+1}}{1-a^{n+1}}e^{-\frac{\lambda x}{a^{n+1}}} + \frac{a^{n+1+(n+1)^2}}{(1-a^{n+1})(1-a^{(n+1)^2})}e^{-\frac{\lambda x}{a^{(n+1)^2}}} - \dots],$$

$x \geq 0.$

Now, for $S(\infty) = \tau_0^{(i)}[u_1 + a^{n+1}u_{n+1} + \dots] + a\tau_1^{(i)}[u_2 + a^{n+2}u_{n+2} + \dots] + \dots + a\tau_n^{(i)}[u_{n+1} + a^{n+1}u_{2n+1} + \dots]$ we have $F_{S(\infty)}(x) = P\{S(\infty) < x\} = P\{a^n\tau_n^{(i)}[u_{n+1} + a^{n+1}u_{2n+1} + \dots] < x - \tau_0^{(i)}[u_1 + a^{n+1}u_{n+1} +$

$\dots] - a\tau_1^{(i)}[u_2 + a^{n+2}u_{n+2} - \dots -] - \dots - a^{n-1}\tau_{n-1}^{(i)}[u_n +$

$a^{n+1}u_{2n} + \dots]\} = P\{[u_{n+1} + a^{n+1}u_{2n+1} + \dots] >$

$\frac{\tau_0^{(i)}[u_1+a^{n+1}u_{n+1}+\dots]+a\tau_1^{(i)}[u_2+a^{n+2}u_4-\dots-]+\dots+a^{n-1}\tau_{n-1}^{(i)}[u_n+a^{n+1}u_{2n}+\dots]-x}{-a^n\tau_n^{(i)}}\} =$

$\int_0^\infty \cdots \int_0^\infty dF(y_1)\dots dF(y_n)[1 - F(\frac{(y_1\tau_0^{(i)}+ay_2\tau_1^{(i)}+\dots+a^{n-1}y_n\tau_{n-1}^{(i)}-x)}{-a^n\tau_n^{(i)}})]$, since all components of $\overline{\tau}_n$ are negative.

The theorem is proven.

4.2. Integral equation for a function from the fading random evolutionary process

In the case of the fading evolutionary process, it is not possible to write a system of Kolmogorov differential equations and use the Kac–Kolesnik–Orsingher technique. However, it turns out that it is possible to write an integral equation for a fading Markov random evolutionary process. By differentiating this equation, we obtain a nonlinear differential equation which describes the fading evolutionary process.

Let us write the integral equations for functions from the fading Markov random evolutionary process similarly to section 3.3. At the same time, we will obtain nonlinear integral equations which describe the movement of a particle under the action of an external force when the speed of movement decreases over time.

Consider the functions from the fading random evolutionary process in R^1 of the form: $u_+(v,x,t) = Ef(x + v\int_0^t(-a)^{\xi(u)}du)$, $u_-(v,x,t) = Ef(x - v\int_0^t(-a)^{\xi(u)}du)$, the first of which is a function from the evolutionary process which starts at the point x

in "positive" directions; the second of which is from the evolutionary process starting at the same point in the "negative" direction.

Let us write the integral equations for these functions, which we will call Kolmogorov's integral equations:

$$u_+(v,x,t) = Ef\left(x + v\int_0^t (-a)^{\xi(u)}du\right) = P(N(t)=0)Ef(x+vt)+$$

$$\int_0^t P(N(ds)=1)Ef\left(x+vs-av\int_s^t(-a)^{\xi(u)}du\right) = e^{-\lambda t}f(x+vt)+$$

$$\int_0^t \lambda e^{-\lambda s}u_-(av, x+vs, t-s)ds.$$

The same for $u_-(v,x,t)$:

$$u_-(v,x,t) = Ef\left(x - v\int_0^t (-a)^{\xi(u)}du\right) = P(N(t)=0)Ef(x-vt)+$$

$$\int_0^t P(N(ds)=1)Ef\left(x-vs+av\int_s^t(-a)^{\xi(u)}du\right) = e^{-\lambda t}f(x-vt)+$$

$$\int_0^t \lambda e^{-\lambda s}u_+(av, x-vs, t-s)ds.$$

We have for $u_+(v,x,t)$:

$$u_+(v,x,t) = e^{-\lambda t}f(x+vt) + \int_0^t \lambda e^{-\lambda s}e^{-\lambda(t-s)}f(x+vs-av(t-$$

$$s))ds + \int_0^t \lambda e^{-\lambda s}\int_0^{t-s}\lambda e^{-\lambda l}u_+(a^2v, x+vs-avl, t-s-$$

$$l)dlds = e^{-\lambda t}f(x+vt) + \lambda e^{-\lambda t}\int_0^t f(x+vs-av(t-s))ds+$$

$$\lambda^2\int_0^t\int_s^t e^{-\lambda m}u_+(a^2v, x+vs-avm+avs, t-m)dmds. \quad [4.5]$$

Similarly:

$$u_-(v,x,t) = e^{-\lambda t}f(x-vt) + \lambda e^{-\lambda t}\int_0^t f(x-vs+av(t-s))ds+$$

$$\lambda^2\int_0^t\int_s^t e^{-\lambda m}u_-(a^2v, x-vs+avm-avs, t-m)dmds. \quad [4.6]$$

Let us consider the question of the existence of solutions of integral equations [4.5] and [4.6] in the space $\pounds$ of continuous bounded functions.

$\pounds$ is the Banach space with respect to the sup-norm, so the principle of compressive mappings can be applied.

Let us write equation [4.5] in the form $u(v,x,t) = Au(v,x,t)$, where $Au(v,x,t)$: the right part of equation [4.5]. Let $f(x), \phi(v,x,t) \in \pounds$. A acts in the space $\pounds$. Really:

$$A\phi(v,x,t) = e^{-\lambda t} f(x) + \lambda e^{-\lambda t} \int_0^t f(x - v(t-2s))ds +$$

$$\lambda^2 \int_0^t \int_0^{t-s} e^{-\lambda(l+s)} \phi(av, x + v(s-l), t-(s+l))dlds \le \sup_x f(x) e^{-\lambda t} +$$

$$\lambda e^{-\lambda t} \int_0^t \sup_x f(x - v(t-2s))ds + \lambda^2 \int_0^t \int_0^{t-s} e^{-\lambda(l+s)} \sup_{v,x,t} \phi(av, x+v(s-l), t-$$

$$(s+l))dlds \le K\left(e^{-\lambda t} + \lambda t e^{-\lambda t} + \lambda^2 \int_0^t \int_0^{t-s} e^{-\lambda(l+s)} dlds\right) = K\left\{e^{-\lambda t} +\right.$$

$$\left.\lambda t e^{-\lambda t} + \lambda^2 \left(-\frac{1}{\lambda} e^{-\lambda t} t - \frac{1}{\lambda^2}(e^{-\lambda t} - 1)\right)\right\} = K$$

where $K = \max\{\sup_x f(x), \sup_{v,x,t} \phi(v,x,t)\}$, thus, $A\phi(v,x,t)$ is a bounded function.

Let us show that A is a compression. We have

$$\rho(A\phi_1, A\phi_2) = \sup_{v,x,t} |\lambda^2 \int_0^t \int_0^{t-s} e^{-\lambda(l+s)} \phi_1(av, x+v(s-l), t-(s+l))dlds -$$

$$\lambda^2 \int_0^t \int_0^{t-s} e^{-\lambda(l+s)} \phi_2(av, x+v(s-l), t-(s+l))dlds \le \lambda^2 \int_0^t \int_0^{t-s} e^{-\lambda(l+s)} \times$$

$$\sup_{v,x,t} |\phi_1(av, x+v(s-l), t-(s+l)) - \phi_2(av, x+v(s-l), t-(s+l))|dlds =$$

$$\rho(\phi_1, \phi_2)[-\lambda t e^{-\lambda t} - e^{-\lambda t} + 1],$$

where $-\lambda t e^{-\lambda t} - e^{-\lambda t} + 1 < 1$. Thus, the solution of equation [4.5] exists and is unique.

Similarly, for equation [4.6], thus we have theorem 4.7.

THEOREM 4.7.– *For $f(x)$ from the space $\pounds$, equations* [4.5] *and* [4.6] *have a unique solution in this space.*

The solution is $\lim_{n\to\infty} u_n(v,x,t) = \lim_{n\to\infty} Au_{n-1}(v,x,t)$, where $u_0(v,x,t)$, an arbitrary function from the space $\pounds$. But the convergence also takes place for functions not belonging to the space $\pounds$.

EXAMPLE 4.2.– *For equation* [4.5] *in the case* $f(x) = x$ *let us put* $u_0(v,x,t) = 0$. *Then,*

$$u_1(v,x,t) = e^{-\lambda t}\left(x + \lambda xt + vt - a\lambda vt^2 + \frac{(1+a)\lambda vt^2}{2}\right),$$

$$u_2(v,x,t) = u_1(v,x,t) + \lambda^2 e^{-\lambda t}\left(\frac{xt^2}{2} + \frac{\lambda xt^3}{6} + \frac{\lambda^2 t^3 v}{6}(1-a+a^2) + \right.$$

$$\left.\frac{\lambda^3 t^4 v}{24}(1-a+a^2-a^3)\right),$$

$$\vdots$$

$$u_n(v,x,t) = e^{-\lambda t}\left(x + \frac{\lambda xt}{1!} + \cdots + x\frac{(\lambda t)^n}{n!}\right) + ve^{-\lambda t}\left(\frac{t}{1!} + \frac{\lambda t^2}{2!}(1-a) + \cdots + \right.$$

$$\left.\frac{\lambda^{n-1}t^n}{n!}(1-a+a^2+\cdots+(-a)^{n-1})\right) = e^{-\lambda t}\left(x + \frac{\lambda xt}{1!} + \cdots + x\frac{(\lambda t)^n}{n!}\right) +$$

$$\frac{v}{(1+a)\lambda}e^{-\lambda t}\left(\frac{\lambda t}{1!}(1+a) + \frac{\lambda^2 t^2}{2!}(1-a^2) + \cdots + \frac{\lambda^n t^n}{n!}(1+(-a)^n)\right),$$

$$\lim_{n\to\infty} u_n(v,x,t) = x + \frac{v}{(1+a)\lambda}(1 - e^{-(1+a)\lambda t}),$$

which coincides with the first moment of the fading random evolutionary process $(p = 1, q = 0; r = 1)$.

REMARK 4.2.– *If* $a = 1$

$$u_+(v,x,t) = e^{-\lambda t} f(x+vt) + \lambda e^{-\lambda t}\int_0^t f(x + v(t-2s))ds +$$

$$\lambda^2 \int_0^t \int_s^t e^{-\lambda m} u_+(v, x + v(2s-m), t-m)dmds.$$

Putting $u_+(v,x,t) = u_+(x,t)$, *we obtain equation* [3.29] *for the random evolutionary process corresponding to the telegraphic process. Similarly, for* $u_-(v,x,t)$.

Equations for functions from multidimensional fading random evolutionary processes have the form:

$$u_i(v,\overline{x},t) = e^{-\lambda t} f(\overline{x} + \overline{\tau}_i vt) + \lambda e^{-\lambda t}\int_0^t f(\overline{x} + \overline{\tau}_i vs_1 + \overline{\tau}_{i+1}av(t-s_1))ds_1 +$$

$$\lambda^2 e^{-\lambda t}\int_0^t \int_0^{t-s_1} f(\overline{x} + \overline{\tau}_i vs_1 + \overline{\tau}_{i+1} avs_2 + \overline{\tau}_{i+2} a^2 v(t - s_1 - s_2)ds_2 ds_1 + \cdots +$$

$\lambda^n e^{-\lambda t}\int_0^t\int_0^{t-s_1}\cdots\int_0^{t-s_1-\cdots-s_{n-1}} f(\overline{x}+\overline{\tau}_i vs_1+\overline{\tau}_{i+1}avs_2+\cdots+\overline{\tau}_{i+n}a^n v(t-$

$s_1-s_2-\cdots-s_n))ds_n\ldots ds_2ds_1+\lambda^{n+1}\int_0^t\int_0^{t-s_1}\int_0^{t-s_2-s_1}\cdots$

$\int_0^{t-s_n-\cdots-s_2-s_1} e^{-\lambda(s_{n+1}+\cdots+s_2+s_1)}u_i(a^{n+1}v,\overline{x}+\overline{\tau}_i vs_1+\overline{\tau}_{i+1}avs_2+\cdots+$

$\overline{\tau}_{i+n}a^n vs_{n+1},t-s_1-s_2-\cdots-s_{n+1})ds_{n+1}\ldots ds_2ds_1.$

EXAMPLE 4.3.– *$n=2$, cyclic change of directions of movement. Then, $S(t)=\overline{x}+v\int_0^t a^{\xi(u)}\overline{\tau}_{\xi(u)}du$, where $\xi(u)\in\{0,1,2\}$.*

We have:

$u_0(v,\overline{x},t)=Ef\left(\overline{x}+v\int_0^t a^{\xi(u)}\overline{\tau}_{\xi(u)+0}du\right)=$
$e^{-\lambda t}f(\overline{x}+\overline{\tau}_0 vt)+\lambda\int_0^t e^{-\lambda s}u_1(av,\overline{x}+\overline{\tau}_0 vs,t-s)ds,$

$u_1(v,\overline{x},t)=Ef\left(av,\overline{x}+v\int_0^t a^{\xi(u)}\overline{\tau}_{\xi(u)+1}du\right)=$
$e^{-\lambda t}f(\overline{x}+\overline{\tau}_1 vt)+\lambda\int_0^t e^{-\lambda s}\times u_2(\overline{x}+\overline{\tau}_1 vs,t-s)ds,$

$u_2(v,\overline{x},t)=Ef\left(\overline{x}+v\int_0^t a^{\xi(u)}\overline{\tau}_{\xi(u)+2}du\right)=e^{-\lambda t}f(\overline{x}+\overline{\tau}_2 vt)+\lambda\int_0^t e^{-\lambda s}\times$
$u_0(av,\overline{x}+\overline{\tau}_2 vs,t-s)ds.$

Sequentially substituting the expressions for $u_1(v,\overline{x},t),u_2(v,\overline{x},t)$ into the first ratio, we get

$u_0(v,\overline{x},t)=e^{-\lambda t}f(\overline{x}+\overline{\tau}_0 vt)+\lambda e^{-\lambda t}\int_0^t f(\overline{x}+\overline{\tau}_0 vs+\overline{\tau}_1 av(t-s))ds+\lambda^2 e^{-\lambda t}\times$

$\int_0^t\int_0^{t-s} f(\overline{x}+\overline{\tau}_0 vs+\overline{\tau}_1 avl+\overline{\tau}_2 a^2 v(t-l-s))dlds+\lambda^3\int_0^t\int_0^{t-s}\int_0^{t-l-s} e^{-\lambda(m+l+s)}\times$

$u_0(a^3v,\overline{x}+\overline{\tau}_0 vs+\overline{\tau}_1 avl+\overline{\tau}_2 va^2 m,t-l-s-m)dmdlds=e^{-\lambda t}f(\overline{x}+\overline{\tau}_0 vt)+$

$\lambda e^{-\lambda t}\int_0^t f(\overline{x}+\overline{\tau}_0 vs+\overline{\tau}_1 av(t-s))ds+\lambda^2 e^{-\lambda t}\int_0^t\int_0^{t-s} f(\overline{x}+\overline{\tau}_0 vs+\overline{\tau}_1 avl+$

$\overline{\tau}_2 a^2 v(t-l-s))dlds-\lambda^3 e^{-\lambda t}\int_0^t\int_0^t\int_0^{t-f-s} e^{\lambda f}u_0(a^3v,\overline{x}+$

$\overline{\tau}_0 vs+\overline{\tau}_1 avl+\overline{\tau}_2 a^2 v(t-f-l-s),f)dldsdf.$

4.3. Equations in partial derivatives for a function of the fading random evolutionary process

Nonlinear differential equations were studied by some authors, for example, in the monograph of Barbu (1976) equations of the hyperbolic type $\frac{\partial}{\partial t}u(t)+Au(t)=f(t)$

are considered, where A is a nonlinear operator in the Banach space; and $\frac{\partial^2}{\partial t^2}u(t) + Au(t) + M(\frac{\partial}{\partial t}u(t)) = f(t), u(0) = u_0, \frac{\partial}{\partial t}u(t)|_{t=0} = v_0$, where M is a nonlinear operator, A is a linear operator. The method proposed below for reducing integral equations, for which the solution is found by the method of successive approximations, to nonlinear hyperparabolic equations allows us to find solutions of high-order nonlinear hyperparabolic equations.

As before, let p be the probability of a "positive direction" start, and q be the probability of a "negative direction", $r = p - q$. Consider the equation:

$$pu_+(v,x,t) + qu_-(v,x,t) = p\{e^{-\lambda t}f(x+vt) + \lambda e^{-\lambda t}\int_0^t f(x+vs-av(t-s))ds + \lambda^2\int_0^t\int_s^t e^{-\lambda m}u_+(a^2v, x+vs-avm+avs, t-m)dmds\} + q\{e^{-\lambda t}f(x-vt) + \lambda e^{-\lambda t}\int_0^t f(x-vs+av(t-s))ds+\lambda^2\int_0^t\int_s^t e^{-\lambda m}u_-(a^2v, x-vs+avm-avs, t-m)dmds\} = p\{e^{-\lambda t}f(x+vt) + \lambda e^{-\lambda t}\int_0^t f(x+vs-av(t-s))ds+ \lambda^2e^{-\lambda t}\int_0^t\int_0^{t-k} e^{\lambda k}u_+(a^2v, x+vs+avs+avk-avt, k)dsdk\} + q\{e^{-\lambda t}f(x-vt) + \lambda e^{-\lambda t}\int_0^t f(x-vs+av(t-s))ds + \lambda^2e^{-\lambda t}\int_0^t\int_0^{t-k} e^{\lambda k}u_-(a^2v, x-vs-avs-avk+avt, k)dsdk\} \quad [4.7]$$

Differentiating both its parts with respect to x and t and expressing integrals over functions and their derivatives, we obtain the Cauchy problem ($u(v,x,t) = pu_+(v,x,t) + qu_-(v,x,t)$):

$$\frac{\partial^2}{\partial x^2}u(v,x,t) = e^{-\lambda t}\frac{d^2}{dx^2}\{pf(x+vt) + qf(x-vt)\} + \lambda e^{-\lambda t}\int_0^t \frac{d^2}{dx^2}\{pf(x+vs-av(t-s)) + qf(x-vs+av(t-s))\}ds + \lambda^2e^{-\lambda t}\int_0^t\int_0^{t-k} e^{\lambda k}\frac{\partial^2}{\partial x^2}u(a^2v, x+vs+av(s+k-t), k)dsdk, \quad \frac{\partial}{\partial t}u(v,x,t) = -\lambda[e^{-\lambda t}\{pf(x+vt) + qf(x-vt)\}+ \lambda e^{-\lambda t}\int_0^t \{pf(x+vs-av(t-s)) + qf(x-vs+av(t-s))\}ds + \lambda^2e^{-\lambda t}\times \int_0^t\int_0^{t-k} e^{\lambda k}u(x+vs+av(s+k-t), k)dsdk] + [ve^{-\lambda t}\frac{d}{dx}\{pf(x+vt) - qf(x-vt)\}- a\lambda ve^{-\lambda t}\int_0^t \frac{d}{dx}\{pf(x+vs-av(t-s)) - qf(x-vs+av(t-s))\}ds - a\lambda^2ve^{-\lambda t}\times$$

$\int_0^t \int_0^{t-k} e^{\lambda k} \frac{\partial}{\partial x} u(a^2 v, x + vs + av(s+k-t), k) ds dk] + \lambda e^{-\lambda t} \times$

$\{pf(x+vt) + qf(x-vt)\} + \lambda^2 e^{-\lambda t} \int_0^t e^{\lambda k} u(a^2 v, x + vt - vk, k) dk = -\lambda u(v, x, t) +$

$[ve^{-\lambda t} \frac{d}{dx} \{pf(x+vt) - qf(x-vt)\} - a\lambda v e^{-\lambda t} \int_0^t \frac{d}{dx} \{pf(x + vs - av(t-s)) -$

$qf(x - vs + av(t-s))\} ds - a\lambda^2 v e^{-\lambda t} \int_0^t \int_0^{t-k} e^{\lambda k} \frac{\partial}{\partial x} u(a^2 v, x + vs + av(s+k-$

$t), k) ds dk] + \lambda e^{-\lambda t} \{pf(x+vt) + qf(x-vt)\} + \lambda^2 e^{-\lambda t} \int_0^t e^{\lambda k} u(a^2 v, x + vt - vk, k) dk,$

$\frac{\partial^2}{\partial t^2} u(v, x, t) = -\lambda \frac{\partial}{\partial t} u(v, x, t) - \lambda [ve^{-\lambda t} \frac{d}{dx} \{pf(x+vt) - qf(x-vt)\} - a\lambda v e^{-\lambda t} \times$

$\int_0^t \frac{d}{dx} \{pf(x + vs - av(t-s)) - qf(x - vs + av(t-s))\} ds - a\lambda^2 v e^{-\lambda t} \int_0^t \int_0^{t-k} e^{\lambda k} \times$

$\frac{\partial}{\partial x} u(a^2 v, x + vs + av(s+k-t), k) ds dk + \lambda e^{-\lambda t} \{pf(x+vt) +$

$qf(x-vt)\} + \lambda^2 e^{-\lambda t} \int_0^t e^{\lambda k} u(a^2 v, x + vt - vk, k) dk] + v^2 [e^{-\lambda t} \frac{d^2}{dx^2} \{pf(x+vt) +$

$qf(x-vt)\} + a^2 \lambda e^{-\lambda t} \int_0^t \frac{d^2}{dx^2} \{pf(x + vs - av(t-s)) + qf(x - vs + av(t-s))\} ds +$

$a^2 \lambda^2 e^{-\lambda t} \int_0^t \int_0^{t-k} e^{\lambda k} \frac{\partial^2}{\partial x^2} u(a^2 v, x + vs + av(s+k-t), k) ds dk] + \lambda v e^{-\lambda t} \frac{d}{dx} \{pf(x+$

$vt) - qf(x-vt)\} + \lambda^2 v e^{-\lambda t} \int_0^t e^{\lambda k} \frac{d}{dx} u(a^2 v, x + vt - vk, k) dk - a\lambda v e^{-\lambda t} \frac{d}{dx} \{pf(x+$

$vt) - qf(x-vt)\} - a\lambda^2 v e^{-\lambda t} \int_0^t e^{\lambda k} \frac{d}{dx} u(a^2 v, x + vt - vk, k) dk + \lambda^2 e^{-\lambda t} e^{\lambda t} \times$

$u(a^2 v, x, t) = -2\lambda \frac{\partial}{\partial t} u(v, x, t) - \lambda^2 u(v, x, t) + \lambda^2 u(a^2 v, x, t) + a^2 v^2 \frac{\partial^2}{\partial x^2} u(v, x, t) -$

$a^2 v^2 e^{-\lambda t} \frac{d^2}{dx^2} \{pf(x+vt) + qf(x-vt)\} + v^2 e^{-\lambda t} \frac{d^2}{dx^2} \{pf(x+vt) + qf(x-vt)\} + (1-$

$a) [\lambda v e^{-\lambda t} \frac{d}{dx} \{pf(x+vt) - qf(x-vt)\} + \lambda^2 v e^{-\lambda t} \int_0^t e^{\lambda k} \frac{\partial}{\partial x} u(a^2 v^2, x + vt - vk, k) dk],$

$\frac{\partial^4}{\partial t^2 \partial x^2} u(v, x, t) = -2\lambda \frac{\partial^3}{\partial t \partial x^2} u(v, x, t) - \lambda^2 \frac{\partial^2}{\partial x^2} u(v, x, t) + \lambda^2 \frac{\partial^2}{\partial x^2} u(a^2 v, x, t) +$

$a^2 v^2 \frac{\partial^4}{\partial x^4} u(v, x, t) - a^2 v^2 e^{-\lambda t} \frac{d^4}{dx^4} \{pf(x+vt) + qf(x-vt)\} + v^2 e^{-\lambda t} \frac{d^4}{dx^4} \{pf(x+$

$vt) + qf(x-vt)\} + (1-a) [\lambda v e^{-\lambda t} \frac{d^3}{dx^3} \{pf(x+vt) - qf(x-vt)\} + \lambda^2 v e^{-\lambda t} \int_0^t e^{\lambda k} \times$

$\frac{\partial^3}{\partial x^3} u(a^2 v, x + vt - vk, k) dk],$

$$\frac{\partial^3}{\partial t^3}u(v,x,t) = -2\lambda\frac{\partial^2}{\partial t^2}u(v,x,t) - \lambda^2\frac{\partial}{\partial t}u(v,x,t) + \lambda^2\frac{\partial}{\partial t}u(a^2v,x,t) + a^2v^2\times$$
$$\frac{\partial^3}{\partial x^2\partial t}u(v,x,t) - (1-a^2)\lambda v^2e^{-\lambda t}\frac{d^2}{dx^2}\{pf(x+vt)+qf(x-vt)\} + (1-$$
$$a)[-\lambda^2ve^{-\lambda t}\frac{d}{dx}\{pf(x+vt)-qf(x-vt)\} + \lambda^3ve^{-\lambda t}\int_0^t e^{\lambda k}\frac{\partial}{\partial x}u(a^2v,x+$$
$$vt-vk,k)dk] + (1-a^2)v^3e^{-\lambda t}\frac{d^3}{dx^3}\{pf(x+vt)-qf(x-vt)\} + (1-a)[\lambda v^2e^{-\lambda t}\times$$
$$\frac{d^2}{dx^2}\{pf(x+vt)+qf(x-vt)\} + \lambda^2v^2e^{-\lambda t}\int_0^t e^{\lambda k}\frac{\partial^2}{\partial x^2}u(a^2v,x+vt-vk,k)dk] + (1-$$
$$a)\lambda^2v\frac{\partial}{\partial x}u(a^2v,x,t) = -3\lambda\frac{\partial^2}{\partial t^2}u(v,x,t) - 3\lambda^2\frac{\partial}{\partial t}u(v,x,t) + \lambda^2\frac{\partial}{\partial t}u(a^2v,x,t)+$$
$$a^2v^2\frac{\partial^3}{\partial x^2\partial t}u(v,x,t) + a^2v^2\lambda\frac{\partial^2}{\partial x^2}u(v,x,t) + (1-a)\lambda^2v\frac{\partial}{\partial x}u(a^2v,x,t) - \lambda^3u(v,x,t)+$$
$$\lambda^3u(a^2v,x,t) + (1-a^2)v^3e^{-\lambda t}\frac{d^3}{dx^3}\{pf(x+vt)-qf(x-vt)\} + (1-a)[\lambda v^2e^{-\lambda t}\frac{d^2}{dx^2}\{p\times$$
$$f(x+vt)+qf(x-vt)\} + \lambda^2v^2e^{-\lambda t}\int_0^t e^{\lambda k}\frac{\partial^2}{\partial x^2}u(a^2v,x+vt-vk,k)dk],$$

$$\frac{\partial^4}{\partial t^4}u(v,x,t) = -3\lambda\frac{\partial^3}{\partial t^3}u(v,x,t) - 3\lambda^2\frac{\partial^2}{\partial t^2}u(v,x,t) + \lambda^2\frac{\partial^2}{\partial t^2}u(a^2v,x,t)+$$
$$a^2v^2\frac{\partial^4}{\partial x^2\partial t^2}u(v,x,t) + a^2v^2\lambda\frac{\partial^3}{\partial x^2\partial t}u(v,x,t) + (1-a)\lambda^2v\frac{\partial^2}{\partial t\partial x}u(a^2v,x,t)-$$
$$\lambda^3\frac{\partial}{\partial t}u(v,x,t) + \lambda^3\frac{\partial}{\partial t}u(a^2v,x,t) - \lambda\{(1-a^2)v^3e^{-\lambda t}\frac{d^3}{dx^3}\{pf(x+vt)-qf(x-vt)\}+$$
$$(1-a)[\lambda v^2e^{-\lambda t}\frac{d^2}{dx^2}\{pf(x+vt)+qf(x-vt)\} + \lambda^2v^2e^{-\lambda t}\int_0^t e^{\lambda k}\frac{\partial^2}{\partial x^2}u(a^2v,x+$$
$$vt-vk,k)dk]\} + v^2\{(1-a^2)v^2e^{-\lambda t}\frac{d^4}{dx^4}\{pf(x+vt)+qf(x-vt)\} + (1-a)[\lambda ve^{-\lambda t}\times$$
$$\frac{d^3}{dx^3}\{pf(x+vt)-qf(x-vt)\} + \lambda^2ve^{-\lambda t}\int_0^t e^{\lambda k}\frac{\partial^3}{\partial x^3}u(a^2v,x+vt-vk,k)dk]\} + (1-$$
$$a)\lambda^2v^2\frac{\partial^2}{\partial x^2}u(a^2v,x,t) = -4\lambda\frac{\partial^3}{\partial t^3}u(v,x,t) - 6\lambda^2\frac{\partial^2}{\partial t^2}u(v,x,t) + \lambda^2\frac{\partial^2}{\partial t^2}u(a^2v,x,t)-$$
$$4\lambda^3\frac{\partial}{\partial t}u(v,x,t) + 2\lambda^3\frac{\partial}{\partial t}u(a^2v,x,t) + (1+a^2)v^2\frac{\partial^4}{\partial x^2\partial t^2}u(v,x,t) + 2(1+a^2)\lambda v^2\times$$
$$\frac{\partial^3}{\partial x^2\partial t}u(v,x,t) + (1-a)\lambda^2v\frac{\partial^2}{\partial x\partial t}u(a^2v,x,t) - a^2v^4\frac{\partial^4}{\partial x^4}u(v,x,t) + (1-a+a^2)\lambda^2\times$$
$$v^2\frac{\partial^2}{\partial x^2}u(v,x,t) + (1-a)\lambda^3v\frac{\partial}{\partial x}u(a^2v,x,t) - \lambda^4u(v,x,t) + \lambda^4u(a^2v,x,t).$$

Initial conditions are, obviously, the following:

$$u(v,x,0)=f(x),\ \frac{\partial}{\partial t}u(v,x,t)|_{t=0}=rv\frac{d}{dx}f(x),$$

$$\frac{\partial^2}{\partial t^2}u(v,x,t)|_{t=0}=-r(1+a)\lambda v\frac{d}{dx}f(x)+v^2\frac{d^2}{dx^2}f(x),$$

$$\frac{\partial^3}{\partial t^3}u(v,x,t)|_{t=0}=\lambda^2 v(1-a+3ra+r)\frac{d}{dx}f(x)+$$

$$\lambda v^2(a^2-a-2)\frac{d^2}{dx^2}f(x)+rv^3\frac{d^3}{dx^3}f(x),$$

where $r=p-q$.

Finally:

$$\frac{\partial^4}{\partial t^4}u(v,x,t)+4\lambda\frac{\partial^3}{\partial t^3}u(v,x,t)+6\lambda^2\frac{\partial^2}{\partial t^2}u(v,x,t)-\lambda^2\frac{\partial^2}{\partial t^2}u(a^2v,x,t)+$$

$$4\lambda^3\frac{\partial}{\partial t}u(v,x,t)-2\lambda^3\frac{\partial}{\partial t}u(a^2v,x,t)-(1+a^2)v^2\frac{\partial^4}{\partial x^2\partial t^2}u(v,x,t)-2(1+a^2)\lambda v^2\times$$

$$\frac{\partial^3}{\partial x^2\partial t}u(v,x,t)-(1-a)\lambda^2v\frac{\partial^2}{\partial x\partial t}u(a^2v,x,t)+a^2v^4\frac{\partial^4}{\partial x^4}u(v,x,t)-(1-a+a^2)\lambda^2\times$$

$$v^2\frac{\partial^2}{\partial x^2}u(v,x,t)-(1-a)\lambda^3v\frac{\partial}{\partial x}u(a^2v,x,t)+\lambda^4u(v,x,t)-\lambda^4u(a^2v,x,t)=0$$

$$u(v,x,0)=f(x),\ \frac{\partial}{\partial t}u(x,t)|_{t=0}=rv\frac{d}{dx}f(x),$$

$$\frac{\partial^2}{\partial t^2}u(x,t)|_{t=0}=-r(1+a)\lambda v\frac{d}{dx}f(x)+v^2\frac{d^2}{dx^2}f(x),\ \frac{\partial^3}{\partial t^3}u(v,x,t)|_{t=0}=\lambda^2v(1-$$

$$a+3ra+r)\frac{d}{dx}f(x)+\lambda v^2(a^2-a-2)\frac{d^2}{dx^2}f(x)+rv^3\frac{d^3}{dx^3}f(x), \qquad [4.8]$$

where $u(v,x,t)=pu_+(v,x,t)+qu_-(v,x,t)$

THEOREM 4.8.– *The Cauchy problem* [4.8] *is equivalent to the integral equation* [4.7], *i.e. if* $u(v,x,t)$ *satisfies equation* [4.7] *and the function* $f(x)$ *in this equation is continuously differentiable, then* $u(v,x,t)$ *satisfies problem* [4.8]. *Vice versa, if* $u(v,x,t)$ *satisfies problem* [4.8] *and* $f(x)$ *is integrable, then* $u(v,x,t)$ *satisfies equation* [4.8].

By substituting the moments of the fading evolutionary process into the equation and the initial conditions, we directly make sure that for $f(x)=x^k$ the corresponding functions $u(v,x,t)$ satisfy the Cauchy problem [4.8].

REMARK 4.3.– *At* $a=1$, *we have* ($u(v,x,t)=u(x,t)$):

$$\frac{\partial^4}{\partial t^4}u(x,t)+4\lambda\frac{\partial^3}{\partial t^3}u(x,t)+5\lambda^2\frac{\partial^2}{\partial t^2}u(x,t)+2\lambda^3\frac{\partial}{\partial t}u(x,t)-2v^2\frac{\partial^4}{\partial t^2\partial x^2}u(x,t)-$$

$$4\lambda v^2 \frac{\partial^3}{\partial t \partial x^2} u(x,t) - \lambda^2 v^2 \frac{\partial^2}{\partial x^2} u(x,t) + v^4 \frac{\partial^4}{\partial x^4} u(x,t) = 0,$$

thus, $\left(\frac{\partial^2}{\partial t^2} + 2\lambda\frac{\partial}{\partial t} + \lambda^2 - v^2\frac{\partial^2}{\partial x^2}\right)\left(\frac{\partial^2}{\partial t^2} + 2\lambda\frac{\partial}{\partial t} - v^2\frac{\partial^2}{\partial x^2}\right) u(x,t) = 0.$

In this equation, the operator is factored and its second component coincides with the operator of the telegraph equation. Accordingly, if $u(x,t)$ *satisfies the telegraph equation, then it satisfies equation* [4.8] *at* $a = 1$.

Note that the last equation is similar to equation [3.38], *obtained for evolutionary processes with the switching process having an Erlang distribution.*

5

Two Models of the Evolutionary Process

In this chapter, we describe two models on a plane.

5.1. Evolution on a complex plane

In this section, an algorithm similar to the algorithm in section 3.2 is described for the case of the Kac model on a complex plane, i.e.

$$\gamma_{r,z}^{\lambda,v}(t) = x + iy + v\int_0^t (-1)^{\xi_r^\lambda(s)}ds +$$

$$iv\int_0^t (-1)^{\xi_r^\lambda(s)}ds = z + (i+1)v\int_0^t (-1)^{\xi_r^\lambda(s)}ds,$$

functions $U_0(z,t) := E_+ f(\gamma_{r,z}^{\lambda,v}(t))$ and $U_1(z,t) := E_- f(\gamma_{r,z}^{\lambda,v}(t))$, where + and - are the starting directions of the evolution, satisfy the Cauchy problem

$$\frac{\partial^2 U}{\partial t^2} + 2\lambda\frac{\partial U}{\partial t} = 2iv^2\frac{\partial^2 U}{\partial z^2}$$

$$U(0,z) = f(z), \frac{\partial}{\partial t}U(t,z)|_{t=0} = rV(1+i)f'(z), \quad [5.1]$$

which means a solution may be developed for complex-analytic initial conditions:

$$\begin{cases} f(x) = \sum_{k=0}^{\infty} f_k z^k, z \in C; \\ g(z) = \sum_{k=0}^{\infty} g_k z^k, z \in C. \end{cases} \quad [5.2]$$

A consequence of this representation of the solution of the Cauchy problem is the following result. We set $\varepsilon = \frac{1}{2\lambda}$ and write equation [5.1] in the form

$$\varepsilon \frac{\partial^2}{\partial t^2} U(t,z) = \left(i \frac{V^2}{2\lambda} \frac{\partial^2}{\partial z^2} - \frac{\partial}{\partial t} \right) U(t,z). \tag{5.3}$$

In the hydrodynamic limit (see Koroliouk and Turbin 1993), when $v \to \infty$, $\lambda \to \infty$ so that $\frac{v^2}{\lambda} \to \sigma^2$ equation [5.3] has the form of a singularly perturbed differential equation with a small parameter for the highest derivative with respect to t. In the limit, we have a Schrödinger-type equation:

$$\frac{\partial}{\partial t} U(t,z) = \sigma^2 i \frac{\partial^2}{\partial z^2} U(t,z).$$

Let us consider the functionals from the process $\gamma_{r,z}^{\lambda,v}(t)$ of the form

$$U_j(t,z) = E_j f(z + (i+1)v \int_0^t (-1)^{\xi_r^\lambda(s)} ds), \tag{5.4}$$

where $j \in \{0,1\}$ is the state of the process $\xi_r^\lambda(s)$ at the moment of time $s = 0$.

THEOREM 5.1.– *Let f be the continuously differentiable function with a compact support. Then, the functions $U_j(t,z)$, defined in equation* [5.4] *satisfy the system of backward Kolmogorov equations:*

$$\begin{cases} \frac{\partial U_0}{\partial t} = (i+1)v \frac{\partial U_0}{\partial z} - \lambda U_0 + \lambda U_1 \\ \frac{\partial U_1}{\partial t} = -(i+1)v \frac{\partial U_0}{\partial z} - \lambda U_1 + \lambda U_0. \end{cases} \tag{5.5}$$

PROOF.– Consider the function $U_0(t,z)$:

$$U_0(t + \Delta t, z) = E_0 f(z + (1+i)v \int_0^{t+\Delta t} (-1)^{\xi_r^\lambda(s)} ds) =$$

$$E f(z + (1+i)v[\int_0^{\Delta t} (-1)^{\xi(s)+0} ds + \int_{\Delta t}^{t+\Delta t} (-1)^{\xi(s)+j} ds]).$$

The probability that the state of the system will change during the time interval Δt is equal to $\lambda \triangle t$, therefore

$$U_0(z, t+\Delta t) = (1 - \lambda \triangle t) E f(z + (i+1)v \int_{\Delta t}^{t+\Delta t} (-1)^{\xi(s)+0} ds +$$

$$(i+1)v \triangle t) + \lambda \triangle t E f(z + (i+1)v \int_{\Delta t}^{t+\Delta t} (-1)(-1)^{\xi(s)} ds + O(\Delta t)) +$$

$$o(\Delta t), \Delta t \to 0.$$

Changing variable $\nu = u - \triangle t$ in the first integral and applying the condition $\xi_{\nu+\triangle t} = \xi_\nu$, since there are no changes over time, and then putting $\nu = u$, we have:

$$U_0(z, t + \triangle t) - U_0(z, t) = Ef(z + (i+1)v \int_0^t (-1)^{\xi(s)+0} ds +$$

$$(i+1)v \triangle t) - Ef(z + (i+1)v \int_0^t (-1)^{\xi(s)+0} ds) - \lambda \triangle t Ef(z +$$

$$(i+1)v \int_0^t (-1)^{\xi(s)+0} ds + (i+1)v \triangle t) + \lambda \triangle t Ef(z +$$

$$(i+1)v \int_{\triangle t}^{t+\triangle t} (-1)^{\xi(s)+1} ds + O(\triangle t)) + o(\triangle t), \triangle t \to 0.$$

Dividing by $\triangle t$ and tending $\triangle t \to 0$, we have:

$$\frac{\partial U_0}{\partial t} = -\lambda U_0 + \lambda U_1 + (i+1)v \frac{\partial U_0}{\partial z}.$$

It is necessary to justify the passage to the limit:

$$\lim_{\triangle t \to 0} \frac{Ef(z + (i+1)v \triangle t + v \int_0^t (-1)^{\xi(s)+0} ds) -}{\triangle t}$$

$$\frac{Ef(z + v \int_0^t (-1)^{\xi(s)+0} ds)}{} = E \lim_{\triangle t \to 0} \frac{f(z + (1+i)v \triangle t +}{}$$

$$\frac{v \int_0^t (-1)^{\xi(s)+0} ds) - f(z + v \int_0^t (-1)^{\xi(s)+0} ds)}{\triangle t} = (i+1)vE_0 f'_z =$$

$$\frac{\partial U_0}{\partial z}(i+1)v.$$

The limit can be carried under the expectation sign due to Lebesgue's theorems on passage to the limit under the integral sign, pointwise convergence of the expression under the sign of mathematical expectations to $(i+1)vf'_z$ (because f is continuously differentiable) and boundedness of the integrand, which is different from 0 on a compact support.

By analogy, we have: $\frac{\partial U_1}{\partial t} = -(i+1)v\frac{\partial U_1}{\partial z} - \lambda U_1 + \lambda U_0$.

Theorem is proven.

By analogy with section 3.1, the functions satisfying system [5.5] satisfy equation:

$$det \begin{pmatrix} \frac{\partial}{\partial t} + \lambda - v(1+i)\frac{\partial}{\partial z} & -\lambda \\ -\lambda & \frac{\partial}{\partial t} + \lambda + v(1+i)\frac{\partial}{\partial z} \end{pmatrix} U(t, z) = 0,$$

where $U(t, z)$ means $U_j(t, z), j = \overline{0, 1}$.

Calculating the determinant, we have:

$$\frac{\partial^2 U}{\partial t^2} + 2\lambda \frac{\partial U}{\partial t} = 2iv^2 \frac{\partial^2 U}{\partial z^2} \qquad [5.6]$$

Let us formulate the Cauchy problem for equation [5.6], the solution of which will be functions $U_j(t,z)$. From the definition of functions, we have: $U_j(t,z) = E_j f(z + (i+1)v \int_0^t (-1)^{\xi(s)} ds)$ and for $t = 0$, we get $U_j(0,z) = E_j f(z) = f(z)$. For initial distribution $P\{\xi(0) = 0\} = p, P\{\xi(0) = 1\} = q$, we get $U(0,z) = pU_0(0,z) + qU_1(0,z) = f(z)$.

From the system of backward Kolmogorov equations, we have:

$$\frac{\partial U_0(t,z)}{\partial t}|_{t=0} = -\lambda U_0(t,z)|_{t=0} + \lambda U_1(t,z)|_{t=0} +$$

$$(i+1)v \frac{\partial U_0(t,z)}{\partial z}|_{t=0} = -\lambda f(z) + \lambda f(z) + (i+1)vE_0 f'_z|_{t=0} =$$

$$(i+1)vE_0 f'_z(z) = (i+1)v f'_z(z).$$

By analogy, $\frac{\partial U_1(t,z)}{\partial t}|_{t=0} = -(i+1)vf'_z(z)$. Taking into account the initial distribution, we have: $U'_t(t,z)|_{t=0} = p(U_0)'_t - q(U_1)'_t = (p-q)(i+1)vf'(z) = (i+1)vrf'(z)$.

Thus, the Cauchy problem for equation [5.6] has the form:

$$U(0,z) = f(z), U'_t(t,z)|_{t=0} = (i+1)vrf'(z). \qquad [5.7]$$

We have proven the following theorem.

THEOREM 5.2.– *Function* $U(t,z) = U_j(t,z), j = \overline{0,1}$ *satisfies equation* [5.6] *with initial conditions* [5.7].

Let $c_r^{\lambda,v}(t,z;n) = E\left(\gamma_{r,z}^{\lambda,v}(t)\right)^n$, then the function $c_r^{\lambda,v}(t,z;n)$ is a solution of equation [5.6] with the initial conditions

$$f(z) = z^n; g(z) = rv(i+1)nz^{n-1}. \qquad [5.8]$$

Then, if in equation [5.2] $g(z) = 0$, the solution $u(t,z)$ of the Cauchy problem

$$U(0,z) = f(z), U'_t(t,z)|_{t=0} = g(z) \qquad [5.9]$$

with a complex analytic function $f(z)$ has the form

$$u_0(t,z) = \sum_{k=0}^{\infty} f_k c_{0,z}^{\lambda,v}(t,z;k).$$

If $r \neq 0$, then the function $(m \geq 1)$ $\frac{1}{rvm}\left[c_{r,z}^{\lambda,v}(t,z;m) - c_{0,z}^{\lambda,v}(t,z;m)\right]$ is a solution of equation [5.6] with the initial conditions

$$f(z) = 0,\ g(z) = z^m$$

and then the function

$$u_r(t,z) = \sum_{m=1}^{\infty} \frac{g_m}{rvm}\left[c_{r,z}^{\lambda,v}(t,z;m) - c_{0,z}^{\lambda,v}(t,z;m)\right]$$

is a solution to equation [5.6] with initial conditions

$$f(z) = 0,\ g(z) = \sum_{m=1}^{\infty} g_m z^m$$

Hence, the function

$$U_0(t,z) + U_r(t,z) = f_0 c_{0,z}^{\lambda,v}(t,z;0) + \sum_{k=1}^{\infty}[f_k c_{0,z}^{\lambda,v}(t,z;k) + \frac{g_k}{rvk}\times$$
$$\left(c_{r,z}^{\lambda,v}(t,z;k) - c_{0,z}^{\lambda,v}(t,z;k)\right)]$$

is a solution [5.6] with initial conditions $f(z) = \sum_{k=0}^{\infty} f_k z^k,\ g(z) = \sum_{k=1}^{\infty} g_k z^k$. Since the function $\frac{g_0}{2\lambda}\left(1 - e^{-2\lambda t}\right)$ is a solution to equation [5.6] with initial conditions $f(z) = 0,\ g(z) = g_0(i+1)$, we arrive at the next result.

THEOREM 5.3.– *Let $c_r^{\lambda,v}(t,z;n)$- solution of equation* [5.6] *with initial conditions* [5.8]. *Then, the solution $U(t,z)$ of the Cauchy problem* [5.9] *with complex analytic conditions* [5.2] *has the form*

$$U(t,z) = f_0 + \frac{g_0}{2\lambda}\left(1 - e^{-2\lambda t}\right) + \sum_{k=1}^{\infty}[f_k c_{0,z}^{\lambda,v}(t,z;k) + \frac{g_k}{rvk}\times$$
$$\left(c_{r,z}^{\lambda,v}(t,z;k) - c_{0,z}^{\lambda,v}(t,z;k)\right)]. \qquad [5.10]$$

The problem of constructing a solution is thus reduced to calculating the moments $c_{r,z}^{\lambda,v}(t,z;k)$ of the process of a one-dimensional complexified Brownian motion.

LEMMA 5.1.– *The following equality holds true:*

$$\lim_{\substack{\lambda\to\infty \\ v\to\infty \\ \frac{v^2}{\lambda}\to\sigma^2}} c_{r,z}^{\lambda,v}(t,z;n) = \sum_{j=0}^{\left[\frac{n}{2}\right]} \binom{n}{2j} z^{n-2j}\mu_{2j}\left(\frac{v^2}{\lambda}t\right)^j (i+1)^j \qquad [5.11]$$

where $[p]$ *is the integer part of* p,

$$\mu_{2j} = \begin{cases} 1 \cdot 3 \cdot \dots \cdot (2j-1) \; if \; j \; is \; an \; even \; number; \\ 0 \; if \; j \; is \; an \; odd \; number. \end{cases}$$

PROOF.– By definition

$$c_{r,z}^{\lambda,v} = E\left(z + v(i+1)\int_0^t (-1)^{\xi_r^\lambda(s)} ds\right)^n =$$

$$\sum_{j=0}^{n} \binom{n}{j} x^{n-j} E\left(v(i+1)\int_0^t (-1)^{\xi_r^\lambda(s)} ds\right)^j .$$

From the weak convergence of the process $v\int_0^t (-1)^{\xi_r^\lambda(s)} ds$ for $\lambda \to \infty$, $v \to \infty$, $\frac{v^2}{\lambda} \to \sigma^2$ to the Wiener process $\sigma w(t)$, $Dw(t) = 1$, it follows that

$$\lim_{\substack{\lambda\to\infty \\ v\to\infty \\ \frac{v^2}{\lambda}\to\sigma^2}} E\left[z + v(i+1)\int_0^t (-1)^{\xi_r^\lambda(s)} ds\right]^n = (i+1)^n \mu_n \left(\frac{v^2}{\lambda} t\right)^n ,$$

which gives equation [5.11].

The lemma is proven.

The lemma allows us to seek a solution to equation [5.6] with initial conditions [5.8] in the form

$$c_r^{\lambda,v}(t,z;n) = z^n + \frac{rvnz^{n-1}}{2\lambda}\left(1 - e^{-2\lambda t}\right)(i+1) +$$

$$\sum_{j=1}^{\left[\frac{n}{2}\right]} \binom{n}{2j} x^{n-2j} \mu_{2j} \left(\frac{v^2}{\lambda} t\right)^j (i+1)^j +$$

$$a_n(t,z) + b_n(t,z)\left(1 - e^{-2\lambda t}\right) \qquad [5.12]$$

where the functions $a_n(t,z)$ and $c_n(t,z)$ are polynomials in z (for a fixed t) and in t (for a fixed x) which degree is at most $n-2$. Since $c_r^{\lambda,v}(0,z;n) = z^n$, then the condition

$$a(0,z) = 0 \qquad [5.13]$$

must be necessarily true. By differentiating [5.12] with respect to t, we find

$$\frac{\partial}{\partial t}c_r^{\lambda,v}(t,z;n) = rv(i+1)nz^{n-1}e^{-2\lambda t}+$$

$$\sum_{j=1}^{\left[\frac{n}{2}\right]}\binom{n}{2j}z^{n-2j}j\mu_{2j}\left(\frac{v^2}{\lambda}\right)^j t^{j-1}(i+1)^j + \frac{\partial}{\partial t}a(t,z)+$$

$$\left(\frac{\partial}{\partial t}b(t,z)\right)\left(1-e^{-2\lambda t}\right) - 2\lambda b(t,z)e^{-2\lambda t}.$$

As soon as $\frac{\partial}{\partial t}c_r^{\lambda,v}(t,z;n)\big|_{t=0} = rv(i+1)z^{n-1}$, we obtain one more condition on $a_n(t,z)$ and $c_n(t,z)$:

$$\binom{n}{2}z^{n-2}\mu_2\left(\frac{v^2}{\lambda}\right)^2(i+1)+$$

$$\frac{\partial}{\partial t}a_n(t,z)\bigg|_{t=0} = 2\lambda b_n(0,z). \qquad [5.14]$$

THEOREM 5.4.– *Functions $a_n(t,z)$ and $b_n(t,z)$ have the form: if n is even:*

$$a_n(t,z) = \sum_{j=1}^{\frac{n}{2}-1}\sum_{k=1}^{\frac{n}{2}-j} l_j^{(k)} z^{n-2(k+j)}t^k(i+1)^{2(k+j)}+$$

$$\sum_{j=0}^{\frac{n}{2}-2}\sum_{k=1}^{\frac{n}{2}-j-1} d_j^{(k)} z^{n-2(k+j)-1}t^k(i+1)^{2(k+j)+1},$$

$$b_n(t,z) = \sum_{j=0}^{\frac{n}{2}-1}\sum_{k=1}^{\frac{n}{2}-j} e_j^{(k)} z^{n-2(k+j)}t^{k-1}(i+1)^{2(k+j)}+$$

$$\sum_{j=1}^{\frac{n}{2}-1}\sum_{k=1}^{\frac{n}{2}-j} f_j^{(k)} z^{n-2(k+j)+1}t^{k-1}(i+1)^{2(k+j)-1} + \sum_{k=2}^{\frac{n}{2}} f_0^{(k)}\times$$

$$z^{n-2k+1}t^{k-1}(i+1)^{2k-1}.$$

if n is odd:

$$a_n(t,z) = \sum_{j=1}^{\left[\frac{n}{2}\right]-1}\sum_{k=1}^{\left[\frac{n}{2}\right]-j} l_j^{(k)} z^{n-2(k+j)}t^k(i+1)^{2(k+j)}+$$

$$\sum_{j=0}^{\left[\frac{n}{2}\right]-2}\sum_{k=1}^{\left[\frac{n}{2}\right]-j-1} d_j^{(k)} z^{n-2(k+j)-1}t^k(i+1)^{2(k+j)+1},$$

$$b_n(t,z) = \sum_{j=0}^{\left[\frac{n}{2}\right]-1} \sum_{k=1}^{\left[\frac{n}{2}\right]-j} e_j^{(k)} z^{n-2(k+j)} t^{k-1} (i=1)^{2(k+j)} +$$

$$\sum_{j=1}^{\left[\frac{n}{2}\right]} \sum_{k=1}^{\left[\frac{n}{2}\right]-j+1} f_j^{(k)} z^{n-2(k+j)+1} t^{k-1} (i+1)^{2(k+j)-1} +$$

$$\sum_{k=2}^{\left[\frac{n}{2}\right]+1} f_0^{(k)} z^{n-2k+1} t^{k-1} (i+1)^{2k-1}.$$

Here,

$$e_j^{(k)} = \frac{l_j^{(1)}}{2\lambda};\ e_j^{(k)} = \frac{1}{2\lambda(k-1)} \left(e_{j-1}^{(k+1)} \cdot k \cdot (k-1) - \right.$$

$$\left. v^2 e_j^{(k-1)} \cdot (n - 2(k+j-1)) \cdot (n - 2(k+j-1) - 1) \right),\ k \neq 1;$$

$$l_j(k) = \frac{1}{2\lambda k} \left(2\lambda e_{j-1}^{(k+1)} \cdot k - l_{j-1}(k+1) \cdot (k+1) \cdot k + e_{j-2}^{(n+1)} \cdot (k+1) \cdot k + \right.$$

$$v^2 l_j^{(k-1)} \cdot (n - 2(k+j-1)) \cdot (n - 2(k+j-1) - 1) - v^2 e_{j-1}^{(k)} \cdot (n - 2(k+j-1)) \times$$

$$\left. (n - 2(k+j-1) - 1) \right);$$

$$f_j^{(k)} = \frac{d_{j-1}^{(1)}}{2\lambda};\ f_j^{(k)} = \frac{1}{2\lambda(k-1)} \left(f_{j-1}^{(k+1)} \cdot k \cdot (k-1) - \right.$$

$$\left. v^2 f_j^{(k-1)} \cdot (n - 2(k+j-1) + 1) \cdot (n - 2(k+j-1)) \right),\ k \neq 1;$$

$$d_j(k) = \frac{1}{2\lambda k} \left(2\lambda f_j^{(k+1)} \cdot k - d_{j-1}(k+1) \cdot (k+1) \cdot k + \right.$$

$$f_{j-1}^{(k+2)} \cdot (k+1) \cdot k + v^2 d_j^{(k-1)} \cdot (n - 2(k+j-1) - 1) \cdot (n - 2(k+j-1)) -$$

$$\left. v^2 f_j^{(k)} \cdot (n - 2(k+j) + 1)(n - 2(k+j)) \right).$$

In doing so, we assume that $b_0^{(k)} = \binom{n}{2k} \mu_{2k} \left(\frac{v^2}{\lambda}\right)^k$, $k = 0, \ldots, \left[\frac{n}{2}\right]$ *and*, $f_0^{(1)} = -\frac{rvn}{2\lambda}$, *and in the case when* k *and* j *go beyond the specified limits of change, we write* $b_j^{(k)} = d_j^{(k)} = e_j^{(k)} = f_j^{(k)} = 0$.

PROOF.– We write $\nu_n(t,z) = \sum_{k=1}^{\left[\frac{n}{2}\right]} \binom{n}{2k} z^{n-2k} \mu_{2k} \left(\frac{v^2}{\lambda} t\right)^k (i++1)^{2k} + a_n(t,z)$, then $c_r^{\lambda,v}(t,z;n) = z^n + \frac{rv(i+1)nz^{n-1}}{2\lambda} \left(1 - e^{-2\lambda t}\right) + \gamma_n(t,z) + b_n(t,z) \left(1 - e^{-2\lambda t}\right)$.

By substituting this expression into equation [5.6], and then grouping and equating the free terms and the terms at $e^{-2\lambda t}$, we get:

$$\frac{\partial^2}{\partial t^2}b_n - 2\lambda\frac{\partial}{\partial t}b_n = (i+1)^2v^2\frac{\partial^2}{\partial z^2}b_n - \frac{n(n-1)(n-2)rv^3(i+1)^3z^{n-3}}{2\lambda} \qquad [5.15]$$

and

$$\frac{\partial^2}{\partial t^2}\nu_n - \frac{\partial^2}{\partial t^2}b_n + 2\lambda\frac{\partial}{\partial t}\nu_n - 2\lambda\frac{\partial}{\partial t}b_n = v^2(i+1)^2(n-1)nz^{n-2}+$$

$$\frac{n(n-1)(n-2)rv^3(i+1)^3z^{n-3}}{2\lambda} + v^2(i+1)^2\frac{\partial^2}{\partial z^2}\nu_n - v^2(i+1)^2\frac{\partial^2}{\partial z^2}b_n. \qquad [5.16]$$

Ratio [5.14] can now be written as:

$$\left.\frac{\partial}{\partial t}\nu_n(t,z)\right|_{t=0} = 2\lambda b_n(0,t). \qquad [5.17]$$

The polynomial $\nu_n(t,z)$ includes the sum $\sum_{k=1}^{\left[\frac{n}{2}\right]}\binom{n}{2k}z^{n-2k}\mu_{2k}\times\left(\frac{v^2}{\lambda}t\right)^k(i+1)^{2k}$, denote the coefficient of $z^{n-2k}t^k(i+1)^{2k}$ by $l_0^{(k)}$. Since in relations [5.15] and [5.16] connecting polynomials ν_n and b_n, differentiation with respect to z is performed twice, the degree of each next term in z will be 2 less than the previous one, so the coefficient of $z^{n-2(k+j)}t^k(i+1)^{2(k+j)}$ is denoted by $l_j^{(k)}$.

It can be seen from equation [5.17] that the polynomial $b_n(t,z)$ contains the term $\frac{l_0^{(1)}}{2\lambda}z^{n-2}$, denoting $e_0^1 = \frac{l_0^{(1)}}{2\lambda}$, and similarly to the previous one, the coefficient for $z^{n-2(k+j)}t^{k-1}(i+1)^{2(k+j)}$ via $e_j^{(k)}$. If in relation [5.15] we collect the coefficients at the powers of z and t coinciding after differentiation, we get:

$$e_{j-1}^{(k+1)}\cdot(k-1)\cdot k - 2\lambda(k-1)e_j^{(k)} = v^2e_j^{(k-1)}\cdot(n-2(k+j-1))\times$$
$$(n-2(k+j-1)-1).$$

Since coefficients with smaller indices can be found earlier, for example, $e_0^{(1)}$ is already known, while $e_{-1}^{(3)}$ is set equal to 0 (j goes beyond the specified limits of change), $e_0^{(2)}$ can be found, we have:

$$e_j^{(k)} = \frac{1}{2\lambda(k-1)}\left(e_{j-1}^{(k+1)}\cdot k\cdot(k-1)-\right.$$
$$\left.v^2e_j^{(k-1)}\cdot(n-2(k+j-1))\cdot(n-2(k+j-1)-1)\right).$$

Since the degree of z is reduced by 2 when differentiating, the term with z^{k-3} does not yet occur, and therefore the presence of the expression $\frac{n(n-1)(n-2)rv^3(i+1)^3 z^{n-3}}{2\lambda}$ in relations [5.15] and [5.16] is taken into account below.

Similarly, collecting the coefficients in equation [5.16], we obtain:

$$l_{j-1}^{(k+1)} \cdot (k+1) \cdot k - e_{j-2}^{(k+1)} \cdot (k+1) \cdot k + 2\lambda l_j^{(k)} k - 2\lambda e_{j-1}^{(k+1)} =$$

$$v^2(i+1)^2 b_j^{(k-1)} \cdot (n - 2(k+j-1)) \cdot (n - 2(k+j-1) - 1) - v^2(i+1)^2 e_{j-1}^{(k)} \times$$

$$(n - 2(k+j-1)) \cdot (n - 2(k+j-1) - 1).$$

Since we know coefficients of lower indices, for example, l_0^k and e_0^k, we have:

$$l_j(k) = \frac{1}{2\lambda k}\Big(2\lambda e_{j-1}^{(k+1)} \cdot k - l_{j-1}(k+1) \cdot (k+1) \cdot k + e_{j-2}^{(k+1)} \cdot (k+1) \cdot k +$$

$$v^2(i+1)^2 l_j^{(k-1)} \cdot (n - 2(k+j-1)) \cdot (n - 2(k+j-1) - 1) - v^2(i+1)^2 e_{j-1}^{(k)} \times$$

$$(n - 2(k+j-1)) \cdot (n - 2(k+j-1) - 1)\Big).$$

Then from equation [5.17], we find $e_j^{(1)} = \frac{l_j^{(1)}}{2\lambda}$ and repeat the same procedure. The limits of k and j can be found from the considerations that polynomials have degree at most $n-2$ and variables z and t cannot have a degree less than 0.

However, relations [5.15] and [5.16] contain terms $\frac{n(n-1)(n-2)rv^3(i+1)^3 z^{n-3}}{2\lambda}$ which will give its contribution to $\nu_n(t,z)$ and $b_n(t,z)$. Denote $f_0^{(1)} = -\frac{rvn}{2\lambda}$ – coefficient of $z^{n-1} \times \left(1 - e^{-2\lambda t}\right)(i+1)$, and in general $f_j^{(k)}$ (the coefficient of $z^{n-2(k+j)+1} \times \; t^{j-1}\left(1 - e^{-2\lambda t}\right)(i+1)^{2(k+j)-1}$, and $d_j^{(k)}$) for $z^{n-2(k+j)-1} t^k (i+1)^{2(k+j)+1}$. Applying the above procedure, we obtain the required relations.

The theorem is proven.

In conclusion, we write equation [5.6] in the form of a singularly perturbed Cauchy problem:

$$\varepsilon^2 \frac{\partial^2}{\partial t^2} U(t,z) = \left(\frac{\sigma^2}{2}\frac{\partial^2}{\partial z^2} - \frac{\partial}{\partial t}\right) U(t,z)$$

$$U(0,z) = f(z), \; \frac{\partial}{\partial t} U(t,z)\Big|_{t=0} = r\frac{\sigma}{\sqrt{2}\varepsilon}(i+1) f'(z), \; r \in R.$$

Using theorem 5.4, we present solutions of this Cauchy problem for conditions of independent interest (in square brackets, the regular part of the solution is distinguished):

$$f(z) = z \ : \ U(t,z) = \left[z + \frac{r}{\sqrt{2}}\sigma\varepsilon(i+1)\right] - \frac{r}{\sqrt{2}}\sigma\varepsilon(i+1)e^{-\frac{t}{\varepsilon^2}};$$

$$f(z) = z^2 \ : \ U(t,z) = \Big[z^2 + \sigma^2 t(i+1)^2 + r\sigma\sqrt{2}\varepsilon z(i+1) -$$

$$\sigma^2\varepsilon^2(i+1)^2\Big] + \left(\sigma^2\varepsilon^2(i+1)^2 - r\sigma\sqrt{2}\varepsilon z(i+1)\right) \times$$

$$e^{-\frac{t}{\varepsilon^2}};$$

$$f(z) = z^3 \ : \ U(t,z) = \Big[z^3 + 3z\sigma^2 t - 3x\sigma^2\varepsilon^2(i+1)^2 +$$

$$\frac{3r}{\sqrt{2}}\sigma\varepsilon z^2(i+1)^2 - \frac{3r}{\sqrt{2}}\sigma^3\varepsilon^3(i+1)^3\Big] +$$

$$(3z\sigma^2\varepsilon^2(i+1)^2 - \frac{3r}{\sqrt{2}}\sigma\varepsilon z^2(i+1) + \frac{3r}{\sqrt{2}}\sigma^3\varepsilon t(i+1)^3 + \frac{3r}{\sqrt{2}}\sigma^3\varepsilon^3(i+1)^3)e^{-\frac{t}{\varepsilon^2}}.$$

5.2. Evolutionary process with infinitely many directions

In the following model of the asymmetric random evolutionary process, the thermodynamic limit is investigated, which describes the increase in the speed of the process under the condition of increasing the intensity of the switching process, similarly to the idea of the Kac model.

The works of Kac (1957), Pinsky (1991), Orsingher (e.g. Orsingher 2002; Orsingher and Sommella 2004) demonstrate this (see also Samoilenko (2001), which contains a more detailed bibliography). Symmetry in this case should be understood as a uniform stationary distribution of the control (switching) Markov process on the symmetric structure in $\mathbf{R}^n$, for example, on the $n+1$-hedra (Samoilenko 2001), or on the unit sphere (Kolesnik 2001, 2003; Samoilenko 2012).

Here, we not only generalize the results of Kolesnik on the multidimensional space, but also solve another problem. We have proven weak convergence of the process of the Markov random evolutionary process, which means we not only have proof of weak convergence of respective distributions (or generators), but we also have proof of the compactness of the process. In the majority of works that deal with random evolutions, compactness of the process is not considered at all. It is also shown that the symmetry of the process is closely connected with the balance condition.

The Markov random evolutionary process in $\mathbf{R}^n$ is studied here using the methods proposed in Korolyuk and Limnios (2005) and developed in Koroliouk and

Samoilenko (2021). We found a solution of the singular perturbation problem for the generator of the evolution and thus the averaging by a stationary measure of the switching process is obtained as a corollary of this solution. At the second stage, we have proven the relative compactness of the family of the Markov random evolutionary process. This method allows us to show weak convergence of the process of the Markov random evolutionary process to the Wiener process in $\mathbf{R}^n$.

5.2.1. *Symmetric case*

We study a particle in the space $\mathbf{R}^n$, which starts at $t = 0$ from the point $x = (x_i, i = \overline{1,n})$. Possible directions of motion are given by the vectors

$$s(\theta) = (\cos\theta_1, \sin\theta_1\cos\theta_2, \sin\theta_1\sin\theta_2\cos\theta_3, ..., \sin\theta_1 ... \sin\theta_{n-2}\cos\theta_{n-1},$$
$$\sin\theta_1 ... \sin\theta_{n-2}\sin\theta_{n-1}), \theta_{n-1} \in [0, 2\pi), \theta_i \in [0, \pi), i = \overline{1, n-2}.$$

These vectors have an initial point in the center of the unit n-dimensional sphere S_n and the terminal point at its surface. Choosing each next direction is random and its time is distributed by the Poisson law. Thus, the switching process is the Poisson one with intensity $\lambda = \varepsilon^{-2}$. The velocity of particle's motion is fixed and equals $v = c\varepsilon^{-1}$, where ε is a small parameter, $\varepsilon \to 0$ $(\varepsilon > 0)$.

Let us define a set $\Theta = \{\theta : s(\theta) \in S_n\}$ and suppose $\theta_t^\varepsilon \in \Theta$ be the switching of the Poisson process.

DEFINITION 5.1.– *Markov symmetrical random evolutionary process is the process* $\xi_t^\varepsilon \in \mathbf{R}^n$, *given by:*

$$\xi_t^\varepsilon := x + v\int_0^t s(\theta_\tau^\varepsilon)d\tau.$$

It is easy to see that when $\varepsilon \to 0$ $(\varepsilon > 0)$, the velocity of the particle and intensity of switching decrease. Our aim is to prove weak convergence of the Markov symmetrical random evolutionary process to the Wiener process when $\varepsilon \to 0$. The main method is the solution of a singular perturbation problem for the generator of the Markov symmetrical random evolutionary process. Let us describe this generator.

A two-component Markov process $(\xi_t^\varepsilon, \theta_t^\varepsilon)$ at the test functions $\varphi(x_1, ..., x_n; \theta) \in C_0^\infty(\mathbf{R}^n \times \Theta)$ can be described by the generator (see, for example, Pinsky (1991))

$$L^\varepsilon\varphi(x_1, ..., x_n; \theta) := \lambda Q\varphi(\cdot; \theta) + vS(\theta)\varphi(x_1, ..., x_n; \cdot) =$$
$$\varepsilon^{-2}Q\varphi(\cdot; \theta) + \varepsilon^{-1}cS(\theta)\varphi(x_1, ..., x_n; \cdot), \qquad [5.18]$$

where

$$S(\theta)\varphi(x_1,...,x_n;\cdot) := -\left(s(\theta),\nabla\right)\varphi(x_1,...,x_n;\cdot),$$

here $\nabla\varphi = (\partial\varphi/\partial x_i, 1 \le i \le n)$,

$$Q\varphi(\cdot;\theta) := (\Pi - I)\varphi(\cdot;\theta) := \frac{1}{N}\int_{S_n}\varphi(\cdot;\theta)\mu(d\theta) - \varphi(\cdot;\theta),$$

and $N = (2\pi)^{n/2}\frac{1}{2\cdot 4\cdot...\cdot(n-2)}$ for even n, $N = (2\pi)^{(n-1)/2}\frac{2}{3\cdot 5\cdot...\cdot(n-2)}$ for odd n; $\mu(d\theta)$ is the element of volume of the sphere S_n, which is equal to

$$\mu(d\theta) := \sin^{n-2}\theta_1 \sin^{n-3}\theta_2 ... \sin\theta_{n-2}d\theta_1...d\theta_{n-1}.$$

Using the well-known formula

$$\int_0^{\pi} sin^{2m}d\theta = 2\cdot\frac{1\cdot 2\cdot ...\cdot(2m-1)}{2\cdot 4\cdot ...\cdot 2m}\cdot\frac{\pi}{2}, \int_0^{\pi} sin^{2m+1}d\theta = 2\cdot\frac{2\cdot 4\cdot ...\cdot 2m}{1\cdot 3\cdot ...\cdot(2m+1)}$$

we can see

$$\int_{S_n}\mu(d\theta) = N.$$

Operator $\Pi\varphi(\cdot;\theta) := \frac{1}{N}\int_{S_n}\varphi(\cdot;\theta)\mu(d\theta)$ is the projector at the null-space of reducibly invertible operator Q, because by definition it maps functions to constants, but constants to itself.

For Π, we have:

$$Q\Pi = \Pi Q = 0.$$

Potential operator R_0 can be defined as:

$$R_0 := \Pi - I.$$

This operator has the following property:

$$R_0 Q = QR_0 = I - \Pi,$$

thus, it is inverse for Q at the range of Q, but for the function ϕ from the null-space of Q, we have

$$R_0\phi = 0.$$

The solution of the singular perturbation problem in the series scheme with the small series parameter $\varepsilon \to 0(\varepsilon > 0)$ (see Korolyuk and Limnios (2005)) for reducibly invertible operator Q and perturbing operator Q_1 consists of the following.

We should find two vectors $\varphi^\varepsilon = \varphi + \varepsilon\varphi_1 + \varepsilon^2\varphi_2$ and ψ that satisfy asymptotic representation

$$[\varepsilon^{-2}Q + \varepsilon^{-1}Q_1]\varphi^\varepsilon = \psi + \varepsilon\theta^\varepsilon$$

with the vector θ^ε, which is uniformly bounded by the norm and such that

$$||\theta^\varepsilon|| \le C, \varepsilon \to 0.$$

The left part of the equation can be rewritten as:

$$[\varepsilon^{-2}Q + \varepsilon^{-1}Q_1](\varphi + \varepsilon\varphi_1 + \varepsilon^2\varphi_2) =$$
$$\varepsilon^{-2}Q\varphi + \varepsilon^{-1}[Q\varphi_1 + Q_1\varphi] + [Q\varphi_2 + Q_1\varphi_1] + \varepsilon Q_1\varphi_2.$$

And as soon as it is equal to the right side, we obtain:

$$\begin{cases} Q\varphi = 0, \\ Q\varphi_1 + Q_1\varphi = 0, \\ Q\varphi_2 + Q_1\varphi_1 = \psi, \\ Q_1\varphi_2 = \theta^\varepsilon. \end{cases}$$

From the last equation, we may see that the function φ_2 should be smooth enough to provide boundedness of $Q_1\varphi_2$. Moreover, from the first equation, we see that any function from the null-space of Q can be taken as φ, and it does not depend on the variable that corresponds to the switching process.

An important condition of solvability for this problem is the balance condition

$$\Pi Q_1 = 0.$$

This condition means that the function $Q_1\varphi$ belongs to the range of Q; thus, we may solve the second equation using the potential operator, which is inverse to Q at its range:

$$\varphi_1 = -R_0Q_1\varphi. \qquad [5.19]$$

Thus, the main problem is to solve the equation

$$Q\varphi_2 = \psi - Q_1\varphi_1 = \psi + Q_1R_0Q_1\varphi.$$

The solvability condition for Q has the view:

$$\Pi Q\Pi\varphi_2 = 0 = \Pi\psi + \Pi Q_1R_0Q_1\Pi\varphi,$$

and we finally obtain

$$\Pi\psi = -\Pi Q_1R_0Q_1\Pi\varphi. \qquad [5.20]$$

For the function φ_2, we obviously have:

$$\varphi_2 = R_0[-\Pi Q_1 R_0 Q_1 \Pi + Q_1 R_0 Q_1]\varphi. \qquad [5.21]$$

Equations [5.19]–[5.21] give the solution of the singular perturbation problem.

In the case of the Markov symmetrical random evolutionary process, the balance condition has the following view:

$$\Pi S(\theta)\mathbf{1}(x) = 0, \qquad [5.22]$$

where $\mathbf{1}(x) = (x_1, ..., x_n)$. Really, every term under the integral contains either $\int_0^\pi \sin^n\theta\cos\theta d\theta = 0$ or $\int_0^{2\pi} \sin\theta d\theta = 0$.

The main result is shown in the following theorem:

THEOREM 5.5.– *Markov symmetrical random evolutionary process ξ_t^ε converges weakly to the Wiener process $w(t) := \xi_t^0$ when $\varepsilon \to 0$:*

$$\xi_t^\varepsilon \Rightarrow \xi_t^0,$$

where $\xi_t^0 \in \mathbf{R}^n$ is defined by the generator

$$L^0\varphi(x_1, ..., x_n) = \frac{c^2}{n}\Delta\varphi(x_1, ..., x_n). \qquad [5.23]$$

Here, $\Delta\varphi := \left(\frac{\partial^2}{\partial x_1^2} + ... + \frac{\partial^2}{\partial x_n^2}\right)\varphi$.

REMARK 5.1.– *The generator* [5.23] *generalizes the generators, obtained in Kolesnik (2003) for the spaces $\mathbf{R}^2$ and $\mathbf{R}^3$.*

We will use the following lemma to prove this theorem.

LEMMA 5.2.– *At the perturbed test functions*

$$\varphi^\varepsilon(x_1, ..., x_n; \theta) = \varphi(x_1, ..., x_n) + \varepsilon\varphi_1(x_1, ..., x_n; \theta) + \varepsilon^2\varphi_2(x_1, ..., x_n; \theta), \qquad [5.24]$$

having bounded derivatives of any degree and compact support, the operator L^ε has the asymptotic representation

$$L^\varepsilon\varphi^\varepsilon(x_1, ..., x_n; \theta) = L^0\varphi(x_1, ..., x_n) + R^\varepsilon(\theta)\varphi(x),$$
$$|R^\varepsilon(\theta)\varphi(x)| \to 0, \varepsilon \to 0, \varphi(x) \in C_0^\infty(\mathbf{R}^d),$$

where L^0 is defined in (5.23), $\varphi_1(x_1, ..., x_n; \theta), \varphi_2(x_1, ..., x_n; \theta)$ and $R^\varepsilon(\theta)\varphi(x)$ are the following:

$$L^0\Pi = -c^2\Pi S(\theta)R_0S(\theta)\Pi, \quad [5.25]$$

$$\begin{aligned}
&\varphi_1 = -cR_0S(\theta)\varphi,\\
&\varphi_2 = c^2R_0S(\theta)R_0S(\theta)\varphi,\\
&R^\varepsilon(\theta)\varphi = \varepsilon c^3S(\theta)R_0S(\theta)R_0S(\theta)\varphi.
\end{aligned}$$

PROOF.– Let us solve the singular perturbation problem for the operator [5.18]. To do this, we use the following correlation:

$$L^\varepsilon\varphi^\varepsilon(x_1, ..., x_n; \theta) = [\varepsilon^{-2}Q + \varepsilon^{-1}cS(\theta)][\varphi + \varepsilon\varphi_1 + \varepsilon^2\varphi_2] = \varepsilon^{-2}Q\varphi +$$
$$\varepsilon^{-1}[Q\varphi_1 + cS(\theta)\varphi] + [Q\varphi_2 + cS(\theta)\varphi_1] + \varepsilon cS(\theta)\varphi_2.$$

Thus, we obtain equations:

$$\begin{cases}
Q\varphi = 0,\\
Q\varphi_1 + cS(\theta)\varphi = 0,\\
L^0\varphi = Q\varphi_2 + cS(\theta)\varphi_1,\\
R^\varepsilon\varphi(\theta) = \varepsilon cS(\theta)\varphi_2.
\end{cases} \quad [5.26]$$

From the first equation, we see that $\varphi(x_1, ..., x_n)$ belongs to the null-space of Q. It is easy to see from the balance condition [5.22] that $S(\theta)\varphi$ belongs to the range of Q; thus, from the second equation of the system [5.26], we have:

$$\varphi_1 = -cR_0S(\theta)\varphi.$$

By substitution into the third equation and using the solvability condition, we can see that:

$$L^0\Pi\varphi + c^2\Pi S(\theta)R_0S(\theta)\Pi\varphi = 0.$$

From the last part of equation [5.22]:

$$R^\varepsilon(\theta)\varphi(x) = \varepsilon c^3S(\theta)R_0S(\theta)R_0S(\theta)\varphi(x) \to 0 \text{ when } \varepsilon \to 0, \varphi(x) \in C_0^\infty(\mathbf{R}^n).$$

Let us find the generator of the limit process L^0 by the formula [5.25]:

$$L^0\varphi = c^2\Pi S(\theta)(I - \Pi)S(\theta)\Pi\varphi = c^2\Pi S^2(\theta)\Pi\varphi - c^2\Pi S(\theta)\Pi S(\theta)\Pi\varphi.$$

The last term equals 0 by the balance condition [5.22]. Thus, finally:

$$L^0 = c^2\Pi S^2(\theta), \quad [5.27]$$

or

$$L^0 = \frac{c^2}{N} \int_{S_n} S^2(\theta)\mu(d\theta).$$

Let us calculate the integral:

$$\frac{c^2}{N} \int_0^{\pi} \cdots \int_0^{\pi} \int_0^{2\pi} \left[\cos^2\theta_1 \frac{\partial^2}{\partial x_1^2} + \sin^2\theta_1 \cos^2\theta_2 \frac{\partial^2}{\partial x_2^2} + ... + \right.$$

$$\sin^2\theta_1 ... \sin^2\theta_{n-2} \cos^2\theta_{n-1} \frac{\partial^2}{\partial x_{n-1}^2} + \sin^2\theta_1 ... \sin^2\theta_{n-2} \sin^2\theta_{n-1} \frac{\partial^2}{\partial x_n^2} +$$

$$\left\{ \sin\theta_1 \cos\theta_1 \cos\theta_2 \frac{\partial^2}{\partial x_1 \partial x_2} + ... + \sin^2\theta_1 ... \sin^2\theta_{n-2} \sin\theta_{n-1} \times \right.$$

$$\left. \left. \cos\theta_{n-1} \frac{\partial^2}{\partial x_{n-1} \partial x_n} \right\} \right] \sin^{n-2}\theta_1 \sin^{n-3}\theta_2 ... \sin\theta_{n-2} d\theta_1 ... d\theta_{n-1} =$$

$$\frac{c^2}{N} \int_0^{\pi} \cdots \int_0^{\pi} \int_0^{2\pi} \left[\cos^2\theta_1 \sin^{n-2}\theta_1 \sin^{n-3}\theta_2 ... \sin\theta_{n-2} \frac{\partial^2}{\partial x_1^2} + \right.$$

$$\sin^n\theta_1 \cos^2\theta_2 \sin^{n-3}\theta_2 ... \sin\theta_{n-2} \frac{\partial^2}{\partial x_2^2} + ... +$$

$$\sin^n\theta_1 \sin^{n-1}\theta_2 ... \sin^3\theta_{n-2} \cos^2\theta_{n-1} \frac{\partial^2}{\partial x_{n-1}^2} +$$

$$\sin^n\theta_1 \sin^{n-1}\theta_2 ... \sin^2\theta_{n-2} \sin^2\theta_{n-1} \frac{\partial^2}{\partial x_n^2} +$$

$$\left\{ \sin^{n-1}\theta_1 \cos\theta_1 \cos\theta_2 \sin^{n-3}\theta_2 ... \sin\theta_{n-2} \frac{\partial^2}{\partial x_1 \partial x_2} + ... + \right.$$

$$\left. \left. \sin^n\theta_1 \sin^{n-1}\theta_2 ... \sin^3\theta_{n-2} \sin\theta_{n-1} \cos\theta_{n-1} \frac{\partial^2}{\partial x_{n-1} \partial x_n} \right\} \right] d\theta_1 ... d\theta_{n-1} =$$

$$\frac{c^2}{N} \int_0^{\pi} \cdots \int_0^{\pi} \int_0^{2\pi} \left[(\sin^{n-2}\theta_1 \sin^{n-3}\theta_2 ... \sin\theta_{n-2} - \sin^n\theta_1 \sin^{n-3}\theta_2 ... \sin\theta_{n-2}) \frac{\partial^2}{\partial x_1^2} + \right.$$

$$(\sin^n\theta_1 \sin^{n-3}\theta_2 ... \sin\theta_{n-2} - \sin^n\theta_1 \sin^{n-1}\theta_2 \sin^{n-4}\theta_3 ... \sin\theta_{n-2}) \frac{\partial^2}{\partial x_2^2} + ... +$$

$$(\sin^n\theta_1 \sin^{n-1}\theta_2 ... \sin^3\theta_{n-2} - \sin^n\theta_1 \sin^{n-1}\theta_2 ... \sin^3\theta_{n-2} \sin^2\theta_{n-1}) \frac{\partial^2}{\partial x_{n-1}^2} +$$

$$\sin^n\theta_1 \sin^{n-1}\theta_2 ... \sin^3\theta_{n-2} \sin^2\theta_{n-1} \frac{\partial^2}{\partial x_n^2} +$$

$$\left\{ \sin^{n-1}\theta_1 \cos\theta_1 \cos\theta_2 \sin^{n-3}\theta_2 ... \sin\theta_{n-2} \frac{\partial^2}{\partial x_1 \partial x_2} + ... + \right.$$

$$\left. \left. \sin^n\theta_1 \sin^{n-1}\theta_2 ... \sin^3\theta_{n-2} \sin\theta_{n-1} \cos\theta_{n-1} \frac{\partial^2}{\partial x_{n-1} \partial x_n} \right\} \right] d\theta_1 ... d\theta_{n-1}.$$

Every term in braces has a multiplier of the type $\int_0^{\pi} \sin^n \theta \cos \theta d\theta = 0$ or $\int_0^{2\pi} \sin \theta \cos \theta d\theta = 0$; thus, the corresponding integral equals 0.

Integration of the correlations in the parentheses gives

$$\int_0^{\pi} ... \int_0^{\pi} \int_0^{2\pi} (\sin^n \theta_1 \sin^{n-1} \theta_2 ... \sin^{n-k+2} \theta_{k-1} \sin^{n-k-1} \theta_k \sin^{n-k-2} \theta_{k+1} ... \sin \theta_{n-2} -$$

$$\sin^n \theta_1 \sin^{n-1} \theta_2 ... \sin^{n-k+2} \theta_{k-1} \sin^{n-k+1} \theta_k \sin^{n-k-2} \theta_{k+1} ... \sin \theta_{n-2}) d\theta_1 ... d\theta_{n-1} =$$

$$N \left(\frac{(2m-1)(2m-2)(2m-3) \cdot ... \cdot (2m-k+1)}{2m(2m-1)(2m-2) \cdot ... \cdot (2m-k+2)} - \right.$$

$$\left. \frac{(2m-1)(2m-2)(2m-3) \cdot ... \cdot (2m-k)}{2m(2m-1)(2m-2) \cdot ... \cdot (2m-k+1)} \right) =$$

$$N \left(\frac{2m-k+1}{2m} - \frac{2m-k}{2m} \right), \text{if } n = 2m$$

$$\text{or } N \left(\frac{(2m)(2m-1)(2m-2) \cdot ... \cdot (2m-k+2)}{(2m+1)2m(2m-1) \cdot ... \cdot (2m-k+3)} - \right.$$

$$\left. \frac{2m(2m-1)(2m-2) \cdot ... \cdot (2m-k+1)}{(2m+1)2m(2m-1) \cdot ... \cdot (2m-k+2)} \right) =$$

$$N \left(\frac{2m-k+2}{2m+1} - \frac{2m-k+1}{2m+1} \right), \text{if } n = 2m+1$$

$$= \frac{N}{n}.$$

Finally, we have:

$$L^0 \varphi(x_1, ..., x_n) = \frac{c^2}{n} \Delta \varphi(x_1, ..., x_n).$$

The lemma is proven.

PROOF OF THEOREM 5.5.– In Lemma 5.2, we proved that $L^{\varepsilon} \varphi^{\varepsilon} \Rightarrow L^0 \varphi$ at the class of functions $C_0^{\infty}(\mathbf{R}^n \times \Theta)$ when $\varepsilon \to 0$. To prove the weak convergence of the process, we should show the relative compactness of the family $(\xi_t^{\varepsilon}, \theta_t^{\varepsilon})$ in $\mathbf{D}_{\mathbf{R}^n \times \Theta}[0, \infty)$. To do this, we use the methods proposed in Stroock and Varadhan (1979), Ethier and Kurtz (1986) and Korolyuk and Limnios (2005). Let us formulate corollary 6.1 from Korolyuk and Limnios (2005) (see also theorem 6.4 in Korolyuk and Limnios (2005)) as the following lemma.

LEMMA 5.3.– *Let the generators $L^{\varepsilon}, \varepsilon > 0$ satisfy the inequalities*

$$|L^{\varepsilon} \varphi(u)| < C_{\varphi}$$

for any real-valued non-negative function $\varphi \in C_0^\infty(\mathbf{R}^n \times \Theta)$, where the constant C_φ depends on the norm of φ, and for $\varphi_0(u) = \sqrt{1+u^2}$,

$$L^\varepsilon \varphi_0(u) \leq C_l \varphi_0(u), |u| \leq l,$$

where the constant C_l depends on the function φ_0, but do not depend on $\varepsilon > 0$.

Then, the family $(\xi_t^\varepsilon, \theta_t^\varepsilon), t \geq 0, \varepsilon > 0$ is relatively compact in $\mathbf{D}_{\mathbf{R}^n \times \Theta}[0, \infty)$.

Let us write the action of the generator [5.18] at the test function $\varphi^\varepsilon(x_1, ..., x_n; \theta) = \varphi(x_1, ..., x_n) + \varepsilon\varphi_1(x_1, ..., x_n; \theta)$, where $\varphi_1(x_1, ..., x_n; \theta) = -cR_0 S(\theta)\varphi(x_1, ..., x_n)$.

We have:

$$L^\varepsilon \varphi^\varepsilon(x_1, ..., x_n; \theta) = \varepsilon^{-2} Q\varphi(x_1, ..., x_n) + \varepsilon^{-1}[Q\varphi_1 + cS(\theta)\varphi(x_1, ..., x_n)] + cS(\theta)\varphi_1(x_1, ..., x_n; \theta).$$

It follows from equation [5.26] that the first two terms equal 0. Let us estimate the last term:

$$cS(\theta)\varphi_1(x_1,..., x_n; \theta) = c^2 S(\theta) R_0 S(\theta)\varphi(x_1,..., x_n) = c^2 S^2(\theta)\varphi(x_1, ..., x_n) = c^2 \left[\cos^2\theta_1 \frac{\partial^2}{\partial x_1^2} + \sin^2\theta_1 \cos^2\theta_2 \frac{\partial^2}{\partial x_2^2} + ... + \sin^2\theta_1 ... \sin^2\theta_{n-2}\cos^2\theta_{n-1} \frac{\partial^2}{\partial x_{n-1}^2} + \sin^2\theta_1 ... \sin^2\theta_{n-2}\sin^2\theta_{n-1} \frac{\partial^2}{\partial x_n^2} + \left\{ \sin\theta_1 \cos\theta_1 \cos\theta_2 \frac{\partial^2}{\partial x_1 \partial x_2} + ... + \sin^2\theta_1 ... \sin^2\theta_{n-2} \sin\theta_{n-1} \times \cos\theta_{n-1} \frac{\partial^2}{\partial x_{n-1}\partial x_n} \right\} \right] \varphi(x_1, ..., x_n) \leq C_{1,\varphi},$$

as soon as all the constants, functions and their derivatives are bounded.

We also have from equation [5.26]:

$$L^\varepsilon \varphi^\varepsilon = L^\varepsilon \varphi + \varepsilon L^\varepsilon \varphi_1 = L^\varepsilon \varphi + \varepsilon c L^\varepsilon R_0 S(\theta)\varphi.$$

Thus,

$$L^\varepsilon \varphi = L^\varepsilon \varphi^\varepsilon - \varepsilon c L^\varepsilon R_0 S(\theta)\varphi \leq C_{1,\varphi} - \varepsilon C_{2,\varphi} < C_\varphi$$

for small ε.

To prove the second condition, it is enough to use the properties of the function $\varphi_0(u) = \sqrt{1+u^2}$, i.e.:

$$|\varphi_0'(u)| \leq 1 \leq \varphi_0(u), |\varphi_0''(u)| \leq \varphi_0(u).$$

So, the proof of the second condition is similar to the previous reasoning.

Thus, the family $(\xi_t^\varepsilon, \theta_t^\varepsilon)$ is relatively compact in $\mathbf{D}_{\mathbf{R}^n \times \Theta}[0, \infty)$.

Now, we may use the following theorem (theorem 6.6 from Korolyuk and Limnios (2005)).

THEOREM 5.6.– *Let random evolution with Markov switching* $(\xi^\varepsilon(t), x^\varepsilon(t)) \in \mathbf{D}_{\mathbf{R}^n \times E}[0, \infty)$ *satisfies the conditions:*

C1: *The family of processes* $(\xi^\varepsilon(t), x^\varepsilon(t)), t \geq 0, \varepsilon > 0$ *is relatively compact.*

C2: *There exists the family of test functions* $\varphi^\varepsilon(u, x) \in C_0^3(\mathbf{R}^n \times E)$*, such that*

$$\lim_{\varepsilon \to 0} \varphi^\varepsilon(u, x) = \varphi(u)$$

uniformly by u, x*.*

C3: *The following uniform convergence is true:*

$$\lim_{\varepsilon \to 0} L^\varepsilon \varphi^\varepsilon(u, x) = L\varphi(u)$$

uniformly by u, x*.*

The family $L^\varepsilon \varphi^\varepsilon, \varepsilon > 0$ *is uniformly bounded; moreover,* $L^\varepsilon \varphi^\varepsilon$ *and* $L\varphi$ *belong to* $C(\mathbf{R}^n \times E)$*.*

C4: *Convergence by the probability of initial values*

$$\xi^\varepsilon(0) \to \widehat{\xi}(0), \varepsilon \to 0,$$

and

$$\sup_{\varepsilon > 0} \mathbf{E}|\xi^\varepsilon(0)| \leq C < +\infty$$

is true.

Then, we have the weak convergence

$$\xi^\varepsilon(t) \Rightarrow \widehat{\xi}(t), \varepsilon \to 0.$$

According to theorem 5.6, we may confirm the weak convergence in $\mathbf{D}_{\mathbf{R}^n}[0, \infty)$

$$\xi_t^\varepsilon \Rightarrow \xi_t^0.$$

Really, all the conditions are satisfied. That is, the family of processes is relatively compact, the generators converge at the test functions belonging to the class $C_0^\infty(\mathbf{R}^n \times \Theta)$, and initial conditions for the limit and pre-limit processes are equal.

The theorem is proven.

5.2.2. *Non-symmetric case*

We study the same particle in $\mathbf{R}^n$, but its velocity is equal to $v(\theta) = c(\theta)\varepsilon^{-1} + c_1(\theta)$, where $\varepsilon \to 0$ $(\varepsilon > 0)$ is the small parameter, the functions $c(\theta), c_1(\theta)$ are bounded.

DEFINITION 5.2.– *Markov non-symmetrical random evolutionary process is the process* $\widetilde{\xi}_t^\varepsilon \in \mathbf{R}^n$, *given by:*

$$\widetilde{\xi}_t^\varepsilon := x + \int_0^t v(\theta_\tau^\varepsilon) s(\theta_\tau^\varepsilon) d\tau.$$

Our aim is to prove the weak convergence of the Markov non-symmetrical random evolutionary process to a diffusion process with drift when $\varepsilon \to 0$.

A two-component Markov process $(\widetilde{\xi}_t^\varepsilon, \theta_t^\varepsilon)$ at the test functions $\varphi(x_1, ..., x_n; \theta) \in C_0^\infty(\mathbf{R}^n \times \Theta)$ is defined by a generator (see, for example, Pinsky (1968))

$$L^\varepsilon \varphi(x_1, ..., x_n; \theta) := \lambda Q \varphi(\cdot; \theta) + v(\theta) S(\theta) \varphi(x_1, ..., x_n; \cdot) =$$

$$\varepsilon^{-2} Q \varphi(\cdot; \theta) + \varepsilon^{-1} c(\theta) S(\theta) \varphi(x_1, ..., x_n; \cdot) + c_1(\theta) S(\theta) \varphi(x_1, ..., x_n; \cdot), \qquad [5.28]$$

where

$$S(\theta) \varphi(x_1, ..., x_n; \cdot) := -\left(s(\theta), \nabla\right) \varphi(x_1, ..., x_n; \cdot).$$

An important condition that let us confirm weak convergence is the balance condition

$$\Pi c(\theta) S(\theta) = 0. \qquad [5.29]$$

REMARK 5.2.– *This is the last condition that defines symmetry or non-symmetry of the process. In the case of the Markov symmetrical random evolutionary process the balance condition* [5.29] *holds true, and* $c_1(\theta) \equiv 0$. *In the case of the Markov non-symmetrical random evolutionary process, the absence of symmetry of the process is caused by the following condition:*

$$\Pi c_1(\theta) S(\theta) = (d, \nabla) \neq 0. \qquad [5.30]$$

EXAMPLE 5.1.– *Condition* [5.29] *can be satisfied for different functions* $c(\theta)$. *That is, in the case of the Markov symmetrical random evolutionary process* $c(\theta) = c = const$. *Then, every term under the integral contains either* $\int_0^\pi \sin^n \theta \cos \theta d\theta = 0$ *or* $\int_0^{2\pi} \sin \theta d\theta = 0$.

Another example is the function $c(\theta) = sin\theta_1$. *Really, we obtain the terms under the integral that are analogical to the previous ones. We note that the dimension of the space in this case should be more than 2, because in* $\mathbf{R}^2$ *this function has no symmetry.*

EXAMPLE 5.2.– *Condition* [5.30] *can also be satisfied for different functions* $c_1(\theta)$. *For example, in* $\mathbf{R}^2$ *for* $c_1(\theta) = sin\theta$, *we obtain:*

$$\frac{1}{2\pi}\int_0^{2\pi} sin\theta \left[cos\theta\frac{\partial}{\partial x_1} + sin\theta\frac{\partial}{\partial x_2}\right] d\theta = \frac{1}{2}\frac{\partial}{\partial x_2}.$$

Another example is the function in $\mathbf{R}^n$:

$$c_1(\theta) = \begin{cases} c_1, \theta_{n-1} \in [\pi, 2\pi), \\ 0, \theta_{n-1} \in [0, \pi). \end{cases}$$

Again, all terms under the integral, except the last one, contain $\int_0^\pi \sin^n \theta \cos \theta d\theta = 0$; *thus, only one term is not trivial*

$$\frac{1}{N}c_1 \int_0^\pi ... \int_0^\pi \int_\pi^{2\pi} sin^{n-1}\theta_1 sin^{n-2}\theta_2 ... sin^2\theta_{n-1} sin\theta_{n-1} d\theta_1 ... d\theta_{n-1}.$$

By simple calculations, we see:

$$\Pi c_1(\theta)S(\theta) = \begin{cases} -\frac{c_1}{2}\frac{3\cdot 5\cdot ...\cdot(n-2)}{2\cdot 4\cdot ...\cdot(n-1)}\frac{\partial}{\partial x_n}, n = 2m+1, \\ -\frac{c_1}{\pi}[1\cdot 2\cdot ...(n-2)]\frac{\partial}{\partial x_n}, n = 2m. \end{cases}$$

We obviously have a wide range of functions that preserve or, on the contrary, do not preserve symmetry. So, we can define the velocity of random evolutionary process in different ways, depending on possible applications.

The main result in this case is the following.

THEOREM 5.7.– *Markov non-symmetrical random evolutionary process* $\widetilde{\xi}_t^\varepsilon$, *converges weakly to the process* $\widetilde{\xi}_t^0$ *when* $\varepsilon \to 0$:

$$\widetilde{\xi}_t^\varepsilon \Rightarrow \widetilde{\xi}_t^0.$$

The limit process $\widetilde{\xi}_t^0 \in \mathbf{R}^n$ *is defined by a generator*

$$L^0\varphi(x_1, ..., x_n) = (d, \nabla)\varphi(x_1, ..., x_n) + (\sigma^2, \Delta)\varphi(x_1, ..., x_n), \qquad [5.31]$$

where $\Delta\varphi(x_1,...,x_n) := \left(\frac{\partial^2}{\partial x_1^2} + ... + \frac{\partial^2}{\partial x_n^2}\right)\varphi(x_1,...,x_n)$,

$$(d,\nabla) := -\frac{1}{N}\int_{S_n} c_1(\theta)(s(\theta),\nabla)\mu(d\theta),$$

$$(\sigma^2,\Delta) := \frac{1}{N}\int_{S_n} c^2(\theta)(s(\theta),\nabla)^2\mu(d\theta).$$

We need the following lemma to prove the theorem.

LEMMA 5.4.– *At the perturbed test functions*

$$\varphi^\varepsilon(x_1,...,x_n;\theta) = \varphi(x_1,...,x_n) + \varepsilon\varphi_1(x_1,...,x_n;\theta) + \varepsilon^2\varphi_2(x_1,...,x_n;\theta), \quad [5.32]$$

having bounded derivatives of any degree and compact support, the operator L^ε *has the asymptotic representation*

$$L^\varepsilon\varphi^\varepsilon(x_1,...,x_n;\theta) = L^0\varphi(x_1,...,x_n) + R^\varepsilon(\theta)\varphi(x),$$

$$|R^\varepsilon(\theta)\varphi(x)| \to 0, \varepsilon \to 0, \varphi(x) \in C^\infty(\mathbf{R}^d),$$

where L^0 *is defined in equation* [5.31], $\varphi_1(x_1,...,x_n;\theta), \varphi_2(x_1,...,x_n;\theta)$ *and* $R^\varepsilon(\theta)\varphi(x)$ *are defined by the correlations:*

$$L^0\Pi = -\Pi c(\theta)S(\theta)R_0c(\theta)S(\theta)\Pi + \Pi c_1(\theta)S(\theta)\Pi\varphi, \quad [5.33]$$

$$\begin{aligned}
&\varphi_1 = -R_0c(\theta)S(\theta)\varphi,\\
&\varphi_2 = R_0c(\theta)S(\theta)R_0c(\theta)S(\theta)\varphi,\\
&R^\varepsilon(\theta)\varphi = \{\varepsilon[c(\theta)S(\theta)R_0c(\theta)S(\theta)R_0c(\theta)S(\theta) + c_1(\theta)S(\theta)R_0c(\theta)S(\theta)] +\\
&\varepsilon^2c_1(\theta)S(\theta)R_0c(\theta)S(\theta)R_0c(\theta)S(\theta)\}\,\varphi.
\end{aligned}$$

PROOF.– We solve the singular perturbation problem for the operator [5.28]. Using the view of test functions [5.32], we have:

$$\begin{aligned}
&L^\varepsilon\varphi^\varepsilon(x_1,...,x_n;\theta) = [\varepsilon^{-2}Q + \varepsilon^{-1}c(\theta)S(\theta) + c_1(\theta)S(\theta)][\varphi + \varepsilon\varphi_1 + \varepsilon^2\varphi_2] =\\
&\varepsilon^{-2}Q\varphi + \varepsilon^{-1}[Q\varphi_1 + c(\theta)S(\theta)\varphi] + [Q\varphi_2 + c(\theta)S(\theta)\varphi_1 + c_1(\theta)S(\theta)\varphi] +\\
&\varepsilon[c(\theta)S(\theta)\varphi_2 + c_1(\theta)S(\theta)\varphi_1] + \varepsilon^2c_1(\theta)S(\theta)\varphi_2.
\end{aligned}$$

Thus, we obtain the following equations:

$$\begin{cases}
Q\varphi = 0,\\
Q\varphi_1 + c(\theta)S(\theta)\varphi = 0,\\
L^0\varphi = Q\varphi_2 + c(\theta)S(\theta)\varphi_1 + c_1(\theta)S(\theta)\varphi,\\
R^\varepsilon\varphi(\theta) = \varepsilon[c(\theta)S(\theta)\varphi_2 + c_1(\theta)S(\theta)\varphi_1] + \varepsilon^2c_1(\theta)S(\theta)\varphi_2.
\end{cases} \quad [5.34]$$

According to the first one, $\varphi(x_1, ..., x_n)$ belongs to the null-space of Q. From the balance condition [5.29], we see that $c(\theta)S(\theta)\varphi$ belongs to the range of Q; thus, from the second equation of equation [5.34], we have

$$\varphi_1 = -R_0 c(\theta)S(\theta)\varphi.$$

By substitution into the third equation, and using the solvability condition, we obtain:

$$L^0\Pi\varphi + \Pi c(\theta)S(\theta)R_0 c(\theta)S(\theta)\Pi\varphi - \Pi c_1(\theta)S(\theta)\Pi\varphi = 0.$$

From the last equation:

$$R^\varepsilon(\theta)\varphi(x) = \{\varepsilon[c(\theta)S(\theta)R_0 c(\theta)S(\theta)R_0 c(\theta)S(\theta) + c_1(\theta)S(\theta)R_0 c(\theta)S(\theta)]+$$
$$\varepsilon^2 c_1(\theta)S(\theta)R_0 c(\theta)S(\theta)R_0 c(\theta)S(\theta)\}\ \varphi(x) \to 0 \text{ when } \varepsilon \to 0, \varphi(x) \in C_0^\infty(\mathbf{R}^n).$$

We calculate the operator L^0 by the formula [5.33]:

$$L^0\varphi = \Pi c(\theta)S(\theta)(I-\Pi)c(\theta)S(\theta)\Pi\varphi + \Pi c_1(\theta)S(\theta)\Pi\varphi = \Pi c^2(\theta)S^2(\theta)\Pi\varphi -$$
$$\Pi c(\theta)S(\theta)\Pi c(\theta)S(\theta)\Pi\varphi + \Pi c_1(\theta)S(\theta)\Pi\varphi.$$

The second term equals 0 by the balance condition [5.29]; the last one is not equal to 0 by equation [5.30]. Thus, we finally have:

$$L^0 = \Pi c^2(\theta)S^2(\theta) + \Pi c_1(\theta)S(\theta). \qquad [5.35]$$

Using the view of $S(\theta)$, we may write:

$$\Pi c_1(\theta)S(\theta) = -\frac{1}{N}\int_{S_n} c_1(\theta)(s(\theta), \nabla)\mu(d\theta) =: (d, \nabla),$$

$$\Pi c^2(\theta)S^2(\theta) = \frac{1}{N}\int_{S_n} c^2(\theta)(s(\theta), \nabla)^2\mu(d\theta) =: (\sigma^2, \Delta).$$

The lemma is proven.

PROOF OF THEOREM 5.7.– We proved in lemma 5.4 that $L^\varepsilon\varphi^\varepsilon \Rightarrow L^0\varphi$ at the class of test functions $C_0^\infty(\mathbf{R}^n \times \Theta)$ when $\varepsilon \to 0$. To prove the weak convergence, we should show the relative compactness of the family of processes $(\widetilde{\xi}_t^\varepsilon, \theta_t^\varepsilon)$ in $\mathbf{D}_{\mathbf{R}^n\times\Theta}[0,\infty)$. To do this, we use lemma 5.3.

We have the following view of the operator [5.28] at the test function $\varphi^\varepsilon(x_1, ..., x_n; \theta) = \varphi(x_1, ..., x_n) + \varepsilon\varphi_1(x_1, ..., x_n; \theta)$, where $\varphi_1(x_1, ..., x_n; \theta) = -R_0 c(\theta)S(\theta)\varphi(x_1, ..., x_n)$:

$$L^\varepsilon\varphi^\varepsilon(x_1, ..., x_n; \theta) = \varepsilon^{-2}Q\varphi(x_1, ..., x_n) + \varepsilon^{-1}[Q\varphi_1 + c(\theta)S(\theta)\varphi(x_1, ..., x_n)]+$$
$$[c(\theta)S(\theta)\varphi_1(x_1, ..., x_n; \theta) + c_1(\theta)S(\theta)\varphi(x_1, ..., x_n; \theta)] + \varepsilon c_1(\theta)S(\theta)\varphi_1(x_1, ..., x_n; \theta).$$

It follows from equation [5.34] that the first two terms equal 0. Let us estimate the third term:

$$c(\theta)S(\theta)\varphi_1(x_1,...,x_n;\theta)+c_1(\theta)S(\theta)\varphi(x_1,...,x_n;\theta)=$$
$$c(\theta)S(\theta)R_0c(\theta)S(\theta)\varphi(x_1,...,x_n)+c_1(\theta)S(\theta)\varphi(x_1,...,x_n;\theta)=$$
$$c^2(\theta)S^2(\theta)\varphi(x_1,...,x_n)+c_1(\theta)S(\theta)\varphi(x_1,...,x_n;\theta)=$$
$$c^2(\theta)\Big[\cos^2\theta_1\frac{\partial^2}{\partial x_1^2}+\sin^2\theta_1\cos^2\theta_2\frac{\partial^2}{\partial x_2^2}+...+$$
$$\sin^2\theta_1...\sin^2\theta_{n-2}\cos^2\theta_{n-1}\frac{\partial^2}{\partial x_{n-1}^2}+\sin^2\theta_1...\sin^2\theta_{n-2}\sin^2\theta_{n-1}\frac{\partial^2}{\partial x_n^2}+$$
$$\Big\{\sin\theta_1\cos\theta_1\cos\theta_2\frac{\partial^2}{\partial x_1\partial x_2}+...+\sin^2\theta_1...\sin^2\theta_{n-2}\sin\theta_{n-1}\times$$
$$\cos\theta_{n-1}\frac{\partial^2}{\partial x_{n-1}\partial x_n}\Big\}\Big]\varphi(x_1,...,x_n)+c_1(\theta)\Big[\cos\theta_1\frac{\partial}{\partial x_1}+\sin\theta_1\cos\theta_2\frac{\partial}{\partial x_2}+...+$$
$$\sin\theta_1...\sin\theta_{n-2}\cos\theta_{n-1}\frac{\partial}{\partial x_{n-1}}+\sin\theta_1...\sin\theta_{n-2}\sin\theta_{n-1}\frac{\partial}{\partial x_n}\Big]\varphi(x_1,...,x_n)\le C_{1,\varphi},$$

as soon as all the constants, functions and their derivatives are bounded.

The last term may be estimated similarly.

From equation [5.34], we also have:

$$L^\varepsilon\varphi^\varepsilon=L^\varepsilon\varphi+\varepsilon L^\varepsilon\varphi_1=L^\varepsilon\varphi+\varepsilon L^\varepsilon R_0c(\theta)S(\theta)\varphi.$$

Thus,

$$L^\varepsilon\varphi=L^\varepsilon\varphi^\varepsilon-\varepsilon cL^\varepsilon R_0S(\theta)\varphi\le C_{1,\varphi}-\varepsilon C_{2,\varphi}<C_\varphi$$

for ε that is small enough.

To prove the second condition of lemma 5.3, we use the following properties of the function $\varphi_0(u)=\sqrt{1+u^2}$:

$$|\varphi_0'(u)|\le 1\le\varphi_0(u),|\varphi_0''(u)|\le\varphi_0(u).$$

We can see again that the proof of the second condition is similar to the previous reasoning.

Thus, the family of the processes $(\widetilde{\xi}_t^\varepsilon,\theta_t^\varepsilon)$ is relatively compact in $\mathbf{D}_{\mathbf{R}^n\times\Theta}[0,\infty)$.

Using theorem 5.6, we confirm the weak convergence in $\mathbf{D}_{\mathbf{R}^n}[0,\infty)$:

$$\widetilde{\xi}_t^{\varepsilon} \Rightarrow \widetilde{\xi}_t^0.$$

Really, all the conditions are satisfied. That is, the family of processes is relatively compact, the generators at the test functions belonging to the class $C_0^{\infty}(\mathbf{R}^n \times \Theta)$ converge, and initial conditions for the limit and pre-limit processes are equal.

The theorem is proven.

EXAMPLE 5.3.– *Let us consider one more variant of evolution in* $\mathbf{R}^2$.

Let

$$c(\theta) = \begin{cases} 1, \theta = 0, \\ 1, \theta = \pi, \end{cases}$$

and

$$c_1(\theta) = 1, \theta = \frac{\pi}{2}.$$

In other cases, both functions equal 0.

The balance condition [5.29] *is true for* $c(\theta)$*; on the contrary, condition* [5.30] *is true for* $c_1(\theta)$.

The limit generator [5.31] *has the view*

$$L^0\varphi(x_1,x_2) = \frac{1}{2\pi}\frac{\partial}{\partial x_2}\varphi(x_1,x_2) + \frac{1}{\pi}\frac{\partial^2}{\partial x_1^2}\varphi(x_1,x_2).$$

Thus, the limit process has two parts: the drift with velocity $\frac{1}{2\pi}$ *in the direction of* x_2 *coordinate and the diffusion part in a one-dimensional subspace, corresponding to the* x_1 *coordinate that is similar to the limit process described in Kac's model.*

6

Diffusion Process with Evolution and Its Parameter Estimation

In this chapter, we consider a discrete Markov process in an asymptotic diffusion environment with a uniformly ergodic embedded Markov chain. It can be approximated by an Ornstein–Uhlenbeck process with evolution. The drift parameter estimation is expressed using the stationarity of the Gaussian limit process.

Let us consider a random evolution $\zeta(t)$, $t \geq 0$, which depends on a random environment $Y(t)$, $t \geq 0$, which, in turn, is switched by an embedded Markov chain X_k, $k \geq 0$. The connection between the continuous-time $t \geq 0$ and the discrete-time $k \geq 0$ will be explained in the sequel.

The purpose of this chapter is to prove the convergence (in distribution) of the process $\zeta(t)$, $t \geq 0$, to the Ornstein–Uhlenbeck process under some scaling of the process and its time parameter.

The limit will be taken by a small series parameter $\varepsilon > 0$, $\varepsilon \to 0$.

6.1. Asymptotic diffusion environment

Consider a discrete Markov process in a semi-Markov asymptotic diffusion environment, determined by a solution of the following scaled stochastic difference equation:

$$\Delta\zeta^\varepsilon(t_{n+1}^\varepsilon) = -\varepsilon^2 V(Y_n^\varepsilon)\zeta^\varepsilon(t_n^\varepsilon) + \varepsilon\sigma(Y_n^\varepsilon)\Delta\mu^\varepsilon(t_{n+1}^\varepsilon), \qquad [6.1]$$

where $t_n^\varepsilon := n\varepsilon^2$, hence $t_{n+1}^\varepsilon = t_n^\varepsilon + \varepsilon^2$, $n > 0$, $\varepsilon > 0$, for the process increments $\Delta\zeta^\varepsilon(t_{n+1}^\varepsilon) := \zeta^\varepsilon(t_{n+1}^\varepsilon) - \zeta^\varepsilon(t_n^\varepsilon)$, $n \geq 0$.

The asymptotic diffusion environment Y_n^ε, $n \geq 0$, is also a random evolutionary process generated by a solution of the following scaled difference evolutionary equation:

$$\Delta Y^\varepsilon(t_{n+1}^\varepsilon) = \varepsilon A_0(Y_n^\varepsilon;\, X_n^\varepsilon) + \varepsilon^2 A(Y_n^\varepsilon;\, X_n^\varepsilon)\,, \quad n \geq 0, \qquad [6.2]$$

with the embedded Markov chain $X_n^\varepsilon := X(t_n^\varepsilon)$, $n \geq 0$.

The terms $A_0(y;\, x)$ and $A(y;\, x)$ are Lipschitz functions, together with the first derivative $A'_{0y}(y;\, x)$.

Here, the predictable evolutional component in equation [6.1] is defined by the following conditional expectation (Koroliouk 2015b):

$$V(Y_n^\varepsilon)\zeta^\varepsilon(t_n^\varepsilon) := E[\Delta\zeta^\varepsilon(t_{n+1}^\varepsilon) \mid Y_n^\varepsilon,\, \zeta^\varepsilon(t_n^\varepsilon)]\zeta^\varepsilon(t_n^\varepsilon),$$

where the drift regression function $V(z)$ is assumed to be positive: $V(z) > 0, \forall z$.

The martingale-difference $\Delta\mu^\varepsilon(t_{n+1}^\varepsilon)$, $n \geq 1$, generated by the process $\Delta\zeta^\varepsilon(t_{n+1}^\varepsilon)$, $n \geq 1$, is determined by the following conditional second moment:

$$-\varepsilon^2\sigma^2(Y_n^\varepsilon) := E\Big[\Big(\Delta\zeta^\varepsilon(t_{n+1}^\varepsilon) + \varepsilon^2 V(Y_n^\varepsilon)\zeta^\varepsilon(t_n^\varepsilon)\Big)^2 \,\Big|\, Y_n^\varepsilon\Big].$$

The embedded Markov chain $X_n^\varepsilon := X(t_n^\varepsilon)$, $t_n^\varepsilon := n\varepsilon^2$, $n \geq 0$, is supposed to be a homogeneous ergodic Markov chain with transition probabilities $P(x, B)$, $x \in E$, $B \in \mathcal{E}$, having a stationary distribution $\rho(B)$, $B \in \mathcal{E}$, which satisfies the condition $\rho(B) = \int_E \rho(dx)P(x, B);\ \rho(E) = 1$.

The stochastic difference equations [6.1] and [6.2] generate a discrete stochastic basis (Borovskikh and Korolyuk 1997, Chapter 1) with filtration $\mathfrak{F}_m(\zeta^\varepsilon, Y^\varepsilon) = \sigma\Big\{\zeta^\varepsilon(t_n^\varepsilon),\, Y^\varepsilon(t_n^\varepsilon)\,,\ n \leq m\Big\}$, $m \geq 0$.

Now, we consider three components $\Big(\zeta^\varepsilon(t_n^\varepsilon),\, Y^\varepsilon(t_n^\varepsilon),\, X_n^\varepsilon\Big)$, $n \geq 0$, as piecewise constant functions with continuous time:

$$\left.\begin{aligned} \zeta^\varepsilon(t) &= \zeta^\varepsilon(t_n^\varepsilon) \\ Y^\varepsilon(t) &= Y^\varepsilon(t_n^\varepsilon) \\ X_t^\varepsilon &= X_n^\varepsilon \end{aligned}\right\} \quad \text{for} \quad n\varepsilon^2 < t \leq (n+1)\varepsilon^2$$

In what follows, a solution for equations [6.1] and [6.2] is given by martingale characterization (Ethier and Kurtz 1986, section 4.4) of a three-component Markov process $\left(\zeta^\varepsilon(t),\, Y^\varepsilon(t),\, X_t\right), t \geq 0$:

$$M^\varepsilon(t) = \varphi\Big(\zeta^\varepsilon(t),\, Y^\varepsilon(t),\, X_t\Big) - \varphi\Big(\zeta^\varepsilon(0),\, Y^\varepsilon(0),\, X_0\Big) - \\ - \int_0^{\varepsilon^2[t/\varepsilon^2]} L^\varepsilon \varphi\Big(\zeta^\varepsilon(s),\, Y^\varepsilon(s),\, X_s^\varepsilon\Big) ds,$$

and the generator of a three-component Markov process $\left(\zeta^\varepsilon(t),\, Y^\varepsilon(t),\, X_t\right), t \geq 0$ is represented as follows (Korolyuk and Limnios 2005, Chapter 5):

$$L^\varepsilon \varphi(c, y, x) := \varepsilon^2 E\Big[\varphi\Big(c + \Delta\zeta^\varepsilon\Big(t_{n+1}^\varepsilon,\, Y^\varepsilon(t_{n+1}^\varepsilon),\, X_{n+1}^\varepsilon\Big)\Big) \Big| \\ \Big| \zeta^\varepsilon(t_n^\varepsilon) = c,\, Y^\varepsilon(t_n^\varepsilon) = y,\, X_n^\varepsilon = x\Big]. \quad [6.3]$$

6.2. Approximation of a discrete Markov process in asymptotic diffusion environment

Let the singular term $A_0(y;\, x)$ satisfies the balance condition:

$$\int_E \rho(dx) A_0(y;\, x) \equiv 0, \quad [6.4]$$

The approximation of a discrete Markov process in asymptotic diffusion environment gives the following.

THEOREM 6.1.– *Let the Markov chain X_n, $n \geq 0$ be uniformly ergodic with the stationary distribution $\rho(E)$, $B \in \mathcal{E}$.*

The finite-dimensional distributions of the discrete Markov process [6.1], *together with asymptotical diffusion $Y^\varepsilon(t)$, $t \geq 0$, converge, as $\varepsilon \to 0$, to a diffusion Ornstein–Uhlenbeck process with evolution:*

$$\left(\zeta^\varepsilon(t),\, Y^\varepsilon(t)\right) \xrightarrow{D} \left(\zeta^0(t),\, Y^0(t)\right), \quad \varepsilon \to 0, \quad 0 \leq t \leq T. \quad [6.5]$$

The limit two-component diffusion process with evolution $\left(\zeta^0(t),\, Y^0(t)\right)$, $t \geq 0$ is set by the generator

$$\mathfrak{L}^0(y)\varphi(c,\, y) = -\, V(y)\, c\, \varphi_c'(c,\, y) + \frac{1}{2}\sigma^2(y)\varphi_c''(c,\, y) + \\ + \widehat{A}(y)\varphi_y'(c,\, y) + \frac{1}{2}\widehat{B}^2(y)\varphi_y''(c,\, y)\,,\; \varphi \in C_0^2(R, \mathcal{B}), \quad [6.6]$$

where by definition

$$\widehat{A}(y) := \int_E \rho(dx)[A(y;\, x) + A_1(y;\, x)], \quad [6.7]$$

$$A_1(y;\, x) := A_0(y;\, x)\, P\, R_0\, A'_{0y}(y;\, x), \quad [6.8]$$

$$\widehat{B}^2(y) = \int_E \rho(dx) B(y;\, x),$$

$$B(y;\, x) = A_0(y;\, x)\, P\, [R_0 + \frac{1}{2}\mathbb{I}]\, A_0(y;\, x). \quad [6.9]$$

Here, $\mathbb{I}$ *is the standard identity matrix,* $\mathbb{P}$ *is the transition operator of the Markov chain* X_t, $t \geq 0$ *and the potential kernel* $\mathbb{R}_0$ *is defined as in (Korolyuk and Limnios 2005, section 5.2):*

$$\mathbb{R}_0 = (\mathbb{Q} + \Pi)^{-1} - \Pi\,, \quad \mathbb{Q} := \mathbb{P} - \mathbb{I}\,, \quad \Pi\varphi(x) := \int_E \rho(dx)\varphi(x). \quad [6.10]$$

REMARK 6.1.– *The limit two-component diffusion process* $\left(\zeta^0(t),\, Y^0(t)\right)$, $t \geq 0$, *set by the generator* [6.6]–[6.10], *has a stochastic representation by the stochastic differential equations:*

$$d\zeta^0(t) = -V(Y^0(t))\zeta^0(t)dt + \sigma(Y^0(t))dW(t),$$

$$dY^0(t) = \widehat{A}(Y^0(t))dt + \widehat{B}(Y^0(t))dW_0(t). \quad [6.11]$$

Consequently, the parameters of the limit diffusion $\zeta^0(t)$, $t \geq 0$, *depend on the diffusion process* $Y^0(t)$, $t \geq 0$.

PROOF OF THEOREM 6.1.– The basic idea is that any Markov process is determined by its generator on the class of real-valued test functions, defined on the set of values of the Markov process (Koroliouk et al. 2014).

First of all, the extended three-component Markov chain is used

$$\left(\zeta^\varepsilon(t_n),\, Y^\varepsilon(t_n),\, X^\varepsilon(t_n) = X_n\right), \quad t_n = n\varepsilon^2\,, \quad \varepsilon > 0, \quad [6.12]$$

with operator characterization in the following form.

LEMMA 6.1.– *The extended Markov chain is determined by the generator*

$$\mathbb{L}^\varepsilon(x)\varphi(c,\, y,\, x) = \varepsilon^{-2}[\Gamma^\varepsilon(y)A^\varepsilon(x)P - \mathbb{I}]\varphi(c,\, y,\, x), \quad [6.13]$$

where the transition operators are defined as follows:

$$\Gamma^\varepsilon(y)\varphi(c) := E[\varphi(c+\Delta\zeta^\varepsilon(t;\, y))\,|\,\zeta^\varepsilon(t) = c,\, Y^\varepsilon(t) = y,\, X^\varepsilon(t) = x],$$
$$\mathbb{A}^\varepsilon(x)\varphi(y) := E[\varphi(y+\Delta Y^\varepsilon(t;\, x))\,|\,Y^\varepsilon(t;\, x) = y,\, X^\varepsilon(t) = x],$$
$$\mathbb{P}\varphi(x) := \int_E P(x,\, dz)\varphi(z). \qquad [6.14]$$

The assertion of lemma 8.1 follows from the next argumentation. The extended three-component Markov chain [6.12], under the additional condition $Y^\varepsilon(t) = y$, $X^\varepsilon(t) = x$, has independent components. So, its transition probabilities are given by the product of the transition probabilities of each component.

An essential step in the proof of theorem 6.1 is realized in the next lemma.

LEMMA 6.2.– *The generator* [6.13]–[6.14] *of the three-component Markov chain* [6.12] *on the class of real-valued test functions* $\varphi(c,\, y,\, x)$, *having bound derivatives up to the third order inclusively, admits an asymptotic representation*

$$\mathbb{L}^\varepsilon(x)\varphi(c,\, y,\, x) = \qquad [6.15]$$
$$\left[\varepsilon^{-2}\mathbb{Q}++\varepsilon^{-1}\mathbb{A}_0(x)P+\mathbb{A}(x)P+\mathbb{L}^0(y)P+\mathbb{R}_\varepsilon(y;\, x)\right]\varphi(c,\, y,\, x); \qquad [6.16]$$

$$\mathbb{A}_0(x)\varphi(y) = A_0(y;\, x)\varphi'(y)\,,\quad \mathbb{A}(x)\varphi(y) = A(y;\, x)\varphi'(y); \qquad [6.17]$$

$$\mathbb{L}^0(y)\varphi(c) = -V(y)c\varphi'(c) + \frac{1}{2}\sigma^2(y)\varphi''(c). \qquad [6.18]$$

The residual term

$$\mathbb{R}_\varepsilon(y;\, x)\varphi(c,\, y,\, x) \to 0\,,\quad \varepsilon \to 0\,,\quad \varphi \in C^3(R^2).$$

Here, we intend the uniform convergence for all the arguments.

PROOF OF LEMMA 6.2.– We use transformation of generator [6.15] by the formula

$$\mathbb{L}^\varepsilon(x)\varphi(c,\, y,\, x) = \qquad [6.19]$$
$$= \varepsilon^{-2}\left[\mathbb{Q} + (A^\varepsilon - \mathbb{I})P + (\Gamma^\varepsilon - \mathbb{I})P + \mathbb{R}_\varepsilon(y;\, x)\right]\varphi(c,\, y,\, x). \qquad [6.20]$$

The residual term

$$\mathbb{R}_\varepsilon(y;\, x)\varphi(c,\, y,\, x) = (\Gamma^\varepsilon - \mathbb{I})(A^\varepsilon - \mathbb{I})P\varphi(c,\, y,\, x).$$

Then, we calculate

$$\varepsilon^{-2}[\Gamma^{\varepsilon}(y) - \mathbb{I}]\varphi(c) = \varepsilon^{-2}\Big\{E[\varphi(c + \Delta\zeta^{\varepsilon}(t;\, y) \,|\, \zeta^{\varepsilon}(t;\, y) = c] - \varphi(c)\Big\} \quad [6.21]$$

$$= [\mathbb{L}^{0}(y) + \mathbb{R}_{\varepsilon}(y;\, c)]\varphi(c). \quad [6.22]$$

The next term in equation [6.19]:

$$\varepsilon^{-2}[A^{\varepsilon}(x) - \mathbb{I}]\varphi(y) = \varepsilon^{-2}\{E[\varphi(y + \Delta Y^{\varepsilon}(t;\, x) \,|\, Y^{\varepsilon}(t;\, x) = y] - \varphi(y)\} = \quad [6.23]$$

$$= \varepsilon^{-2}\left[E[\Delta Y^{\varepsilon}(t;\, x)]\varphi'(y) + \frac{1}{2}E[\Delta Y^{\varepsilon}(t;\, x)]^{2}\varphi''(y) + \varepsilon^{2}\mathbb{R}_{\varepsilon}(x)\varphi(y)\right] = \quad [6.24]$$

$$= \left[\varepsilon^{-1}\mathbb{A}_0(y;\, x) + \mathbb{A}(y;\, x)\right]\varphi'(y) + \frac{1}{2}\mathbb{A}_0^{2}(y;\, x)\varphi''(y) + \mathbb{R}_{\varepsilon}(x)\varphi(y). \quad [6.25]$$

gives the asymptotic expansion in lemma 6.2:

$$\mathbb{L}^{\varepsilon}(x)\varphi(c,\, y,\, x) = [\varepsilon^{-2}\mathbb{Q} + \varepsilon^{-1}\mathbb{A}_0(x)\, P + \mathbb{A}(x)\, P + \quad [6.26]$$

$$+ \frac{1}{2}(\mathbb{A}_0(x)\, P)^{2} + \mathbb{L}^{0}(y)]\varphi(c,\, y,\, x) + \mathbb{R}_{\varepsilon}(y;\, x)\varphi(c,\, y,\, x). \quad [6.27]$$

□

Next, we use the solution of the singular perturbation problem for the truncated operator (Korolyuk and Limnios 2005).

LEMMA 6.3.– *The solution of the singular perturbation problem for the truncated operator is realized on perturbed test functions:*

$$\mathbb{L}_0^{\varepsilon}(x)\varphi^{\varepsilon}(c,\, y,\, x) \doteq \Big[\varepsilon^{-2}\mathbb{Q} + \varepsilon^{-1}\mathbb{A}_0(x)\,\mathbb{P} + \mathbb{A}(x)\,\mathbb{P} + \quad [6.28]$$

$$+ \frac{1}{2}(\mathbb{A}_0(x)\,\mathbb{P})^{2} + \mathbb{L}^{0}(y)\Big][\varphi(c,\, y) + \varepsilon\varphi_1(c,\, y,\, x) + \varepsilon^{2}\varphi_2(c,\, y,\, x)] = \quad [6.29]$$

$$= \mathfrak{L}^{0}(y)\varphi(c,\, y) + \mathbb{R}_{\varepsilon}(x)\varphi(c,\, y). \quad [6.30]$$

The averaging parameters are determined by the formulas [6.6]–[6.10].

The limit operator is calculated by the formula

$$\mathfrak{L}^{0}(y)\varphi(c,\, y) = \mathbb{L}^{0}(y)\varphi(c,\, y) + \widehat{A}(y)\varphi_y'(c,\, y) + \frac{1}{2}\widehat{B}^{2}(y)\varphi_y''(c,\, y). \quad [6.31]$$

PROOF OF LEMMA 6.3.– To solve the singular perturbation problem for the truncated operator, consider the asymptotic representation by the powers of ε:

$$\mathbb{L}_0^\varepsilon(x)\varphi^\varepsilon(c,\, y,\, x) = \varepsilon^{-2}\mathbb{Q}\varphi(c,\, y) + \varepsilon^{-1}[\mathbb{Q}\varphi_1(c,\, y,\, x) + \tag{6.32}$$

$$+ \mathbb{A}_0(x)\varphi(c,\, y)] + \Big[\mathbb{Q}\varphi_2(c,\, y,\, x) + \mathbb{A}_0(x)\,\mathbb{P}\,\varphi_1(c,\, y,\, x) + \tag{6.33}$$

$$+ [\mathbb{A}(x) + \frac{1}{2}(\mathbb{A}_0(x)\mathbb{P})^2 + \mathbb{L}^0(y)]\varphi(c,\, y)\Big] + \mathbb{R}_\varepsilon(x)\varphi(c,\, y). \tag{6.34}$$

Obviously, that $\mathbb{Q}\varphi(c,\, y) = 0$.

The balance condition [6.4] is then used. The solution of the equation

$$\mathbb{Q}\varphi_1(c,\, y,\, x) + \mathbb{A}_0(x)\varphi(c,\, y) = 0$$

is given by the formula (Korolyuk and Limnios 2005, section 5.4):

$$\varphi_1(c,\, y,\, x) = \mathbb{R}_0\mathbb{A}_0(x)\varphi(c,\, y).$$

Using this result in the following equation:

$$\mathbb{Q}\varphi_2(c,\, y,\, x) + \big[\mathbb{B}(x) + \mathbb{A}(x) + \mathbb{L}^0(y)\big]\varphi(c,\, y) = \mathfrak{L}^0(y)\varphi(c,\, y). \tag{6.35}$$

Here, by definition:

$$\mathbb{B}(x) := \mathbb{A}_0(x)PR_0\mathbb{A}_0(x) + \frac{1}{2}(\mathbb{A}_0(x)P)^2$$

The limit operator is calculated using the balance condition:

$$\mathfrak{L}^0(y)\varphi(c,\, y) = \Big\{\Pi\Big[\mathbb{B}(x) + \mathbb{A}(x)\Big]\Pi + \mathbb{L}^0(y)\Big\}\varphi(c,\, y). \tag{6.36}$$

Recall the projector's operation:

$$\Pi\mathbb{B}(x)\Pi = \int_E \rho(dx)B(y,\, x)\,,\quad B(y,\, x) = A_0(y,\, x)\mathbb{P}\mathbb{R}_0A_0(y,\, x) + \frac{1}{2}(A_0(y,\, x))^2.$$

Taking into account the definition of evolutionary operators [6.17], the limit generator is determined by formula [6.31]. □

The limit operator [6.36] provides a solution of equation [6.35], which is a function of $\varphi_2(c, y, x)$. The existence of perturbing functions $\varphi_i(\cdot)$, $i = 1, 2$, ensures the asymptotical representation [6.28]. That completes the proof of theorem 6.1. □

The volatility is generated by the introduction of a random environment $Y^0(t)$, $t \geq 0$ into the diffusion parameter of the Ornstein–Uhlenbeck diffusion process $\zeta^0(t)$, $t \geq 0$ (see Koroliouk (2016)).

6.3. Parameter estimation of the limit process

The limit Ornstein–Uhlenbeck diffusion process parameter estimation is substantiated in this section without the assumption of volatility, which greatly changes the kind of estimates (Koroliouk 2016). The stationarity of the Gaussian statistical experiment is essentially used (Koroliouk 2016).

It is known (Cohen and Elliott 2015) that diffusion-type processes are given by stochastic differential

$$d\xi_t = \alpha_t(\xi_t)dt + dW_t. \tag{6.37}$$

The predictable component satisfies the conditions:

$$P\Big(\int_0^T \alpha_t^2(\xi_t)dt < \infty\Big) = 1\ ,\ \ T < \infty, \tag{6.38}$$

$$P\Big(\int_0^\infty \alpha_t^2(\xi_t)dt = \infty\Big) = 1, \tag{6.39}$$

which ensures the absolute continuity of the measure $\mu_\xi(B) := P\{\omega : \xi \in B\}$ and the measure $\mu_W(B) := P\{\omega : W \in B\}$ for all $B \in \mathcal{B}_T{=}\sigma(\xi_t : 0 \leq t \leq T)$.

The Radon–Nicodemus derivative specifies the density of the measure

$$\zeta_T(\xi) := \frac{d\mu_\xi}{d\mu_W}(\xi, T), \tag{6.40}$$

which for processes of diffusion type [6.37] has the following representation.

THEOREM 6.2.– *For Cohen and Elliott (2015), the measure density* [6.40] *for processes of diffusion type* [6.37] *with additional conditions* [6.38] *is given by exponential martingale*

$$\frac{d\mu_\xi}{d\mu_W}(\xi_t, T) = \exp\Big[\int_0^T \alpha_t(\xi_t)d\xi_t - \frac{1}{2}\int_0^T \alpha_t^2(\xi_t)dt\Big]. \tag{6.41}$$

In particular, the exponential martingale [6.40] is determined by a solution of the stochastic Doléans–Dade equation (Borovskikh and Korolyuk 1997)

$$d\zeta_T(\xi) = \zeta_T(\xi)\alpha_T(\xi)d\xi_T\ ,\ \ \zeta_0(\xi) = 1, \tag{6.42}$$

or in equivalent form:

$$\zeta_T(\xi) - 1 = \zeta_T(\xi)\alpha_T(\xi)d\xi_T. \tag{6.43}$$

The relationship of the density [6.41] with the stochastic Doléans–Dade equation [6.42] is explained using the Ito formula for the exponential function $\varphi(\xi) = \exp[\eta_T(\xi) - \frac{1}{2}\langle\eta(\xi)\rangle_T]$, with $\eta_T(\xi) := \int_0^T \alpha_t(\xi)dt$, $\langle\eta(\xi)\rangle_T := \int_0^T \alpha_t^2(\xi)dt$, namely (see Borovskikh and Korolyuk 1997):

$$d\varphi(\xi_T) = \varphi'(\xi_T)[d\eta_T(\xi) - \frac{1}{2}d\langle\eta(\xi)\rangle_T] + \frac{1}{2}\varphi''(\xi_T)d\langle\eta(\xi)\rangle_T. \qquad [6.44]$$

Taking into account equality $\varphi(\xi_T) = \varphi'(\xi_T) = \varphi''(\xi_T)$ for exponential function $\varphi(\xi)$, we have a stochastic Doléans–Dade differential equation for exponential martingale [6.41].

According to the results of the previous section, the limit diffusion process for normalized discrete Markov processes is the Ornstein–Uhlenbeck process with a linear predictable component

$$d\alpha_t = -V_0\alpha_t dt + \sigma dW_t \ , \quad 0 \leq t \leq T. \qquad [6.45]$$

Without limiting of generality, let us put $\sigma = 1$.

The maximum likelihood method for estimating the parameter V_0 of a diffusion process with a stochastic differential [6.37] ($\sigma = 1$) is realized for the logarithm of the measure density [6.41]:

$$L(V,T) := \ln\zeta_T(\xi) = -V\int_0^T \alpha_t dt - \frac{V^2}{2}\int_0^T \alpha_t^2 dt. \qquad [6.46]$$

Therefore, the equation for estimating the maximum likelihood method is:

$$\max_{0\leq V\leq 2} \partial L(V,T)/\partial V = -\int_0^T \alpha_t dt - V_T\int_0^T \alpha_t^2 dt = 0, \qquad [6.47]$$

and the estimate of the maximum likelihood method has the following form:

$$V_T = -\int_0^T \alpha_t d\alpha_t \Big/ \int_0^T \alpha_t^2 dt. \qquad [6.48]$$

The least squares method estimation of parameter V_0 of the diffusion process with stochastic differential [6.37] ($\sigma = 1$) is implemented using equality:

$$\int_0^T \alpha_t d\alpha_t = -V_0\int_0^T \alpha_t^2 dt + \int_0^T \alpha_t dW_t. \qquad [6.49]$$

So, we have a relationship

$$V_0 - V_T = \int_0^T \alpha_t dW_t \Big/ \int_0^T \alpha_t^2 dt. \qquad [6.50]$$

The estimation of the least squares method has a representation

$$V_T^0 = -\int_0^T \alpha_t d\alpha_t \Big/ \int_0^T \alpha_t^2 dt. \qquad [6.51]$$

COROLLARY 6.1.– *The estimates of maximum likelihood and least squares coincide:* $V_T = V_T^0$.

COROLLARY 6.2.– *Estimation by the least squares method and hence estimation by the method of maximum likelihood of the parameter* V_0 *are strongly consistent:*

$$P1 \lim_{T \to \infty} V_T^0 = V_0. \qquad [6.52]$$

REMARK 6.2.– *In the presence of volatility (see Koroliouk et al. (2016)), the maximum likelihood estimate and the least squares estimate are different, but the property of strong consistency* [6.52] *is retained.*

7

Filtration of Stationary Gaussian Statistical Experiments

The filtration of stationary Gaussian statistical experiments is determined by a solution of the equation of optimum filtration, which is characterized by the two-dimensional matrix of covariances. The parameters of a filtered signal are set by empiric covariances.

The solution of filtration problems for sequences with a Gaussian (normal) distribution is based on the normal correlation theorem (Liptser and Shiryaev 2001, theorem 13.1), which provides the linear filtration.

In the studies of the stochastic sequences with discrete time under the additional conditions of stationarity and Gaussian property, the covariance characteristics of the sequence α_t, $t \geqslant 0$, and its increments $\Delta\alpha_{t+1} := \alpha_{t+1} - \alpha_t$, $t \geqslant 0$, are essentially used.

7.1. Introduction

In the present chapter, the problem of filtration of stationary Gaussian statistical experiments is considered for a two-component stationary Gaussian sequence of the statistical experiment $(\alpha_t, \Delta\alpha_{t+1})$, $t \geqslant 0$, which is characterized by the two-dimensional matrix of covariances

$$\mathbb{R}_\alpha = \begin{bmatrix} R_\alpha & R_\alpha^0 \\ R_\alpha^0 & R_\alpha^\Delta \end{bmatrix}, \qquad [7.1]$$

$$R_\alpha := E\alpha_t^2\,, \;\; R_\alpha^0 := E(\alpha_t\, \Delta\alpha_{t+1})\,, \;\; R_\alpha^\Delta := E(\Delta\alpha_t)^2.$$

In the calculation of the covariances in equation [7.1], we use the stochastic difference equation

$$\Delta\alpha_{t+1} = -V_0\alpha_t + \sigma_0\Delta W^0_{t+1}, \qquad [7.2]$$

which defines the sequence of statistical experiment α_t, $t \geqslant 0$, and its increments $\Delta\alpha_{t+1} := \alpha_{t+1} - \alpha_t$, $t \geqslant 0$, for a given α_0.

It turns out that a filtered stationary Gaussian statistical experiment is determined by a solution of the equation of optimum filtration (see theorem 7.3), which is characterized by the two-dimensional matrix of covariances with the stochastic component, which sets a renewing sequence.

The stationarity of the statistical experiment α_t, $t \geqslant 0$ in a wide sense is ensured by the additional conditions (Koroliouk 2016, theorem 1):

THEOREM 7.1 (THEOREM OF STATIONARITY).– *The statistical experiment α_t, $t \geqslant 0$, which is determined by a solution of the stochastic difference equation* [7.2], *is a sequence stationary in a wide sense, if the relation*

$$R_\alpha =: E\alpha_t^2 = \sigma_0^2/V_0(2 - V_0)\ , \ \ E\alpha_t = 0\ , \ \ t \geqslant 0, \qquad [7.3]$$

is valid, and the initial value α_0 is a normally distributed random variable uncorrelated with the stochastic component ΔW_{t+1}: $E(\alpha_0\,\Delta W_{t+1}) = 0$.

It is known (see, for example, Nevelson and Hasminskii 1973) that the solution of the stochastic difference equation [7.2] has a Markov property.

Moreover, it turns out that the two-component stationary Gaussian sequence $(\alpha_t, \Delta\alpha_{t+1})$, $t \geqslant 0$, which is set by the matrix of covariances [7.1], is also determined by a solution of the stochastic difference equation [7.2] under the additional condition of Markov property. This result is presented in Koroliouk (2016, theorem 5) for multivariant statistical experiments.

THEOREM 7.2 (THEOREM OF EXISTENCE OF STOCHASTIC DIFFERENCE EQUATION).– *The stationary Gaussian–Markovian statistical experiment, which is characterized by the matrix of covariances* [7.1], *satisfies the stochastic difference equation* [7.2] *with normally distributed stochastic component $\sigma_0\Delta W^0_{t+1}$, $t \geqslant 0$.*

In this case, the variance of the stochastic component is set by the coefficient of stationarity $\mathcal{E}_0$:

$$\sigma_0^2 = R_\alpha\,\mathcal{E}_0\ , \ \ \mathcal{E}_0 := 2V_0 - V_0^2.$$

7.2. Stochastic difference equation of the process of filtration

The problem of filtration of stationary Gaussian statistical experiments is considered for the solution of the *stochastic difference equation*

$$\Delta\alpha_{t+1} = -V_0\alpha_t + \sigma_0\Delta W^0_{t+1}\ ,\quad t \geqslant 0, \qquad [7.4]$$

which determines a useful signal.

The signal α_t, $t \geqslant 0$ is registered with the use of a filter β_t, $t \geqslant 0$, which is also a solution of the stochastic difference equation

$$\Delta\beta_{t+1} = -V\beta_t + \sigma\Delta W_{t+1}\ ,\quad t \geqslant 0. \qquad [7.5]$$

The process (observable) of filtration is set by the sum

$$\xi_t = \alpha_t + \beta_t\ ,\quad t \geqslant 0, \qquad [7.6]$$

with a signal and a filter, which are uncorrelated: $E(\alpha_t\,\beta_t) = 0$.

Hence, the process of filtration ξ_t, $t \geqslant 0$, is also set by the stochastic difference equation

$$\Delta\xi_{t+1} = -V\xi_t - C\alpha_t + \sigma_0\Delta W^0_{t+1} + \sigma\Delta W_{t+1}\ ,\quad C := V_0 - V. \qquad [7.7]$$

In view of the conditions of stationarity of the solutions of the stochastic difference equations [7.4] and [7.5], the variances of stochastic components ΔW^0_{t+1} and ΔW_{t+1} are given by the relations

$$\sigma_0^2 = (2V_0 - V_0^2)\cdot R_\alpha\ ,\quad \sigma^2 = (2V - V^2)\cdot R_\beta; \qquad [7.8]$$

$$E(\Delta W^0_{t+1})^2 = E(\Delta W_{t+1})^2 = 1. \qquad [7.9]$$

The validity of the stochastic difference equations [7.4]–[7.7] for a signal and a filter allows us to characterize the problem of filtration by the two-dimensional matrices of covariances

$$\mathbb{R}_\alpha = \begin{bmatrix} R_\alpha & R^0_\alpha \\ R^0_\alpha & R^\Delta_\alpha \end{bmatrix}\ ,\quad \mathbb{R}_\beta = \begin{bmatrix} R_\beta & R^0_\beta \\ R^0_\beta & R^\Delta_\beta \end{bmatrix}\ ,\quad \mathbb{R}_\xi = \begin{bmatrix} R_\xi & -R^0_\xi \\ -R^0_\xi & 2R^0_\xi \end{bmatrix}. \qquad [7.10]$$

Elements of the matrices of covariances $\mathbb{R}_\alpha$ and $\mathbb{R}_\beta$ are given by the formulas:

$$R^0_\alpha := E[\alpha_t\Delta\alpha_{t+1}] = -V_0R_\alpha\ ,\quad R^0_\beta := E[\beta_t\Delta\beta_{t+1}] = -VR_\beta,$$

$$R^\Delta_\alpha := E[\Delta\alpha_t]^2 = 2V_0R_\alpha\ ,\quad R^\Delta_\beta := E[\Delta\beta_t]^2 = 2VR_\beta. \qquad [7.11]$$

Since a signal and a filter are uncorrelated, relation [7.6] ensures a representation of the matrix of covariances $\mathbb{R}_\xi$ and its inversion:

$$\mathbb{R}_\xi = \mathbb{R}_\alpha + \mathbb{R}_\beta,$$
$$\mathbb{R}_\xi^{-1} = (\mathbb{R}_\alpha + \mathbb{R}_\beta)^{-1} = \mathbb{R}_\alpha^{-1}(\mathbb{I} + \mathbb{R}_\alpha^{-1}\mathbb{R}_\beta)^{-1}, \quad [7.12]$$

and

$$R_{\xi\alpha} := E(\xi_t\alpha_t) = E(\alpha_t)^2 = \mathbb{R}_\alpha.$$

The calculation of the elements of the matrix of covariances $\mathbb{R}_\xi$ with regard to the stochastic difference equation [7.7] and relations [7.8] yields

$$R_\xi^0 := -E(\xi_t\,\Delta\xi_{t+1}) = VR_\xi + CR_\alpha = VR_\beta + V_0R_\alpha = -(R_\alpha^0 + R_\beta^0),$$
$$R_\xi^\Delta := E(\Delta\xi_{t+1})^2 = 2(VR_\xi + CR_\alpha) = -2(R_\alpha^0 + R_\beta^0). \quad [7.13]$$

7.3. Coefficient of filtration

By the theorem of normal correlation (Liptser and Shiryaev 2001, theorem 13.1), the matrix of covariances of the coefficients of filtration is set by the relations

$$\Phi = \mathbb{R}_\alpha\mathbb{R}_\xi^{-1} = (\mathbb{I} + \mathbb{R}_\alpha^{-1}\mathbb{R}_\beta)^{-1}. \quad [7.14]$$

LEMMA 7.1.– *The elements of the matrix of the coefficients of filtration have the following representation:*

$$\Phi_{11} = d^{-1}(2-V_0)R_\alpha[VR_\xi + CR_\alpha] = d^{-1}(2-V_0)R_\alpha[VR_\beta + V_0R_\alpha]$$
$$= -d^{-1}(2-V_0)R_\alpha[R_\alpha^0 + R_\beta^0],$$
$$\Phi_{22} = d^{-1}V_0R_\alpha[(2-V)R_\xi + (V-V_0)R_\alpha] \quad [7.15]$$
$$= d^{-1}V_0R_\alpha[(2-V_0)R_\alpha + 2R_\beta],$$
$$\Phi_{12} = d^{-1}C(R_\alpha^2 - R_\xi R_\alpha) = -d^{-1}V_0R_\alpha(2R_\xi + R_\xi^0)\,, \quad \Phi_{21} = 0. \quad [7.16]$$

Here, by definition,

$$d := \det\mathbb{R}_\xi = V(2-V)R_\xi^2 - 2CR_\xi R_\alpha - C^2R_\alpha^2. \quad [7.17]$$

At the same time, the following relation between elements of the matrix of the coefficients of filtration holds:

$$\Phi_{22} = \Phi_{11} - 2\Phi_{12}. \quad [7.18]$$

REMARK 7.1.– *The presence of zero* ($\Phi_{21} = 0$) *in the matrix of the coefficients of filtration* [7.15] *ensures the optimum filtration of stationary Gaussian statistical experiments with the use of only increments of the process of filtration, which is set by equation* [7.7].

PROOF OF LEMMA 7.1.– We use the representation of the inverse matrix [7.1]:

$$\mathbb{R}_\xi^{-1} = \begin{bmatrix} 2R_\xi^0 & R_\xi^0 \\ R_\xi^0 & R_\xi \end{bmatrix} d^{-1}. \qquad [7.19]$$

Now, the multiplication of matrices [7.14] gives representation [7.15].

The calculation of the determinant of the matrix $\mathbb{R}_\xi$

$$\det \mathbb{R}_\xi = 2R_\xi R_\xi^0 - (R_\xi^0)^2,$$

gives formula [7.17] taking into account [7.13].

To prove [7.18], we consider the difference, by changing the parameter $V_0 = V + C$:

$$\begin{aligned}\Phi_{11} - \Phi_{22} &= [-2CR_\xi R_\alpha + 2CR_\alpha^2]/d \\ &= [-2CR_\alpha(R_\xi - R_\alpha)]/d = [-2CR_\alpha R_\beta]/d = 2\Phi_{12}.\end{aligned} \qquad [7.20]$$

□

7.4. Equation of optimal filtration

To construct the equation of optimal filtration, we use the stochastic difference equation [7.4], a signal α_t, $t \geq 0$, and the observable process of filtration ξ_t, $t \geq 0$, which is set by sum [7.6] and is determined by a solution of the stochastic difference equation [7.7]. In this case, we essentially use the covariance characteristics [7.10] with regard for lemma 7.1, in which elements of the matrix of the coefficients of filtration are represented, as well as relation [7.18].

The equation of optimal filtration for the two-component a posteriori means $\widehat{\alpha}_t$, $\Delta\widehat{\alpha}_{t+1}$, $t \geq 0$: reads

$$\widehat{\alpha}_t := E[\alpha_t \,|\, \mathcal{F}_t^\xi]\,, \quad \Delta\widehat{\alpha}_{t+1} := E[\Delta\alpha_{t+1} \,|\, \mathcal{F}_{t+1}^\xi]\,, \quad t \geq 0, \qquad [7.21]$$

It is constructed by the scheme described in Liptser and Shiryaev (2001, Chapter XIII) with the use of the theorem of normal correlation (Liptser and Shiryaev 2001, theorem 13.1).

The mean square error of the optimal filtration is determined by the matrix of covariances:

$$\mathbf{\Gamma} = \begin{bmatrix} \Gamma_{11} & \Gamma_{12} \\ \Gamma_{21} & \Gamma_{22} \end{bmatrix} \qquad [7.22]$$

The elements of the matrix $\mathbb{\Gamma}$ are as follows:

$$\begin{aligned}\Gamma_{11} &= E[(\alpha_t - \widehat{\alpha}_t)^2 \,|\, \mathcal{F}_t^\xi],\\ \Gamma_{12} &= E[(\alpha_t - \widehat{\alpha}_t)(\Delta\alpha_{t+1} - \Delta\widehat{\alpha}_{t+1}) \,|\, \mathcal{F}_{t+1}^\xi],\\ \Gamma_{21} &= E[(\Delta\alpha_{t+1} - \Delta\widehat{\alpha}_{t+1})(\alpha_t - \widehat{\alpha}_t) \,|\, \mathcal{F}_{t+1}^\xi]\\ \Gamma_{22} &= E[(\Delta\alpha_{t+1} - \Delta\widehat{\alpha}_{t+1})^2 \,|\, \mathcal{F}_{t+1}^\xi].\end{aligned} \qquad [7.23]$$

The matrix of errors $\mathbb{\Gamma}$ has the representation (Liptser and Shiryaev 2001, theorem 13.1):

$$\mathbb{\Gamma} = \mathbb{R}_\alpha - \mathbb{R}_\alpha \mathbb{R}_\xi^{-1} \mathbb{R}_\alpha = \mathbb{R}_\alpha[\mathbb{I} - \Phi^*]. \qquad [7.24]$$

We will formulate the equation of optimal filtration for the two-component filtered signal [7.21]. Namely, the following proposition takes place.

THEOREM 7.3.– *The filtered signal ($\widehat{\alpha}_t$, $\Delta\widehat{\alpha}_{t+1}$) is determined by the equation of optimal filtration for increments:*

$$\Delta\widehat{\alpha}_{t+1} + V_0\widehat{\alpha}_t = \Phi_{22}[\Delta\xi_{t+1} + V\xi_t + C\widehat{\alpha}_t]. \qquad [7.25]$$

The mean square error of the optimal filtration for the increments has the representation:

$$E[(\Delta\widehat{\alpha}_{t+1} - \Delta\alpha_{t+1})^2 \,|\, \mathcal{F}_{t+1}^\xi] = 2V_0(1 - \Phi_{22})R_\alpha. \qquad [7.26]$$

PROOF OF THEOREM 7.3.– We use the representation of filtered increments of a signal [7.7] (see Liptser and Shiryaev (2001, formulas (13.60)–(13.61)))

$$\begin{aligned}E[\Delta\alpha_{t+1} \,|\, \mathcal{F}_t^\xi, \xi_{t+1}] - E[\Delta\alpha_{t+1} \,|\, \mathcal{F}_t^\xi] &=\\ = \Phi_{22}[\Delta\xi_{t+1} - E[\Delta\xi_{t+1} \,|\, \mathcal{F}_t^\xi]].\end{aligned} \qquad [7.27]$$

In view of the relations

$$\Delta\widehat{\alpha}_{t+1} := E[\Delta\alpha_{t+1} \,|\, \mathcal{F}_t^\xi] = -V_0\,\widehat{\alpha}_t\,, \quad E[\Delta\xi_{t+1} \,|\, \mathcal{F}_t^\xi] = -(V\xi_t + C\widehat{\alpha}_t), \qquad [7.28]$$

we get assertion [7.25] of theorem 7.3. The mean square error [7.26] of the equation of optimal filtration is proved with the use of the coefficients of filtration

$$\begin{aligned}E[(\widehat{\alpha}_t - \alpha_t)^2 \,|\, \mathcal{F}_t^\xi] &= (1 - \Phi_{11} - V_0\Phi_{12})R_\alpha,\\ E[(\Delta\widehat{\alpha}_{t+1} - \Delta\alpha_{t+1})^2 \,|\, \mathcal{F}_{t+1}^\xi] &= 2V_0(1 - \Phi_{22})R_\alpha,\\ E[(\widehat{\alpha}_t - \alpha_t)(\Delta\widehat{\alpha}_{t+1} - \Delta\alpha_{t+1}) \,|\, \mathcal{F}_{t+1}^\xi] &= -V_0(1 - \Phi_{11} + 2\Phi_{12})R_\alpha =\\ &= -V_0(1 - \Phi_{22})R_\alpha,\end{aligned} \qquad [7.29]$$

and representation [7.15]. □

By definition [7.23], the matrix $\mathbb{\Gamma}$ is symmetric. The symmetry of matrices on the right-hand side of representation [7.26] is ensured by relation [7.18] of lemma 7.1.

7.5. Characterization of a filtered signal

To construct the equation of optimal filtration, we use the stochastic difference equation [7.4] for a signal and the observable process of filtration [7.25]. Then, we use the representation of a filter with regard to a posteriori means of a two-component signal $(\widehat{\alpha}_t, \Delta\widehat{\alpha}_{t+1})$, $t \geq 0$:

$$\Delta\xi_{t+1} + V\xi_t + C\widehat{\alpha}_t = \sigma_0 \Delta W^0_{t+1} + \sigma\Delta W_{t+1} - C(\alpha_t - \widehat{\alpha}_t). \qquad [7.30]$$

For the characterization of a filtered signal, we note, first of all, that the left-hand side of the equation of optimal filtration,

$$\widehat{\varrho}_t = \Delta\widehat{\alpha}_{t+1} + V_0\widehat{\alpha}_t \qquad [7.31]$$

sets a stationary Gaussian–Markovian process characterized by the variance

$$\widehat{\sigma}^2 := E\widehat{\varrho}_t^2 = \sigma_0^2 + \sigma^2 + C^2\Gamma_{11}. \qquad [7.32]$$

Here, the mean square error of Γ_{11} has representation [7.29].

At the same time, we calculate the covariance $\widehat{R}_\alpha$, by using formula [7.32]:

$$\widehat{\sigma}^2 = V_0(2 - V_0) \cdot \widehat{R}_\alpha \ , \ \ \widehat{R}_\alpha =: E(\widehat{\alpha}_t)^2. \qquad [7.33]$$

Hence, the filtered two-component signal $(\widehat{\alpha}_t, \Delta\widehat{\alpha}_{t+1})$, $t \geq 0$ is a stationary Gaussian process, which is characterized by the matrix of covariances

$$\widehat{\mathbb{R}}_\alpha = \begin{bmatrix} \widehat{R}_\alpha & \widehat{R}^0_\alpha \\ \widehat{R}^0_\alpha & \widehat{R}^\Delta_\alpha \end{bmatrix} \ , \ \ \widehat{R}^0_\alpha = -V_0\widehat{R}_\alpha \ , \ \ \widehat{R}^\Delta_\alpha = 2V_0\widehat{R}_\alpha. \qquad [7.34]$$

The covariance of a filter $\widehat{R}_\alpha$ is given by equations [7.32] and [7.33].

The equation for a filtered signal [7.30] means that the following equality holds (see Liptser and Shiryaev (2001, theorem 13.5)):

$$E[\Delta\xi_{t+1} + V\xi_t + C\widehat{\alpha}_t]^2 = \widehat{\sigma}^2. \qquad [7.35]$$

Moreover, by theorem 13.5 in Liptser and Shiryaev (2001), we have

$$E[\Delta\xi_{t+1} + V\xi_t + C\widehat{\alpha}_t]^2 = \mathrm{cov}(\Delta\xi_{t+1}, \Delta\xi_{t+1} \,|\, \mathcal{F}^\xi_t]). \qquad [7.36]$$

Thus, the equation of optimal filtration [7.25] becomes

$$\Delta\widehat{\alpha}_{t+1} + V_0\widehat{\alpha}_t = \Phi_{22}[\Delta\xi_{t+1} + V\xi_t + C\widehat{\alpha}_t], \qquad [7.37]$$

with regard to the result in Liptser and Shiryaev (2001, formula (13.85)), passes into the stochastic difference equation

$$\Delta\widehat{\alpha}_{t+1} + V_0\widehat{\alpha}_t = \widehat{\sigma}\Delta\widehat{W}_{t+1}\ , \quad t \geq 0, \qquad [7.38]$$

where the sequence $\Delta\widehat{W}_{t+1}, t \geq 0$ of standard normally distributed random variables is called a renewing sequence. In this case, the variance $\widehat{\sigma}^2$ is given by formula [7.33].

CONCLUSION 7.1.– The filtered signal $(\widehat{\alpha}_t,\, \Delta\widehat{\alpha}_{t+1}),\ t \geq 0$, determined by the equation of optimal filtration [7.25], is characterized also by a stationary solution of equation [7.38] with the renewing sequence of the stochastic component, which is normally distributed with zero mean and the variance $\widehat{\sigma}^2$ and is characterized by the two-dimensional matrix of covariances [7.34].

Now, we have the possibility to evaluate the parameters of a filtered signal by the trajectories of an observable process.

The validity of the equation of optimal filtration [7.38] for a filtered statistical experiment allows us to use the optimal estimates (see Koroliouk (2016)) of the parameters of a shift V_0 and the variance $\widehat{\sigma}^2$ of a filtered statistical experiment with the use of empiric covariances of a filtered process.

CONCLUSION 7.2.– The optimum estimates of the parameters V_0, $\widehat{\sigma}$ of the filtered signal [7.38] are given by the relations (Koroliouk 2016):

$$\widehat{V}_T^0 = -\widehat{R}_T^0/\widehat{R}_T\ , \quad \widehat{\sigma}_T^2 = \mathcal{E}_T^0\widehat{R}_T\ , \quad \mathcal{E}_T^0 = 2V_T^\Delta - (V_T^0)^2, \qquad [7.39]$$

where the empiric covariances $\widehat{R}_T$, $\widehat{R}_T^0$, $\widehat{R}_T^\Delta$ are determined on the trajectories of the filtered signal $(\widehat{\alpha}_t,\, \Delta\widehat{\alpha}_{t+1}), t \geq 0$:

$$\widehat{R}_T := \frac{1}{T}\sum_{t=0}^{T-1}\widehat{\alpha}_t^2\ , \quad \widehat{R}_T^0 = \frac{1}{T}\sum_{t=0}^{T-1}\widehat{\alpha}_t\Delta\widehat{\alpha}_t\ , \quad \widehat{R}_T^\Delta := \frac{1}{T}\sum_{t=0}^{T-1}(\Delta\widehat{\alpha}_t)^2. \qquad [7.40]$$

8

Adapted Statistical Experiments with Random Change of Time

Here, we study statistical experiments with random change of time, which transforms a discrete stochastic basis into a continuous one. The adapted stochastic experiments are studied in a continuous stochastic basis in the series scheme. The transition to limit by the series parameter generates an approximation of adapted statistical experiments by a diffusion process with evolution.

The average intensity parameter of renewal times is estimated in three different cases: the Poisson renewal process, a stationary renewal process with delay and the general renewal process with Weibull–Gnedenko renewal time distribution.

8.1. Introduction

Statistical experiments are defined as averaged sums of random variables with a finite number of possible values. In particular, the average sum of binary values ± 1 determines the average content of a certain feature in the elements that make up some complex systems.

Statistical experiments are defined in a discrete stochastic basis:

$$\mathfrak{B}_{\mathbb{N}} = (\Omega,\ \mathfrak{F},\ (\mathfrak{F}_k,\ k \in \mathbb{N}),\ \mathcal{P})$$

with filtration $(\mathfrak{F}_k,\ k \in \mathbb{N} = \{0, 1, ...\})$ on the probability space $(\Omega,\ \mathfrak{F},\ \mathcal{P})$.

This chapter deals with adapted statistical experiments defined by a random change of time (Jacod and Shiryaev 1987), which transforms a discrete stochastic basis $\mathfrak{B}_{\mathbb{N}}$ into a continuous one:

$$\mathfrak{B}_T = (\Omega,\ \mathfrak{G},\ (\mathfrak{G}_t,\ t \in \mathbb{R}_+),\ \mathcal{P})$$

The adapted statistical experiments in a continuous stochastic basis $\mathfrak{B}_T$ are considered in the series scheme with the series parameter $N \to \infty$. The limit passage, by $N \to \infty$, generates an approximation of adapted statistical experiments by a diffusion process with evolution (Jacod and Shiryaev 1987, Chapter I).

8.2. Statistical experiments and evolutionary processes

Statistical experiments in a discrete stochastic basis $\mathfrak{B}_{\mathbb{N}}$ are defined as averaged sums of the sample random variables $(\delta_n(k),\ 1 \le n \le N),\ k \ge 0$, identically distributed and jointly independent by different $n \in [1, N]$, for a fixed $k \ge 0$, with two possible values ± 1:

$$S_N(k) := \frac{1}{N} \sum_{n=1}^{N} \delta_n(k)\,, \quad k \ge 0, \qquad [8.1]$$

The variation of the discrete parameter of time $k \in \mathbb{N}$ (which is called also the stages) defines step-to-step evolution of the process [8.1].

The binary statistical experiment [8.1] is defined by the difference of the positive frequencies:

$$S_N(k) = S_N^+(k) - S_N^-(k)\,, \quad k \ge 0,$$

$$S_N^\pm(k) := \frac{1}{N} \sum_{n=1}^{N} \delta_n^\pm(k)\,, \quad \delta_n^\pm(k) := I\{\delta_n(k) = \pm 1\}.$$

The predictive component of binary and frequency statistical experiments is defined by the corresponding conditional expectations:

$$C(k+1) := E[\delta_n(k+1) \,|\, S_N(k) = C(k)]\,, \quad 1 \le n \le N\,, \quad k \ge 0,$$

$$P_\pm(k+1) := E[\delta_n^\pm(k+1) \,|\, S_N^\pm(k) = P_\pm(k)]\,, \quad 1 \le n \le N\,, \quad k \ge 0.$$

and does not depend on the sample size N.

The dynamics, by k of the predictable components of statistical experiment $S_N(k)$ and $S_N^\pm(k)$, are determined by *evolutionary processes*:

$$C(k+1) = E[S_N(k+1) \,|\, S_N(k) = C(k)]\,, \quad k \ge 0, \qquad [8.2]$$

$$P_\pm(k+1) = E[S_N^\pm(k+1) \,|\, S_N^\pm(k) = P_\pm(k)]\,, \quad k \ge 0. \qquad [8.3]$$

The following obvious identities take place:

$$C(k) = P_+(k) - P_-(k)\,, \quad P_+(k) + P_-(k) \equiv 1\,, \quad k \ge 0.$$

Hence, the relations:

$$P_{\pm}(k) = \frac{1}{2}\left[1 \pm C(k)\right], \quad k \geq 0. \qquad [8.4]$$

defines the relationship between evolutionary processes [8.2] and [8.3].

The evolutionary process $C(k)$, $k \geq 0$, defined by the conditional expectation [8.2], is determined by the dynamics of increments:

$$\Delta C(k+1) := C(k+1) - C(k), \quad k \geq 0.$$

The basic assumption (Koroliouk 2015). The evolutionary equation for the increments
$\Delta C(k+1)$ is given by the difference evolution equation:

$$\Delta C(k+1) = -V_0(C(k)), \quad k \geq 0, \qquad [8.5]$$

with the regression function of increments:

$$V_0(c) = V(1 - c^2)(c - \rho), \quad |c| \leq 1. \qquad [8.6]$$

The numerical parameters have natural limitations: $V > 0$, $|\rho| < 1$.

The regression function of increments is characterized by two absorbing points ± 1 and by equilibrium value ρ.

8.3. Stochastic dynamics of statistical experiments

The stochastic component is expressed by martingale-differences:

$$\Delta\mu_N(k+1) := \Delta S_N(k+1) - E[\Delta S_N(k+1) \mid S_N(k)], \quad k \geq 0. \qquad [8.7]$$

Given the difference evolution equation [8.5]–[8.6], the martingale-differences [8.7] have the following representation:

$$\Delta\mu_N(k+1) = \Delta S_N(k+1) + V_0(S_N(k)), \quad k \geq 0, \quad \mu_N(0) = 0. \qquad [8.8]$$

CONCLUSION.– The statistical experiment increments are determined by the sum two components:

$$\Delta S_N(k+1) = -V_0(S_N(k)) + \Delta\mu_N(k+1), \quad k \geq 0. \qquad [8.9]$$

The predictable component $V_0(S_N(k))$, $k \geq 0$, is given by the regression function of increments [8.6].

Martingale-differences [8.7] are characterized by the first two moments

$$E\Delta\mu_N(k+1) = 0, \quad E[(\Delta\mu_N(k+1))^2 \mid S_N(k)] = \sigma^2(S_N(k))/N, \quad k \geq 0. \qquad [8.10]$$

The dispersion of the stochastic component Korolijouk (2015a), Korolijouk (2015b) has the following representation:

$$\sigma^2(c) = 1 - V^2(c)\,, \quad V(c) = c - V_0(c)\,, \quad |c| \le 1. \tag{8.11}$$

The stochastic dynamics of statistical experiments $S_N(k)$, $k \ge 0$ is specified by the stochastic difference equations [8.9]–[8.11].

The properties of the stochastic component allow the next specification.

LEMMA 8.1.– *The stochastic component, defined by martingale-differences* [8.8], *has the following representation:*

$$\Delta\mu_N(k+1) = \frac{1}{N}\sum_{n=1}^{N}\beta_n(k+1)\,, \quad k \ge 0. \tag{8.12}$$

The sample variables $\beta_n(k+1)$, $0 \le n \le N$, $k \ge 0$, take two values:

$$\beta_n(k+1) = \Big\{\pm 1 - V(C(k))\,, \text{ with probability } \; P_\pm(k+1)\Big\}\,, \quad k \ge 0, \tag{8.13}$$

where:

$$P_\pm(k+1) = \frac{1}{2}\big[1 \pm C(k+1)\big] = \frac{1}{2}\big[1 \pm V(C(k))\big].$$

The latter equality provides the predictability of evolutionary process $C(k)$, $k \ge 0$.

CONCLUSION.– The stochastic component [8.12] has the Bernuolli distribution:

$$\begin{aligned} B_N(\nu; V(C(k))) &= P\{\Delta\mu_N(k+1) = \nu - V(C(k)) \,|\, S_N(k) = C(k)\} \\ &= \frac{N!}{N_+!N_-!}P_+^{N_+}(k+1)P_-^{N_-}(k+1), \end{aligned} \tag{8.14}$$

where:

$$N_\pm/N = \frac{1}{2}[1 \pm \nu]\,, \quad \nu = \nu_+ - \nu_-\,, \quad \nu_\pm = N_\pm/N.$$

with first two moments:

$$E[\beta_n(k+1) \,|\, S_N(k)] = 0\,, \quad \forall k \ge 0,$$

$$E[\beta_n^2(k+1) \,|\, S_N(k)] = \sigma^2(S_N(k)) = 1 - V^2(S_N(k)).$$

Now, the statistical experiment dynamics have the next two interpretations:

– the increments $\Delta S_N(k)$ are defined by difference equation [8.9], in which the stochastic component has the Bernoulli distribution [8.14];

– the probabilities [8.13] are defined Bernoulli distribution [8.14] of the stochastic component at a fixed k-th stage.

8.4. Adapted statistical experiments in series scheme

The properties of the stochastic component, given in lemma 8.1, make it possible to represent the adapted statistical experiments as a special semimartingale (Jacod and Shiryaev 1987). The normalized series scheme ($N \to \infty$) makes it possible to study the limit process.

The passage from the discrete stochastic basis $\mathfrak{B}_{\mathbb{N}} = (\Omega, \mathfrak{F}, (\mathfrak{F}_k, k \in \mathbb{N}), \mathcal{P})$ to the continuous one $\mathfrak{B}_T = (\Omega, \mathfrak{G}, (\mathfrak{G}_t, t \in \mathbb{R}_+), \mathcal{P})$ is realized by a random change of time:

$$\nu(t), t \geq 0 , \quad \nu(0) = 0. \qquad [8.15]$$

The counting renewal process $\nu(t), t \geq 0$, that is everywhere right-continuous and has left limits, is determined by the Markov renewal moments:

$$\tau_k := \inf\{t : \nu(t) \geq k\} , \quad k \geq 0. \qquad [8.16]$$

The regularity of the counting renewal process $\nu(t)$, $t \geq 0$ is provided by the following condition:

$$P\{\tau_k < +\infty\} = 1 , \quad \forall k > 0. \qquad [8.17]$$

The renewal intervals:

$$\theta_{k+1} := \tau_{k+1} - \tau_k , \quad k \geq 0 , \quad \tau_0 = 0. \qquad [8.18]$$

are determined by the distribution function:

$$\Phi(t) = P\{\theta_{k+1} < t\} , \quad \overline{\Phi}(t) := 1 - \Phi(t) = P\{\theta_{k+1} \geq t\} , \quad t \geq 0. \qquad [8.19]$$

The normalized counting renewal process $\nu_N(t), t \geq 0$, in the series scheme, by $N \to \infty$, is determined by the series parameter time stretching:

$$\nu_N(t) := \nu(tN) , \quad t \geq 0. \qquad [8.20]$$

The normalized renewal moments:

$$\tau_k^N := \inf\{t : \nu_N(t) \geq k\} , \quad k \geq 0, \qquad [8.21]$$

are scaled by the sample volume parameter N:

$$\tau_k^N = \tau_k / N , \quad k \geq 0. \qquad [8.22]$$

DEFINITION 8.1.– *A random change of time in discrete stochastic basis $\mathfrak{B}_{\mathbb{N}}$ is given by the filtration:*

$$\mathfrak{G}_t^N = \mathfrak{F}_{\nu_N(t)} , \quad t \geq 0. \qquad [8.23]$$

DEFINITION 8.2.– *The adapted statistical experiments with random change of time* [8.16] *is determined by its increments in the Markov renewal moments:*

$$\Delta\alpha_N(\tau_{k+1}^N) := \alpha_N(\tau_{k+1}^N) - \alpha_N(\tau_k^N)\,, \quad k \geq 0, \qquad [8.24]$$

by the normalized regression functions of increments:

$$\Delta\alpha_N(\tau_{k+1}^N) = -V_0(\alpha_N(\tau_k^N))/N + \Delta\mu_N(\tau_{k+1}^N)/\sqrt{N}\,, \quad k \geq 0, \qquad [8.25]$$

using the notations:

$$\alpha_k^N := \alpha_N(\tau_k^N)\,, \quad \mu_k^N := \mu_N(\tau_k^N), \qquad [8.26]$$

the stochastic difference equation [8.25] is simplified as follows:

$$\Delta\alpha_{k+1}^N = -\frac{1}{N}V_0(\alpha_k^N) + \frac{1}{\sqrt{N}}\Delta\mu_{k+1}^N\,, \quad k \geq 0. \qquad [8.27]$$

CONCLUSION.– The adapted statistical experiment $\alpha_N(t)$, $t \geq 0$, is a special semimartingale (Jacod and Shiryaev 1987), defined by two components:

– the predictable component defined by the regression function of increments with bounded variation $V_0(c)$, $|c| \leq 1$;

– the stochastic component defined by the Bernoulli distribution [8.14] of increments $\Delta\mu_N(k+1)$, $k \geq 0$.

Namely, the adapted statistical experiment is represented as follows:

$$\alpha_N(t) = \alpha_N(0) + V_N(t) + M_N(t)\,, \quad t \geq 0, \qquad [8.28]$$

$$V_N(t) := -\frac{1}{N}\sum_{k=0}^{\nu_N(t)-1} V_0(\alpha_k^N)\,, \quad M_N(t) := \frac{1}{\sqrt{N}}\sum_{k=0}^{\nu_N(t)-1} \Delta\mu_{k+1}^N.$$

LEMMA 8.2.– *The adapted statistical experiment $\alpha_N(t)$, $t \geq 0$, is characterized, as a special semimartingale, by the three predictable characteristics (Jacod and Shiryaev 1987, Chapter 2):*

– *evolutionary component:*

$$V_t^N = -\frac{1}{N}\sum_{k=0}^{\nu_N(t)-1} V_0(\alpha_k^N)\,, \quad t \geq 0; \qquad [8.29]$$

– *variation of the stochastic component:*

$$\sigma_t^N = \frac{1}{\sqrt{N}}\sum_{k=0}^{\nu_N(t)-1} \sigma^2(\alpha_k^N)\,, \quad \sigma^2(c) := 1 - V^2(c)\,, \quad t \geq 0; \qquad [8.30]$$

– *compensating measure of jumps:*

$$\Gamma_t^N(g) = \sum_{k=0}^{\nu_N(t)-1} E\big[g(-V_0(\alpha_k^N)/N + \Delta\mu_{k+1}^N/\sqrt{N}) \,|\, \mathfrak{F}_k^N\big], \qquad [8.31]$$

$$g(c) \in \mathcal{C}_3(R), \quad t \geq 0. \qquad [8.32]$$

PROOF 8.1.– The statement of the lemma 8.2 provides the following definition of the triplet of predictable characteristics of the special semimartingale (Jacod and Shiryaev 1987, Chapter 2), as a solution of the stochastic difference equation [8.27] in the random moments of time τ_k^N, $k \geq 0$:

$$V_t^N := \sum_{k=0}^{\nu_N(t)-1} E[\Delta\alpha_{k+1}^N \,|\, \mathfrak{F}_k^N], \quad t \geq 0;$$

$$\sigma_t^N := \sum_{k=0}^{\nu_N(t)-1} E[(\Delta\alpha_{k+1}^N)^2 \,|\, \mathfrak{F}_k^N], \quad t \geq 0; \qquad [8.33]$$

$$\Gamma_t^N(g) := \sum_{k=0}^{\nu_N(t)-1} E[g(\Delta\alpha_{k+1}^N) \,|\, \mathfrak{F}_k^N], \quad t \geq 0. \qquad [8.34]$$

□

Therefore, the predictable characteristics of adapted statistical experiments [8.16] are represented as sums of random variables defined on the sequences $\alpha_k^N = \alpha_N(\tau_k^N)$, $k \geq 0$, stopped at the moment $\tau_N(t) = \tau_{\nu(tN)}$.

8.5. Convergence of the adapted statistical experiments

The limit theorem for the adapted statistical experiments is based on the canonical representation for semimartingales by the triplet of predictable characteristics [8.29], [8.30], and [8.31]. It is implemented in the following two stages:

Stage 1. The compactness of the adapted statistical experiments [8.28] in series scheme with the parameter $N \to \infty$ is established by using the approach (Ethier and Kurtz 1986) (see also Liptser (1994), Limnios and Samoilenko (2013)).

Stage 2. By additional conditions for predictable characteristics: the functions $V_0(c)$, $\sigma^2(c)$, $|c| \leq 1$ identify the limiting process, defined by the limit predictable characteristics.

At the first stage the approach proposed in Liptser (1994) is used (see also Limnios and Samoilenko (2013) and Korolyuk and Limnios (2005)). That is, the first condition set is the *compact containmentness*.

LEMMA 8.3.– *By the condition of the initial value boundedness* $E|\alpha_0^N| \leq c_0$ *with a constant, independent of* N, *there takes place the compact containment condition:*

$$\lim_{c\to\infty} \sup_{N>0} P\{ \sup_{0\leq t\leq T} |\alpha_t^N| > c\} = 0. \qquad [8.35]$$

PROOF 8.2.– We use semimartingale representation of the adapted statistical experiments:

$$\alpha_N(t) = \alpha_N(0) + V_N(t) + M_N(t)\ , \quad t \geq 0. \qquad [8.36]$$

The evolutionary component $V_N(t)$, $t \geq 0$ is given by the sum [8.18], and the stochastic component is characterized by the modified component σ_t^N (see [8.19]).

The regularity condition of the counting renewal process [8.15] provides the boundedness of the components:

$$\sup_{0\leq t\leq T} |V_N(t)|^2 \leq C_1\ , \quad \sup_{0\leq t\leq T} |\sigma_t^N|^2 \leq C_2.$$

Consequently, by the boundedness of the initial values, the following inequality takes place:

$$E \sup_{0\leq t\leq T} |\alpha_N(t)|^2 \leq C$$

with a constant C, independent of N.

Now Kolmogorov's inequality for adapted statistical experiments $\alpha_N(t)$, $0 \leq t \leq T$, establishes the condition of compact containment [8.21]. □

REMARK 8.1.– *Another approach of establishment the compact containment condition* [8.21] *is presented in the monograph (Ethier and Kurtz 1986, Chapter 4, section 5).*

CONCLUSION.– Under the conditions of lemma 8.2, the following estimate takes place:

$$E|\alpha_n(t) - \alpha_N(t')|^2 \leq C_T|t - t'|\ , \quad 0 \leq t, t' \leq T. \qquad [8.37]$$

Under conditions [8.21] and [8.23], the compactness of the process $\alpha_N(t)$, $0 \leq t \leq T$, takes place.

At the second stage, under the compactness condition of the adapted statistical experiments in the series scheme $\alpha_N(t)$, $0 \leq t \leq T$, $N > 0$, the verification of the limiting process boils down to the study of convergence (as $N \to \infty$) of the predictable characteristics [8.18]–[8.20].

Firstly, we need to verify the convergence of the compensating measures of jumps [8.20]:

$$\sup_{0\le t\le T} \Gamma_t^N(g) \xrightarrow{D} 0\,, \quad N \to \infty, \tag{8.38}$$

or, equivalently,

$$\sup_{0\le t\le T} \Gamma_t^N(g) = \sup_{0\le t\le T} \sum_{k=1}^{\nu_N(t)} E\big[g(-V_0(\alpha_k^N)/N + \Delta\mu_{k+1}^N/\sqrt{N}) \,|\, \mathfrak{F}_k^N\big] \xrightarrow{D} 0\,,\ N \to \infty, \tag{8.39}$$

for $g(c) \in \mathcal{C}_3\,(R)$ (see (Jacod and Shiryaev 1987, Chapter VII, section 2a)).

The properties of the test functions: $g(c) = o(c^2)$, as $c \to 0$, provides the convergence of the compensating measures of jumps:

$$\sup_{0\le t\le T} \Gamma_t^N(g) = o_N(1) \to 0\,, \quad N \to \infty. \tag{8.40}$$

Next, we established the convergences of the evolutionary component [8.29] and of the variation of the stochastic component [8.30].

LEMMA 8.4.– *There are convergences in distribution, as $N \to \infty$, under the conditions of lemma 8.3:*

$$V_t^N \xrightarrow{D} V_t^0 = -\int_0^{qt} V_0(\alpha^0(s))ds\,, \quad 0 \le t \le T, \tag{8.41}$$

$$\sigma_t^N \xrightarrow{D} \sigma_t^0 = \int_0^{qt} \sigma^2(\alpha^0(s))ds\,, \quad 0 \le t \le T, \tag{8.42}$$

$$\sigma^2(c) = 1 - V^2(c).$$

Here, the limit process $\alpha^0(t), t \ge 0$ is determined by the condition of compactness (see lemma 8.3):

$$\alpha^{N_r}(t) \xrightarrow{D} \alpha^0(t)\,, \quad N_r \to 0\,, \quad r \to \infty.$$

PROOF 8.3.– Since both predictable characteristics [8.18] and [8.19] have the same structure of the integral functional on the process $\alpha_N(t), t \ge 0$, so enough to explore the convergence of one of them, for example, the evolutionary component [8.18].

It used the martingale characterization:

$$\mu_V^N(t) = \varphi(\alpha_N(t)) - \varphi(\alpha_N(0)) - \frac{1}{N} \sum_{k=0}^{\tau_N(t)-1} \theta^{k+1} \mathbb{L}_V^N \varphi(\alpha_k^N)\,, \quad \varphi(c) \in C^2(R), \tag{8.43}$$

with normalized generator:

$$\mathbb{L}_V^N \varphi(c) =: qNE[\varphi(c + \Delta V_{k+1}^N) - \varphi(c) \,|\, \alpha_k^N = c] \qquad [8.44]$$

which does not depend on k. Here, the normalizing factor is:

$$q := 1/E\theta_{k+1} \,, \quad k \geq 0.$$

It is easy to verify the martingale property in Markov renewal moments τ_k^N, $k \geq 0$.

The normalized generator admits asymptotic representation at the class of test functions $\varphi(c) \in C^2(\mathbb{R})$:

$$\mathbb{L}_V^N \varphi(c) = \mathbb{L}_V^0 \varphi(c) + R_N \varphi(c) \,, \quad \varphi(c) \in C^2(\mathbb{R}).$$

with the neglecting term:

$$R_N \varphi(c) \to 0 \,, \quad N \to \infty \,, \quad \varphi(c) \in C^2(\mathbb{R}).$$

The limit operator $\mathbb{L}_V^0$ sets the evolution:

$$\mathbb{L}_V^0 \varphi(c) = -qV_0(c)\varphi'(c) \,, \quad \varphi(c) \in C^2(\mathbb{R}).$$

The limit evolution is given by the following relation:

$$V_t^0 = -\int_0^{qt} V_0(\alpha^0(u))du \,, \quad t \geq 0.$$

Similarly, we have established the quadratic characteristic convergence [8.19] using the martingale characterization:

$$\mu_\sigma^N(t) = \varphi(\alpha_N(t)) - \varphi(\alpha_N(0)) - \frac{1}{N} \sum_{k=0}^{\tau_N(t)-1} \theta^{k+1} \mathbb{L}_\sigma^N \varphi(\alpha_k^N) \,, \quad \varphi(c) \in C^2(R), \qquad [8.45]$$

with generator:

$$\mathbb{L}_\sigma^N \varphi(c) =: qNE[\varphi(c + \Delta\sigma_{k+1}^N) - \varphi(c) \,|\, \alpha_k^N = c] \,, \quad \varphi(c) \in C^2(\mathbb{R}),$$

with increments:

$$\Delta\sigma_{k+1}^N := \frac{1}{N}\sigma^2(\alpha_{k+1}^N)$$

The asymptotic representation for the class of test functions $\varphi(c) \in C^2(\mathbb{R})$ is the following:

$$\mathbb{L}_\sigma^N \varphi(c) = q\sigma_0^2(c)\varphi'(c) + R_N \varphi(c) \,, \quad \varphi(c) \in C^2(\mathbb{R}).$$

with neglecting term:

$$R_N\varphi(c) \to 0\,, \quad N \to \infty\,, \quad \varphi(c) \in C^2(\mathbb{R}).$$

Therefore, the limiting quadratic characteristic has the following representation:

$$\sigma_t^0 = \int_0^{qt} \sigma^2(\alpha_0(u))du\,, \quad t \geq 0\,, \quad \sigma^2(c) = 1 - V^2(c).$$

At the final stage, we use the unambiguity condition for semimartingale characterization of diffusion Markov process with evolution $\alpha^0(t)$, $t \geq 0$, given by the generator (Jacod and Shiryaev 1987, Chapter IX):

$$\mathbb{L}_V^0\varphi(c) = -V_0(c)\varphi'(c) + \frac{1}{2}\sigma^2(c)\varphi''(c)\,, \quad \varphi(c) \in C^2(\mathbb{R}). \qquad \square$$

THEOREM 8.1.– *The adapted statistical experiments $\alpha_N(t)$, $t \geq 0$ in series scheme with the series parameter $N \to \infty$, determined by the predictable characteristics* [8.18]–[8.20] *with additional condition of convergence of initial values:*

$$\alpha_N(0) \xrightarrow{D} \alpha_0\,, \quad E\alpha_N(0) \to E\alpha_0\,, \quad N \to \infty.$$

converge, in distribution, to the diffusion process with evolution with scale change of time

$$\alpha_N(t) \xrightarrow{D} \alpha_0(t)\,, \quad 0 \leq t \leq T\,, \quad N \to \infty.$$

The predictable characteristics of the limiting process $\alpha_0(t)$, $t \geq 0$ have the following representation:

$$V_t^0 = \int_0^{qt} V_0(\alpha^0(u))du\,, \quad \sigma_t^0 = \int_0^{qt} \sigma^2(\alpha_0(u))du\,, \quad 0 \leq t \leq T.$$

and the compensating measure of jumps is absent:

$$\Gamma_t^N(g) \to 0\,, \quad N \to \infty\,, \quad g(c) \in C_3(\mathbb{R}).$$

CONCLUSION.– The limiting diffusion process with evolution $\alpha_0(t)$, $t \geq 0$ is given by the stochastic differential equation:

$$d\alpha(t) = -V_0(\alpha(t))dt + \sigma(\alpha(t))dW_t\,, \quad t \geq 0,$$

with the linear time scaling:

$$\alpha_0(t) = \alpha(qt)\,, \quad t \geq 0.$$

8.6. Scaling parameter estimation

According to the conclusion of theorem 8.1, the limiting adapted statistical experiment $\alpha_0(t)$, $t \geq 0$, is described by diffusion processes with evolution $\alpha(t)$, $t \geq 0$, with the time scaling.

The scaling parameter is determined by the renewal intensity $q = 1/E\theta_{k+1}$, $k \geq 0$.

The main statistical problem for the adapted statistical experiments is to estimate the scaling parameter q using the theory of renewal processes Korolyuk and Limnios (2005), Feller (1971) and Shurenkov (1984).

Firstly, the renewal function for the counting renewal process $\nu(t)$, $t \geq 0$, can be used. It is known (Feller 1971, Chapter 6) that the renewal function is defined as follows:

$$U(t) := \sum_{n=0}^{\infty} \Phi^{n*}(t) \, , \quad t \geq 0. \qquad [8.46]$$

Here, by induction:

$$\Phi^{(n+1)*}(t) = \Phi^{n*}(t) * \Phi(t) \, , \quad \Phi^{0*}(t) = 1 \, , \ \forall t \geq 0.$$

It is assumed that $\Phi(0) = 0$. The finiteness of the renewal function $U(t)$, $\forall t \geq 0$ is a consequence of regularity condition [8.17] and of statistical equality:

$$U(t) = E\nu(t) \, , \quad t \geq 0. \qquad [8.47]$$

Moreover, the renewal function [8.46] can be used to represent a solution of the renewal equation:

$$Z(t) - \int_0^t Z(t-s)\Phi(ds) = g(t) \, , \quad t > 0. \qquad [8.48]$$

with a predetermined function $g(t)$ at the right-hand side that is absolutely integrable on positive real semiline $R_+ = [0, +\infty)$. It is useful to note that we can consider the class of bounded non-decreasing functions $g(t)$ that are just absolutely integrated. Here, $\Phi(t)$ is the renewal interval distribution function.

Therefore, a solution of the renewal equation [8.48] is represented as follows:

$$Z(t) = \int_0^t g(t-s)U(ds) \, , \quad t \geq 0. \qquad [8.49]$$

The central role in renewal theory plays the nodal limit renewal theorem in Smith (1958) (see also Shurenkov (1984)), which, in our terms, is formulated as follows:

$$\lim_{t\to\infty} Z(t) = \lim_{t\to\infty} \int_0^t g(t-s)U(ds) = q \int_0^{\infty} g(t)dt. \qquad [8.50]$$

In this particular case, the elementary limit renewal theorem means the convergence:

$$\lim_{t\to\infty} U(t+h) - U(t) = qh\,, \quad h > 0. \qquad [8.51]$$

Other particular case is the Poisson renewal process with exponential distribution of renewal times:

$$\overline{\Phi}_q(t) = \exp[-qt] = P\{\theta_{k+1} \geq t\}\,, \quad k \geq 0\,, \quad t \geq 0. \qquad [8.52]$$

In this case,

$$E\nu(t) = qt. \qquad [8.53]$$

The natural question: in which other situation does the "stationary" equality [8.51] take place? The positive answer, as it is known (Feller 1971, Chapter XI, section 3), is for renewal process with delay, determined by the initial distribution function of limit overjumps:

$$\Phi_0(t) = q \cdot \int_0^t \overline{\Phi}(s)ds, \qquad [8.54]$$

which provides equality [8.51].

The limit overjump distribution [8.52] can be obtained using the nodal renewal theorem [8.50] using the renewal equation [8.48] with the given right-hand side function:

$$g_s(t) = \overline{\Phi}(t+s)\,, \quad t \geq 0\,, \quad s \geq 0. \qquad [8.55]$$

Moreover, the scaling parameter q can be estimated by the nodal renewal theorem (Shiryaev 2018, Chapter IV, section 3):

$$\nu(T)/T \xrightarrow{P1} q\,, \quad T \to \infty. \qquad [8.56]$$

8.7. Statistical estimations of the renewal intensity parameter

The renewal theory discussed in the previous section leads to the following conclusion.

The simplest Poisson renewal process, as well as the stationary renewal process with delay, is characterized by the equality:

$$E\nu(T) = qT\,, \quad T > 0. \qquad [8.57]$$

At the same time, for a process with arbitrarily distributed renewal intervals:

$$\Phi(t) = P\{\theta_{k+1} \leq t\}\,, \quad k \geq 0, \qquad [8.58]$$

the parameter q has estimation by using the strong law of large numbers (Shiryaev 2018, Chapter IV, section 3):

$$\widehat{q} \approx \nu(T)/T \qquad [8.59]$$

The above-mentioned statistical estimations have been numerically verified on the simulated trajectories of the renewal processes with previously fixed parameters in the cases discussed above.

8.7.1. *Poisson's renewal process with parameter* $q = 2$

In this case, the nodal formula $E\nu(t) = qt$ and its statistical interpretation $E\widehat{\nu}(t) = \widehat{q}t$ imply the statistical estimates $\widehat{q}_T = \frac{1}{M}\sum_{m=1}^{M}\nu_m(T)/T$. The use of simulation calculations based on exponential renewal interval generation $\theta_i = -(1/q)\ln(1-x_i)$, where $x_i \in U(0,1)$ is a uniformly distributed random number on a unit interval, we obtain the values indicated in Table 8.1 of the level T hitting times for the renewal process τ_i, $i \geq 1$. Then, the corresponding estimates $\widehat{q}t$ are given in Table 8.2 for different parameters T.

	m=1	m=2	m=3	m=4	m=5	m=6	m=7	m=8	m=9	m=10
T=5	17	5	6	3	11	14	10	8	8	10
T=10	31	19	20	14	22	21	20	26	24	17
T=20	48	45	46	34	46	43	37	41	36	38
T=40	77	80	89	81	88	81	70	73	74	77
T=70	144	138	154	145	142	150	136	135	132	138
T=100	213	212	207	208	195	214	205	191	192	198
T=150	322	327	297	294	302	315	308	285	288	297
T=200	404	433	384	387	389	425	416	364	374	403

Table 8.1. *Hitting times* $\nu_m(T)$

	T=5	T=10	T=20	T=40	T=70	T=100	T=150	T=200
M=10	1.88	2.18	2.07	1.985	2.005714286	2.028	2.018	1.9685

Table 8.2. *Estimated parameter* $q = 2$

8.7.2. *Stationary renewal process with delay, determined by the initial distribution function of the limit overjumps*

Here, a particular case is considered, with the initial renewal intervals calculated by the overjump of level T for a big enough T. The other renewal intervals have the

Weibull–Gnedenko distribution function $W(1/2, 1/2)$: $\Phi(t) = 1 - e^{-\sqrt{2t}}$, $t \geq 0$. The strong law of large numbers provides the statistical estimation $\widehat{q} \approx \nu(T)/T$.

Considering that $1/q = E\theta_k = (1/2)\Gamma(3) = 1$, hence $q = 1$.

By the corresponding simulation calculations, we obtain Table 8.3, which indicates the level T hitting times $\nu_m(T)$, $m = 1, 2, \ldots$ for the renewal process τ_k, $k \geq 1$. The corresponding estimates $\widehat{q}t$ are given in Table 8.4 for different parameters T.

	m=1	m=2	m=3
T=200	200	187	204
T=300	299	279	322
T=400	430	378	415

Table 8.3. *Hitting times* $\nu_m(T)$

	m=1	m=2	m=3
T=200	1	0.935	1.02
T=300	0.996666667	0.93	1.073333333
T=400	1.075	0.945	1.0375

Table 8.4. *Estimated parameter* $q = 1$

8.7.3. *Renewal processes with arbitrarily distributed renewal intervals*

Here, a particular case is considered, with the Weibull–Gnedenko distribution function $W(2, 2)$: $\Phi(t) = 1 - e^{-t^2/4}$, $t \geq 0$. The strong law of large numbers provides the statistical estimation $\widehat{q} \approx \nu(T)/T$.

	m=1	m=2	m=3
T=300	169	168	171
T=450	243	243	249
T=580	311	318	321
T=725	390	402	401

Table 8.5. *Hitting times* $\nu_m(T)$

Considering that $1/q = E\theta_k = \lambda\Gamma(1,5) = \sqrt{\pi}$, we have $q = 1/\sqrt{\pi} = 0.564189584$. Using W(2,2) renewal interval generation $\theta_k = 2 \cdot (-\ln(x_k))^{1/2}$, $x_k \in U(0, 1)$, we obtain, by mean of simulation calculations, the level T hitting times $\nu_m(T)$, $m = 1, 2, ...$ for the renewal process τ_k, $k \geq 1$ which values are given in Table 8.5. The corresponding estimates $\widehat{q}t$ are given in Table 8.6 for different parameters T.

	m=1	m=2	m=3
T=300	0.563333333	0.56	0.57
T=450	0.566666667	0.557777778	0.566666667
T=580	0.574137931	0.565517241	0.565517241
T=725	0.569655172	0.55862069	0.56137931

Table 8.6. *Estimated parameter* $q = 0.564189584$

CONCLUSION.– The convergence of the adapted statistical experiments with random change of time to a limit diffusion process with evolution $\alpha_0(t)$, $t \geq 0$, given by the stochastic difference equation with the linear time scaling, reduces the problem of the random change of time to a statistical estimation of only the average renewal intensity parameter q.

Other approach on the stochastic experiments parameter estimation is given in Koroliouk (2016).

9

Filtering of Stationary Gaussian Statistical Experiments

This chapter proposes a new filtering model for stationary Gaussian–Markov stochastic evolutionary systems, determined by diffusion-type stochastic difference equations.

9.1. Stationary statistical experiments

The *statistical experiment (SE)* is defined as the averaged sums:

$$S_N(k) = \frac{1}{N}\sum_{r=1}^{N}\delta_r(k), \; k \geq 0, \qquad [9.1]$$

in which the random variables $\delta_r(k)$, $1 \leq r \leq N$, $k \geq 0$, are equally distributed and independent of each fixed $k \geq 0$, which take binary values 0 or 1.

In particular, let us consider

$$\delta_r(k) = I(A) = \begin{cases} 1, & \text{if event } A \text{ occurs;} \\ 0, & \text{if event } A \text{ does not occur.} \end{cases}, \quad 1 \leq r \leq N\,, \quad k \geq 0.$$

In this case, the random amount $S_N(k)$, $k \geq 0$, describes the relative frequencies of the presence of the attribute A in a sample of fixed volume N at each time instant $k \geq 0$.

Introducing the normalized fluctuations $\zeta_N(k) := \sqrt{N}(S_N(k) - \rho)$, where ρ be the equilibrium of statistical experiment (Koroliouk et al. 2014; Koroliouk 2015a), we get its important representation.

Namely, some natural conditions (Koroliouk 2015b, proposition 5.2), the statistical experiment [9.1] has the following diffusion approximation:

$$\Delta\zeta(k+1) = -V\zeta(k) + \sigma\Delta W(k+1)\,, \quad 0 \le V \le 2\,, \quad \sigma \ge 0, \tag{9.2}$$

where the increments $\Delta\zeta(k+1) := \zeta(k+1) - \zeta_N(k)$ and $\Delta W(k+1)$ are the standard normally distributed martingale differences. The solution of the stochastic difference equation [9.2] is called *discrete Markov diffusion* (Koroliouk et al. 2016). The next theorem (Koroliouk 2016) gives the necessary and sufficient conditions of the stationarity, in wide sense, of the discrete Markov diffusion [9.2].

THEOREM 9.1 (THEOREM ON STATIONARITY).– *The discrete Markov diffusion* [9.2] *is a stationary random sequence in wide sense if and only if the following relations take place:*

$$E\zeta(0) = 0\,, \quad E\zeta^2(0) = R_\zeta = \sigma^2/(2V - V^2). \tag{9.3}$$

Now, consider a stationary, in wide sense, two-component random sequence $\big(\zeta(k),\ \Delta\zeta(k+1)\big)$, $k \ge 0$, with the following joint covariances:

$$R_\zeta = E\big[\zeta(k)\big]^2\,, \quad R_\zeta^0 = E\big[\zeta(k)\Delta\zeta(k+1)\big]\,, \quad R_\zeta^\Delta = E\big[\Delta\zeta(k+1)\big]^2. \tag{9.4}$$

In filtering problem of Gaussian stationary discrete Markov diffusion, the equivalence formulated in the following theorem (see Koroliouk (2016)) is essentially used.

THEOREM 9.2 (THEOREM ON EQUIVALENCE).– *Let the two-component Gaussian–Markov random sequence* $\big(\zeta(k),\ \Delta\zeta(k+1)\big)$, $k \ge 0$, *with the mean value* $E[\zeta(k)] = 0$, $k \ge 0$, *and the joint covariances* [9.4] *that satisfy the stationarity condition*

$$\sigma^2 = \big(2V - V^2\big)R_\zeta. \tag{9.5}$$

Then, the random sequence $\big(\zeta(k),\ \Delta\zeta(k+1)\big)$, $k \ge 0$, *is a solution of the stochastic difference equation* [9.2], *which is a discrete Markov diffusion.*

PROOF 9.1.– By theorem on normal correlation (Liptser and Shiryaev 2001, theorem 13.1), we have:

$$E\big[\Delta\zeta(k+1) \,|\, \zeta(k)\big] = R_\zeta^0 R_\zeta^{-1}\zeta(k). \tag{9.6}$$

Hence,

$$R_\zeta^0 = -VR_\zeta \quad \text{and} \quad R_\zeta^\Delta = 2VR_\zeta. \tag{9.7}$$

Consider the martingale differences

$$\Delta W(k+1) = \frac{1}{\sigma}\Big(\Delta\zeta_N(k+1) + V\zeta(k)\Big). \qquad [9.8]$$

and calculate its first two moments. We have

$$E\Big[\Delta W(k+1)\Big] = \frac{1}{\sigma} E\Big[\Delta\zeta_N(k+1) + V\zeta(k)\Big] = 0, \qquad [9.9]$$

$$E\Big[\Delta W(k+1)\Big]^2 = 1. \qquad [9.10]$$

Now, it remains to prove that the stochastic part covariations are:

$$E\Big[\Delta W(k+1)\Delta W(r+1)\Big] = \begin{cases} 1, & \text{if } k = r, \\ 0, & \text{otherwise.} \end{cases} \qquad [9.11]$$

Suppose for determination that $r < k$. Using the Markov property of the sequence $(\zeta(k), k \geq 0$, and the relation [9.9], we obtain:

$$E\Big[\Delta W(k+1) \,|\, \zeta(r), \zeta(k)\Big] = E\Big[\Big(\Delta\zeta(k+1) + V\zeta(k)\Big) \,|\, \zeta(k)\Big] = 0. \qquad [9.12]$$

Theorem 9.2 is proven. □

9.2. Filtering of discrete Markov diffusion

The filtering and extrapolation problem is considered by many authors (e.g. Moklyachuk et al. (2018, 2019)). In our constructions of the new filter, we proceed from the following basic principle: the presence of two normally distributed random sequences implies the presence of their covariances, which contain information about the filtering.

The task is to estimate the unknown parameters of a stationary Gaussian–Markov signal process $\alpha(k)$ by using the trajectories of the signal $(\alpha(k),\ \Delta\alpha(k+1))$, and a stationary Gaussian–Markov filtering process $(\beta(k),\ \Delta\beta(k+1))$, $k \geq 0$.

The signal with unknown parameters is determined by the next equation:

$$\Delta\alpha(k+1) = -V_0\alpha(k) + \sigma_0\Delta W^0(k+1)\,, \quad k \geq 0. \qquad [9.13]$$

The filtering process by the equation:

$$\Delta\beta(k+1) = -V\beta(k) + \sigma\Delta W(k+1)\,, \quad k \geq 0. \qquad [9.14]$$

It is known that the best estimate (in the mean square sense) of the signal $(\alpha(k), \Delta\alpha(k+1))$, by observing the filtering process $(\beta(k), \Delta\beta(k+1))$, coincides with the conditional expectation

$$(\widehat{\alpha}(k), \Delta\widehat{\alpha}(k+1)) = E\left[(\alpha(k), \Delta\alpha(k+1)) \,\middle|\, (\beta(k), \Delta\beta(k+1))\right]. \quad [9.15]$$

The next calculation of filtering matrix $\mathbf{\Phi}_\beta$, determined by the conditional expectation [9.15], essentially uses theorem 9.2 on equivalence and is based on theorem on normal correlation by Liptser and Shiryaev (2001).

THEOREM 9.3.– *The estimate* [9.15] *is determined by the filtering equation*

$$\big(\widehat{\alpha}(k), \Delta\widehat{\alpha}(k+1)\big) = \mathbf{\Phi}_\beta \cdot \begin{pmatrix} \beta(k) \\ \Delta\beta(k+1) \end{pmatrix}, \quad [9.16]$$

with the filtering matrix

$$\mathbf{\Phi}_\beta = \begin{bmatrix} 1 & 0 \\ -V_0 & 0 \end{bmatrix} R_{\alpha\beta} R_\beta^{-1}. \quad [9.17]$$

where

$$R_{\alpha\beta} := E\big[\alpha(k)\beta(k)\big] \ , \ \ R_\beta := E\big[\beta^2(k)\big]. \quad [9.18]$$

COROLLARY 9.1.– *The interpolation of the signal $\alpha(k)$ by observing the filtering process $\beta(k)$ is*

$$\widehat{\alpha}(k) = \mathbf{\Phi}_{11}\beta(k) \ , \ \ \mathbf{\Phi}_{11} := R_{\alpha\beta}R_\beta^{-1};$$

$$\Delta\widehat{\alpha}(k+1) = \mathbf{\Phi}_{21}\beta(k) = -V_0\mathbf{\Phi}_{11}\Delta\beta(k+1).$$

COROLLARY 9.2.– *We have the following statistical parameter estimation:*

$$V_0 \approx V_0^T = -\frac{\mathbf{\Phi}_{21}^T}{\mathbf{\Phi}_{11}^T}. \quad [9.19]$$

COROLLARY 9.3.– *We have the following statistical parameter estimation:*

$$\sigma_\alpha \approx \sigma_\alpha^T = \mathcal{E}_0^T \cdot R_\alpha^T \ , \ \ \mathcal{E}_0^T := 2V_0^T - \left(V_0^T\right)^2. \quad [9.20]$$

PROPOSITION 9.1.– *Under the assumption of mutual uncorrelatedness* [9.23] *(see further on by numbering), the statistical estimates* [9.19][1]–[9.20] *are unbiased and strongly consistent, as $T \to \infty$.*

1 For the filtering parameter estimation, see the section 9.4 below.

PROOF OF THEOREM 9.3.– By the theorem on normal correlation (Liptser and Shiryaev 2001, theorem 13.1), the filtering matrix introduced in equation [9.16] has the following form:

$$\mathbf{\Phi}_\beta = \mathbb{R}_{\alpha\beta}\mathbb{R}_\beta^{-1}, \tag{9.21}$$

where

$$\mathbb{R}_{\alpha\beta} := \begin{bmatrix} R_{\alpha\beta} & R^0_{\alpha\beta} \\ R^0_{\beta\alpha} & R^\Delta_{\alpha\beta} \end{bmatrix}, \quad \mathbb{R}_\beta := \begin{bmatrix} R_\beta & R^0_{\beta}, \\ R^0_\beta & R^\Delta_\beta \end{bmatrix}, \tag{9.22}$$

and the covariances are defined as follows:

$$R^0_{\alpha\beta} := E[\alpha(k)\Delta\beta(k+1)],$$

$$R^0_{\beta\alpha} := E[\beta(k)\Delta\alpha(k+1)], \quad R^\Delta_{\alpha\beta} := E[\Delta\alpha(k+1)\Delta\beta(k+1)],$$

$$R^0_\beta := E[\beta(k)\Delta\beta(k+1)], \quad R^\Delta_\beta := E[(\Delta\beta(k+1))^2].$$

Under the assumption of mutual uncorrelatedness

$$E[\alpha(k)\cdot W(k)] = 0, \quad E[\beta(k)\cdot W^0(k)] = 0, \qquad E[W(k)\cdot W^0(k)] = 0, \quad k \geq 0, \tag{9.23}$$

the equations [9.13]–[9.14] imply the following representations:

$$R^0_{\alpha\beta} = -VR_{\alpha\beta}, \quad R^0_{\beta\alpha} = -V_0R_{\alpha\beta}, \quad R^\Delta_{\alpha\beta} = VV_0R_{\alpha\beta}; \tag{9.24}$$

$$R^0_\beta = -VR_\beta, \quad R^\Delta_\beta := 2VR_\beta.$$

So, the matrix

$$\mathbb{R}_\beta = \begin{bmatrix} R_\beta & -VR_\beta \\ -VR_\beta & 2VR_\beta \end{bmatrix} \tag{9.25}$$

has the following inversion:

$$\mathbb{R}_\beta^{-1} = \begin{bmatrix} 2VR_\beta & VR_\beta \\ VR_\beta & R_\beta \end{bmatrix} \cdot d_\beta^{-1}, \quad d_\beta := (2V - V^2)R^2_\beta. \tag{9.26}$$

Now, let us calculate the elements of the filtering matrix

$$\mathbf{\Phi}_\beta = \begin{bmatrix} \Phi_{11} & \Phi_{12} \\ \Phi_{21} & \Phi_{22} \end{bmatrix} \tag{9.27}$$

By equation [9.21], taking into account equation [9.26], we have:

$$\mathbf{\Phi}_\beta = \begin{bmatrix} R_{\alpha\beta} & -VR_{\alpha\beta} \\ -V_0R_{\alpha\beta} & VV_0R_{\alpha\beta} \end{bmatrix} \cdot \begin{bmatrix} 2VR_\beta & VR_\beta \\ VR_\beta & R_\beta \end{bmatrix} \cdot d_\beta^{-1}. \tag{9.28}$$

Hence, taking into account the relation $d_\beta := (2V - V^2)R_\beta^2$, we obtain

$$\begin{aligned} \Phi_{11} &= R_{\alpha\beta}R_\beta^{-1}, \\ \Phi_{21} &= -V_0 R_{\alpha\beta}R_\beta^{-1}, \\ \Phi_{12} &= \Phi_{22} = 0. \end{aligned} \qquad [9.29]$$

So, the matrix

$$\mathbf{\Phi}_\beta = \begin{bmatrix} R_{\alpha\beta}R_\beta^{-1} & 0 \\ -V_0 R_{\alpha\beta}R_\beta^{-1} & 0 \end{bmatrix}, \qquad [9.30]$$

which is equivalent to equation [9.17]. Theorem 9.3 is proven. □

9.3. The filtering error

Let us denote the filtering mean square estimation error

$$\Gamma(k) = E\Big[\alpha(k) - \widehat{\alpha}(k)\Big]^2 + E\Big[\Delta\alpha(k+1) - \Delta\widehat{\alpha}(k+1)\Big]^2. \qquad [9.31]$$

By stationarity of the processes $\alpha(k)$ and $\beta(k)$, $k \geq 0$, we shall skip the parameter k where it is considered possible and convenient.

By the normal correlation theorem (Liptser and Shiryaev 2001, theorem 13.3), the mean square error of the filtering is expressed as the trace of the following error matrix:

$$\begin{aligned} \mathbf{\Gamma} &= \begin{bmatrix} \Gamma_{11} & \Gamma_{12} \\ \Gamma_{21} & \Gamma_{22} \end{bmatrix} = cov[\alpha(k), \Delta\alpha(k+1) \,|\, \beta(k), \Delta\beta(k+1)] \\ &= \mathbb{R}_\alpha - \mathbb{R}_{\alpha\beta}\mathbb{R}_\beta^{-1}\mathbb{R}_{\alpha\beta}^* = \mathbb{R}_\alpha[\mathbb{I} - \underbrace{\mathbb{R}_\alpha^{-1}\mathbb{R}_{\alpha\beta}}_{\mathbf{\Phi}_\alpha}\underbrace{\mathbb{R}_\beta^{-1}\mathbb{R}_{\alpha\beta}^*}_{\mathbf{\Phi}_\beta^*}], \quad \forall k \geq 0. \end{aligned} \qquad [9.32]$$

Let us denote $\mathcal{F}_k^\beta$ the natural increasing sequence of σ-algebras of events, generated by the trajectories of the filtering discrete Markov diffusion $\beta(k)$, $k \geq 0$. Then, the elements of error matrix $\mathbf{\Gamma}$ are defined as:

$$\left.\begin{aligned} \Gamma_{11} &= E\big[\big(\alpha(k) - \widehat{\alpha}(k)\big)^2 \,|\, \mathcal{F}_k^\beta\big], \\ \Gamma_{12} &= E\big[(\alpha(k) - \widehat{\alpha}(k))(\Delta\alpha(k+1) - \Delta\widehat{\alpha}(k+1)) \,|\, \mathcal{F}_k^\beta\big], \\ \Gamma_{21} &= E\big[(\Delta\alpha(k+1) - \Delta\widehat{\alpha}(k+1))(\alpha(k) - \widehat{\alpha}(k)) \,|\, \mathcal{F}_k^\beta\big], \\ \Gamma_{22} &= E\big[\big(\Delta\alpha(k+1) - \Delta\widehat{\alpha}(k+1)\big)^2 \,|\, \mathcal{F}_k^\beta\big], \end{aligned}\right\}, \quad \forall k \geq 0,$$

and

$$\mathbb{R}_\alpha = \begin{bmatrix} 1 & -V_0 \\ -V_0 & 2V_0 \end{bmatrix} \cdot R_\alpha^2,$$

the covariation matrix $\mathbb{R}_{\alpha\beta}$ is defined in equation [9.20] and the term Φ_β is defined in formula [9.30].

Let us calculate the term Φ_α.

$$\Phi_\alpha = \mathbb{R}_\alpha^{-1}\mathbb{R}_{\alpha\beta} = \begin{bmatrix} R_\alpha^\Delta & R_\alpha^0 \\ R_\alpha^0 & R_\alpha \end{bmatrix} \cdot \begin{bmatrix} R_{\alpha\beta} & R_{\alpha\beta}^0 \\ R_{\alpha\beta}^0 & R_{\alpha\beta}^\Delta \end{bmatrix} \cdot d_\alpha^{-1}, \quad [9.33]$$

$$d_\alpha := V_0(2 - V_0)R_\alpha^2.$$

So that

$$\Phi_\alpha = \begin{bmatrix} 2V_0 R_\alpha & V_0 R_\alpha \\ V_0 R_\alpha & R_\alpha \end{bmatrix} \cdot \begin{bmatrix} R_{\alpha\beta} & -V R_{\alpha\beta} \\ -V_0 R_{\alpha\beta} & R_{\alpha\beta} \end{bmatrix} \cdot d_\alpha^{-1} =$$

$$= \begin{bmatrix} 2V_0 - V_0^2 & -V(2V_0 - V_0^2) \\ 0 & 0 \end{bmatrix} \cdot R_{\alpha\beta} R_\alpha \cdot \frac{1}{R_\alpha^2 V_0(2 - V_0)}, \quad [9.34]$$

and finally

$$\Phi_\alpha = \begin{bmatrix} 1 & -V \\ 0 & 0 \end{bmatrix} \cdot R_{\alpha\beta} R_\alpha^{-1}. \quad [9.35]$$

Next, using equation [9.17], we obtain

$$\Phi_\beta^* = \mathbb{R}_\beta^{-1}\mathbb{R}_{\alpha\beta}^* = \begin{bmatrix} 1 & -V_0 \\ 0 & 0 \end{bmatrix} \cdot R_{\alpha\beta} R_\beta^{-1}. \quad [9.36]$$

So,

$$\Phi_\alpha \cdot \Phi_\beta^* = \begin{bmatrix} 1 & -V \\ 0 & 0 \end{bmatrix} \cdot \begin{bmatrix} 1 & -V_0 \\ 0 & 0 \end{bmatrix} \cdot R_{\alpha\beta}^2 R_\alpha^{-1} R_\beta^{-1} =$$

$$= \begin{bmatrix} 1 & -V_0 \\ 0 & 0 \end{bmatrix} \cdot R_{\alpha\beta}^2 R_\alpha^{-1} R_\beta^{-1}. \quad [9.37]$$

Hence,

$$\mathbb{I} - \Phi_\alpha \Phi_\beta^* = \begin{bmatrix} 1 & 0 \\ 0 & 1 \end{bmatrix} - \begin{bmatrix} 1 & -V_0 \\ 0 & 0 \end{bmatrix} \underbrace{R_{\alpha\beta}^2 R_\alpha^{-1} R_\beta^{-1}}_{=:\Gamma_{\alpha\beta}} = \quad [9.38]$$

$$= \begin{bmatrix} 1 - \Gamma_{\alpha\beta} & V_0 \Gamma_{\alpha\beta} \\ 0 & 1 \end{bmatrix}.$$

So, the filtering error matrix [9.30] has the following form:

$$\mathbb{\Gamma} = \mathbb{R}_\alpha(\mathbb{I} - \mathbb{\Phi}_\alpha \mathbb{\Phi}^*_\beta) = \begin{bmatrix} 1 & -V_0 \\ -V_0 & 2V_0 \end{bmatrix} R^2_\alpha \cdot \begin{bmatrix} 1-\Gamma_{\alpha\beta} & V_0\Gamma_{\alpha\beta} \\ 0 & 1 \end{bmatrix} =$$

$$= \begin{bmatrix} 1-\Gamma_{\alpha\beta} & -V_0(1-\Gamma_{\alpha\beta}) \\ -V_0(1-\Gamma_{\alpha\beta}) & V_0(2-V_0\Gamma_{\alpha\beta}) \end{bmatrix} \cdot R^2_\alpha. \qquad [9.39]$$

Using the trivial identity $2 - V_0\Gamma = 2 - V_0 + V_0(1-\Gamma)$, we have:

$$\mathbb{\Gamma} = R^2_\alpha \cdot (1-\Gamma_{\alpha\beta}) \cdot \begin{bmatrix} 1 & -V_0 \\ -V_0 & V_0^2 \end{bmatrix} + R^2_\alpha \cdot \begin{bmatrix} 0 & 0 \\ 0 & V_0(2-V_0) \end{bmatrix}. \qquad [9.40]$$

and considering the stationarity condition $\sigma_0^2 = R_\alpha V_0(2 - V_0)$, we obtain the following equivalence of equation [9.39]:

$$\mathbb{\Gamma} = R^2_\alpha \cdot (1-\Gamma_{\alpha\beta}) \cdot \begin{bmatrix} 1 & -V_0 \\ -V_0 & V_0^2 \end{bmatrix} + R_\alpha \cdot \begin{bmatrix} 0 & 0 \\ 0 & \sigma_0^2 \end{bmatrix}. \qquad [9.41]$$

Hence,

$$\Gamma_{11} = R^2_\alpha \cdot (1-\Gamma_{\alpha\beta}), \quad \Gamma_{12} = -V_0 R^2_\alpha \cdot (1-\Gamma_{\alpha\beta}), \qquad [9.42]$$

$$\Gamma_{21} = -V_0 R^2_\alpha \cdot (1-\Gamma_{\alpha\beta}), \quad \Gamma_{22} = V_0^2 R^2_\alpha \cdot (1-\Gamma_{\alpha\beta}) + R^2_\alpha \cdot (2V_0 - V_0^2).$$

9.4. The filtering empirical estimation

In real physical observations, the condition of mutual uncorrelatedness [9.23] is practically not satisfied. Therefore, the covariance characteristics [9.23] should be taken into account in the covariance analysis of filtering, if they are nonzero. The corresponding correction terms are subject to estimates, based on the filtering equation [9.16].

We will explore the best estimate (in the mean square sense), determined by the following empirical filtering equation:

$$\left(\widehat{\alpha}(k), \Delta\widehat{\alpha}(k+1)\right) = \mathbb{\Phi}^T_\beta \cdot \begin{pmatrix} \beta(k) \\ \Delta\beta(k+1) \end{pmatrix}, \quad k \geq 0, \qquad [9.43]$$

with the empirical filtering matrix

$$\mathbb{\Phi}^T_\beta = \mathbb{R}^T_{\alpha\beta}(\mathbb{R}^T_\beta)^{-1}, \qquad [9.44]$$

where

$$\mathbb{R}^T_{\alpha\beta} := \begin{bmatrix} R^T_{\alpha\beta} & R^{0T}_{\alpha\beta} \\ R^{0T}_{\beta\alpha} & R^{\Delta T}_{\alpha\beta} \end{bmatrix}, \quad \mathbb{R}^T_\beta := \begin{bmatrix} R^T_\beta & R^{0T}_\beta, \\ R^{0T}_\beta & R^{\Delta T}_\beta \end{bmatrix}. \qquad [9.45]$$

The following empirical covariances are used here:

$$R^T_{\alpha\beta} := \frac{1}{T}\sum_{k=0}^{T-1}[\alpha(k)\beta(k)]\ , \quad R^{0T}_{\alpha\beta} := \frac{1}{T}\sum_{k=0}^{T-1}[\alpha(k)\Delta\beta(k+1)],$$

$$R^{0T}_{\beta\alpha} := \frac{1}{T}\sum_{k=0}^{T-1}(\beta(k)\Delta\alpha(k+1))\ , \quad R^{\Delta T}_{\alpha\beta} := \frac{1}{T}\sum_{k=0}^{T-1}(\Delta\alpha(k+1)\Delta\beta(k+1)),$$

$$R^T_{\beta} := \frac{1}{T}\sum_{k=0}^{T-1}(\beta(k)^2)\ , \quad R^{0T}_{\beta} := \frac{1}{T}\sum_{k=0}^{T-1}(\beta(k)\Delta\beta(k+1)), \qquad [9.46]$$

$$R^{\Delta T}_{\beta} := \frac{1}{T}\sum_{k=0}^{T-1}[(\Delta\beta(k+1))^2].$$

Note that for one-component correlations, we have the representation

$$R^{0T}_{\beta} = -VR^T_{\beta}\ , \quad R^{\Delta}_{\beta} := 2VR^T_{\beta}. \qquad [9.47]$$

So, the factor matrix

$$\mathbb{R}^T_{\beta} = \begin{bmatrix} R^T_{\beta} & -VR^T_{\beta} \\ -VR^T_{\beta} & 2VR^T_{\beta} \end{bmatrix} \qquad [9.48]$$

has the following inversion:

$$(\mathbb{R}^T_{\beta})^{-1} = \begin{bmatrix} 2VR^T_{\beta} & VR^T_{\beta} \\ VR^T_{\beta} & R^T_{\beta} \end{bmatrix} \cdot (d^T_{\beta})^{-1}\ , \quad d^T_{\beta} := (2V - V^2)(R^T_{\beta})^2. \qquad [9.49]$$

Supposing that the mutual correlations [9.23] in reality are not null, the empirical covariances are connected by more complex relations, namely

$$R^{0T}_{\alpha\beta} = -VR^T_{\alpha\beta} + \sigma\frac{1}{T}\sum_{k=0}^{T-1}(\alpha(k)\Delta W(k+1)),$$

$$R^{0T}_{\beta\alpha} = -V_0R^T_{\alpha\beta} + \sigma_0\frac{1}{T}\sum_{k=0}^{T-1}(\beta(k)\Delta W^0(k+1)), \qquad [9.50]$$

$$R^{\Delta T}_{\alpha\beta} = VV_0R^T_{\alpha\beta} - \sigma\frac{1}{T}\sum_{k=0}^{T-1}(\alpha(k)\Delta W(k+1)) -$$

$$-\sigma_0\frac{1}{T}\sum_{k=0}^{T-1}(\beta(k)\Delta W^0(k+1)) + \sigma\sigma_0\frac{1}{T}\sum_{k=0}^{T-1}(\Delta W(k+1)\Delta W^0(k+1)).$$

Taking into account equations [9.45] and [9.48], we have

$$\mathbb{R}^T_{\alpha\beta} = \begin{bmatrix} R^T_{\alpha\beta} & -VR^T_{\alpha\beta} + A^T \\ -V_0 R^T_{\alpha\beta} + B^T & VV_0 R^T_{\alpha\beta} + C^T \end{bmatrix}, \tag{9.51}$$

where

$$A^T := \sigma \frac{1}{T} \sum_{k=0}^{T-1} (\alpha(k)\Delta W(k+1)),$$

$$B^T := \sigma_0 \frac{1}{T} \sum_{k=0}^{T-1} (\beta(k)\Delta W^0(k+1)), \tag{9.52}$$

$$C^T := -\sigma \frac{1}{T} \sum_{k=0}^{T-1} (\alpha(k)\Delta W(k+1)) - \sigma_0 \frac{1}{T} \sum_{k=0}^{T-1} (\beta(k)\Delta W^0(k+1)) + \tag{9.53}$$

$$+ \sigma\sigma_0 \frac{1}{T} \sum_{k=0}^{T-1} (\Delta W(k+1)\Delta W^0(k+1)).$$

Now, our task is to express the filtering matrix in terms of empirical covariances. By the definition [9.44], we have

$$\Phi^T_\beta = \begin{bmatrix} R^T_{\alpha\beta} & -VR^T_{\alpha\beta} + A^T \\ -V_0 R^T_{\beta\alpha} + B^T & VV_0 R^T_{\alpha\beta} + C^T \end{bmatrix} \cdot \begin{bmatrix} 2VR^T_\beta & VR^T_\beta, \\ VR^T_\beta & R^T_\beta \end{bmatrix} \cdot d^{-1}_\beta. \tag{9.54}$$

So, we have

$$\begin{aligned}
(d^T_\beta) \cdot \Phi^T_{11} &= \mathcal{E} R^T_{\alpha\beta} R^T_\beta + VA^T R^T_\beta \,, \quad \mathcal{E} := 2V - V^2; \\
(d^T_\beta) \cdot \Phi^T_{12} &= \quad 0 \quad + A^T R^T_\beta; \\
(d^T_\beta) \cdot \Phi^T_{21} &= -V_0 \mathcal{E} R^T_{\alpha\beta} R^T_\beta + V(2B^T + C^T) R^T_\beta; \\
(d^T_\beta) \cdot \Phi^T_{22} &= \quad 0 \quad + (VB^T + C^T) R^T_\beta.
\end{aligned} \tag{9.55}$$

Taking into account the relation $d^T_\beta = \mathcal{E}(R^T_\beta)^2 = \sigma \cdot R^T_\beta$, we obtain:

$$\begin{aligned}
\Phi^T_{11} &= R^T_{\alpha\beta}(R^T_\beta)^{-1} + VA^T \cdot \left(\sigma R^T_\beta\right)^{-1}; \\
\Phi^T_{12} &= A^T \cdot (\mathcal{E} R^T_\beta)^{-1}; \\
\Phi^T_{21} &= -V_0 R^T_{\alpha\beta}(R^T_\beta)^{-1} + V(2B^T + C^T) \cdot (\sigma R^T_\beta)^{-1}; \\
\Phi^T_{22} &= VB^T + C^T) \cdot (\sigma R^T_\beta)^{-1},
\end{aligned} \tag{9.56}$$

which we can rewrite in the matrix form as

$$\Phi_\beta^T = \begin{bmatrix} 1 & 0 \\ -V_0 & 0 \end{bmatrix} R_{\alpha\beta}^T (R_\beta^T)^{-1} + \begin{bmatrix} VA^T & A^T, \\ V(2B^T + C^T) & VB^T + C^T \end{bmatrix} (\sigma R_\beta^T)^{-1}. \quad [9.57]$$

The empirical matrix representation [9.57] contains two terms. The first addendum defines the filtering matrix under conditions of uncorrelatedness [9.23] of the stochastic components of signal and filter. The second addendum defines additional statistical estimates, generated by the correlation of the stochastic components of signal and filter.

10

Asymptotic Large Deviations for Markov Random Evolutionary Process

10.1. Asymptotic large deviations

Asymptotic large deviations are the study of distributing a random time of entering a region by asymptotically decreasing the probability of hitting it.

Let us consider, as a significant example of the Markov random evolutionary process, a recurrent Markov chain.

Our aim is to obtain the necessary and sufficient conditions for the convergence of the distributions of normalized first entry times into asymptotically receding domains for ergodic Markov chains with arbitrary state space.

Consider a homogeneous Markov chain $\eta_n, n = 0, 1, ...$, with a measurable state space $(X, \mathfrak{B})$, and transition probabilities $P(x, A)$.

Hereinafter, the following conditions are satisfied:

A) The σ-algebra is separable.

B) η_n is a φ-recurrent chain in the sense of Harris, i.e. there exists a σ-finite measure φ such that $P_x\{\tau(R) < \infty\} = 1$ for any φ-positive set R and for all $x < X$. Here, $\tau(R) = min(n : n \geq 1, \eta_n \in R)$ is the first time of entry of the chain η_n into the set $(R \in \mathfrak{B})$.

C) The Markov chain η_n, has a probability invariant measure π.

By virtue of conditions A–C, the measure π is unique.

Let $D = \{D_\varepsilon, \varepsilon > 0\}$ be a system of domains satisfying the following conditions:

D) $\varphi(D_\varepsilon) > 0$ for $\varepsilon > 0$ (the enterability condition).

E) $P(x, D_\varepsilon) \to 0$ as $\varepsilon \to 0$ for all $x \in X$ (the asymptotic remoteness condition).

The condition E is necessary and sufficient for $\tau(D_\varepsilon) \to \infty$ as $\varepsilon \to 0$ for all $x \in X$ (here and elsewhere, the symbols $\xrightarrow{P1_x}$, $\xrightarrow{P_x}$ and $\xrightarrow[weakly]{x}$ denote, respectively, convergence with probability 1, the convergence in probability and weak convergence of joint distributions of random functionals defined on the paths of the Markov chain η_n with the initial state at the point x. The problem thus arises of the possible limit distributions for the normalized variables $\tau(D_\varepsilon)$.

Next, we introduce *normalizing functions* for the hitting moments $\tau(D_\varepsilon)$.

A chain $\eta_n, n \geq 0$ is called uniformly φ-recurrent if

$$\sup_{x \in X} P_x\{\tau(S) > n\} \longrightarrow 0 \ as \quad n \to \infty$$

for any φ-positive S.

For a φ-positive R, define recursively for $n \geq 0$

$$\tau(0, R) = 0, \quad \text{and} \quad \tau(n, R) = \min(k : \ k > \tau(n-1, R), \ \eta_k \in R)$$

time points of successive return to R.

Condition A provides the property

$$P_x\{\tau(n, R < \infty\} = 1, \quad x \in X, \quad n \geq 1$$

The random sequence

$$\eta_n^R = \eta_{\tau(n+1, R)}$$

represents a homogeneous Markov chain with a measurable state space $(R, \mathfrak{B}'_R)$ and transition probabilities

$$P_R(x, A) = P_x\{\eta_{\tau(R) \in A}\}.$$

Here, $\mathfrak{B}'_R$ is a σ-algebra generated by sets of type $B \bigcap R, \ B \in \mathfrak{B}$. Denote by $\mathfrak{L}_D$ the class of sets R with $0 < \varphi(R) < \infty$, for which:

– the chain η_n^R is uniformly φ-recurrent (with respect to the restriction of the measure φ to $\mathfrak{B}'_R$);

– $\sup_{x \in R} f_R(x, D_\varepsilon) \to 0$ as $\varepsilon \to 0$, where

$$f_R(x, D) = P_x\{\tau(D) \leq \tau(R)\}.$$

The functions

$$f_R(D_\varepsilon) = \int_R \pi(dx) f_R(x, D_\varepsilon)$$

play the role of normalizing functions for $\tau(D)$, where $R \in \mathfrak{L}_D$ (the structure of the class $\mathfrak{L}_D$ will be described in the sequel; in particular, its non-emptiness is proven there under conditions A, B, D and E).

The asymptotic large deviation problem is solved by the following result.

THEOREM 10.1.– *Let conditions A–D hold.*

– *If condition E holds, then for any $R \in \mathfrak{L}_D$, we have*

$$f_R(D_\varepsilon) \downarrow 0 \text{ and } P_x\{f_R(D_\varepsilon)\tau(D_\varepsilon) > t\} \longrightarrow e^{-t} \qquad [10.1]$$

as $\varepsilon \to 0$, $r \geq 0$ for all $x \in X$.

– *If for some non-random function a_ε, $0 \leq a_\varepsilon \to 0$ as $\varepsilon \to 0$, the convergence*

$$P_x\{a_\varepsilon \tau(D_\varepsilon) < \cdot\} \xrightarrow[weakly]{x} F(\cdot) \qquad [10.2]$$

holds , as $\varepsilon \to 0$, for all $x \in X$, where F is a nonsingular distribution function on $[0, \infty)$, continuous at zero, then condition E is satisfied, $a_\varepsilon \sim a f_R(D_\varepsilon)$, for some constant $a > 0$, and F is the exponential distribution function with parameter a^{-1}. Here, the symbol $a_\varepsilon \sim b_\varepsilon$ means that $a_\varepsilon b_\varepsilon^{-1} \to 1$ as $\varepsilon \to 0$.

PROOF OF THEOREM 10.1.– We will assume that $\mathfrak{L}_D \neq \varnothing$. Choose a fixed $R \in \mathfrak{L}_D$. Define the variables

$$\chi_n(R, D_\varepsilon) = 1 - \prod_{k=\tau(n-1,R)+1}^{\tau(n,R)} \chi(\eta_k \notin D_\varepsilon), \; n \geq 1$$

$$\mu(R, D_\varepsilon) = \min(n : \; n \geq 1, \; \chi_n(R, D_\varepsilon) = 1), \quad \chi_{nR} = \tau(n, R) - \tau(n-1, R).$$

The following estimate holds for $\tau(D_\varepsilon)$:

$$\chi_{1R} + \ldots + \chi_{\mu(R,D_\varepsilon)-1R} \leq \tau(D_\varepsilon) \leq \chi_{1R} + \ldots + \chi_{\mu(R,D_\varepsilon)R}. \qquad [10.3]$$

Under conditions A–C, the strong law of large numbers holds for the Markov chain η_n, i.e.

$$n^{-1}[f(\eta_1) + \ldots + f(\eta_n)] \xrightarrow{P1_x} \int f(x)\pi(dx) \; , \; n \to \infty \; , \; x \in X,$$

for any function f integrable with respect to the measure π. Choosing the indicator of the set R to be f and using the known dual relation connection between the hitting frequencies and the sums of recurrence time at the set R, we obtain

$$\pi(R)n^{-1}\sum_{k=1}^{[nt]}\chi_{kR} \xrightarrow{P1_x} t \text{ as } n\to\infty,\ x\in X. \qquad [10.4]$$

LEMMA 10.1.– *For each $\mathfrak{L}_D$, there exists a $b_{\varepsilon R}\downarrow 0$ such that for $t\geq 0$*

$$P_x\{\mu(R,D_\varepsilon) > b_{\varepsilon r}^{-1}t \to e^{-t}\} \text{ as } \varepsilon\to 0 \qquad [10.5]$$

for all $x\in X$ uniformly in $x\in R$.

Let us assume that lemma 10.1 has been proven. We can use (Sil'vestrov 1972, theorem 1) on the weak convergence of distributions of superpositions of random functions. By virtue of degeneracy of the limit distribution in equations [10.4] and [10.5], we have, for each $x\in X$ which has placed the weak convergence, as $\varepsilon\to 0$:

$$\left(b_{\varepsilon R}\mu(R,D_\varepsilon),\ \pi(R)b_{\varepsilon R}\sum_{k=1}^{[tb_{\varepsilon R}^{-1}]}\varkappa_{kR}\right) \xrightarrow[weakly]{x} (L(1),t)\ ,\ \ t\geq 0. \qquad [10.6]$$

Here and elsewhere, $L(a)$ is a random variable having an exponential distribution with parameter a. We also note that the pre-limit processes of step sums of random variables on the left in equation [10.6] are monotonically nondecreasing, while the corresponding limit process on the right in equation [10.6] is continuous. Thus, all the conditions of (Sil'vestrov 1972, theorem 1) are satisfied and its application yields

$$\pi(R)b_{\varepsilon R}(\varkappa_{1R}+\ldots+\varkappa_{\mu(R,D_\varepsilon)R}) \xrightarrow[weakly]{x} L(1) \text{ as } \varepsilon\to 0,$$

and similarly

$$\pi(R)b_{\varepsilon R}(\varkappa_{1R}+\ldots+\varkappa_{\mu(R,D_\varepsilon)-1R}) \xrightarrow[weakly]{x} L(1) \text{ as } \varepsilon\to 0.$$

From the estimates in equation [10.3] and the last two relations, it follows in an obvious way that

$$\pi(R)b_{\varepsilon R}\tau(D_\varepsilon) \xrightarrow[weakly]{x} L(1) \text{ as } \varepsilon\to 0,\ x\in X. \qquad [10.7]$$

It is still necessary to prove lemma 10.1 and obtain the asymptotic representation for the normalizing factor $b_{\varepsilon R}$.

First, let $x\in R$. By condition B) in the definition of the class $\mathfrak{L}_D$, we may assume without the loss of generality that $\sup_{x\in R} f_R(x,D_\varepsilon) < 1$ for all $\varepsilon > 0$. Using the definition of $\mu(R,D_\varepsilon)$, we obtain the representation

$$P_x\{\mu(R,D_\varepsilon) > b_{\varepsilon R}^{-1}t\} = E_x\exp\{-\xi_\varepsilon(> b_{\varepsilon R}^{-1}t)\}, \qquad [10.8]$$

where

$$\xi_\varepsilon(t) = \sum_{n=1}^{[t]} -\log(1 - f_R(\eta^R_{\varepsilon n-1}, D_\varepsilon)).$$

Here, $\eta^R_{\varepsilon n}$, $n \geq 0$, is a homogeneous Markov chain with a measurable phase space $(R, \mathfrak{B}'_R)$ and transition probabilities

$$P_{\varepsilon R}(x, A) = P_x\{\eta_{\tau(R)} \in A,\ \tau(R) < \tau(D_\varepsilon)\}(1 - f_R(x, D_\varepsilon))^{-1}. \qquad [10.9]$$

Later on, we will require a version of the weak law of large numbers which is uniform with respect to the initial conditions for the so-called cyclic exponentially ergodic Markov chains in a series scheme. A Markov chain η_n is said to be cyclic exponentially ergodic if positive integers $d, h_0, ..., h_d$, numbers $0 < d, \rho_1, ..., \rho_d < 1$, and sets $C_0, ..., C_d \in \mathfrak{B}$ exist, such that:

a) $C_k \bigcap C_j = \emptyset,\ \ k \neq j$;

b) $\bigcup_k C_k = X$;

c) $P(x, C_{k+1}) = 1$ for $x \in C_k$, $k = 1, 2, ..., d$, $C_{d+1} = C_1$;

d) $|P^{(dh_k)}(x, A) - P^{(dh_k)}(y, A| \leq \rho_k$ for $x, y \in C_k$, $A \in \mathfrak{B} \bigcap C_k$, $k = 1, 2, ..., d$;

e) $P^{(h_0)} \leq \rho_0$ for $x \in C_0$.

We call the set of elements $\{d, h_k, \rho_k, C_k, k = 0, ..., d\}$ the defining set of the cyclic exponentially ergodic Markov chain, and the number d its period. For $d = 1$ and $C_0 = \emptyset$, a cyclic exponentially ergodic chain is simply exponentially ergodic (Loéve 1977, 1978). A cyclic exponentially ergodic chain η_n, $n \geq 0$ has a unique invariant probability measure

$$\pi = d^{-1}(\pi_1 + ... + \pi_d)$$

where π_k is the invariant measure of the exponentially ergodic Markov chain with phase space C_k, $\mathfrak{B} \bigcap C_k$ and one-step transition probabilities $P^{(d)}(x, A)$, $x \in C_k$, $A \in \mathfrak{B} \bigcap C_k$ extended to be identically zero on $X \setminus C_k$. The inequality

$$\sup_A \left| d^{-1} \sum_{k=0}^{d-1} P^{(n+k)}(x, A) - \pi(A) \right| \leq$$

$$\leq \begin{cases} \rho^{[n/hd]}, & \text{for } X \setminus C_0 \\ \rho^{[n(1-c)/hd]} + \rho_0^{[nc/h_0]}, & \text{for } C_0, \end{cases} \qquad [10.10]$$

holds for the rate of convergence in the ergodic theorem for the transition probabilities of cyclic exponentially ergodic Markov chains, where $p = \max_k p_k$, $h = \max_k h_k$, $k = 1, ..., d$, $0 < c < 1$. When the separability condition A is verified, every uniformly φ-recurrent Markov chain η_n is cyclic exponentially ergodic with a period

d. Moreover, the period d, the class of inessential states C_0 and the cyclic classes $C_1, ..., C_d$ in the sense of the definitions by Sil'vestrov (1972) coincide with the period d and the corresponding classes $C_0, ..., C_d$, appearing in the definition given above of a cyclic exponentially ergodic Markov chain.

LEMMA 10.2.– *For each $\varepsilon > 0$, let $\eta_{\varepsilon n}$ be a homogeneous Markov chain with measurable state space $(X, \mathfrak{B})$ and transition probabilities $P_\varepsilon(x, A)$, which is cyclic exponentially ergodic with a defining set $\{d_\varepsilon, h_{\varepsilon k}, \rho_{\varepsilon k}, C_{\varepsilon k}, k = 0, ..., d_\varepsilon\}$. Let π_ε be the invariant probability measure of the chain $\eta_{\varepsilon n}$ and $f_\varepsilon(x)$ be a non-negative $\mathfrak{B}$-measurable function.*

If the following conditions hold:

a) $\lim_{\varepsilon\to 0}(d_\varepsilon h_\varepsilon + h_{\varepsilon 0} + (1-\rho_\varepsilon)^{-1} + (1-\rho_{\varepsilon 0})^{-1}) < \infty$, where $h_\varepsilon = \max_k h_{\varepsilon k}$, $\rho_\varepsilon = \max_k \rho_{\varepsilon k}$, $k = 0, ..., d_\varepsilon$;

b) $\delta_\varepsilon = \sup_{x\in X} f_\varepsilon(x) \to 0$, $\varepsilon \to 0$;

c) $b_\varepsilon = \int_X f_\varepsilon(x)\pi_\varepsilon(dx) > 0$

for all sufficiently small ε, then

$$\lim_{\varepsilon\to 0} \sup_{x\in X} P_x\{|\zeta_\varepsilon(t) - t| > \sigma\} = 0, \quad t, \delta > 0, \qquad [10.11]$$

where

$$\zeta_\varepsilon(t) = \sum_{k=1}^{[b_\varepsilon{}^{-1}t]} f_\varepsilon(\eta_{\varepsilon k-1}).$$

PROOF 10.1.– Using [10.10], and conditions a) and b), we have:

$$\sup_{x\in X} |E_x\zeta_\varepsilon(t) - t| \le |[b_\varepsilon{}^{-1}t]]b_\varepsilon - t| +$$

$$+ \sup_{x\in X} d_\varepsilon \sum_{r<d_\varepsilon^{-1}[b_\varepsilon^{-1}t]} \left| E_x d_\varepsilon^{-1} \sum_{k=0}^{d_\varepsilon - 1} f_\varepsilon(\eta_{\varepsilon r d_{\varepsilon+k}}) - b_\varepsilon \right| + 2\delta_\varepsilon d_\varepsilon \le$$

$$\le |[b_\varepsilon{}^{-1}t]]b_\varepsilon - t| + \sup_{x\in X} d_\varepsilon \sum_{r<d_\varepsilon^{-1}[b_\varepsilon^{-1}t]} 2\delta_\varepsilon\{\rho_\varepsilon^{[r(1-c)/h_\varepsilon]} + \rho_{\varepsilon 0}^{[rd_\varepsilon c/h_{\varepsilon 0}]}\} + 2\delta_\varepsilon d_\varepsilon \le$$

$$\le |[b_\varepsilon{}^{-1}t]]b_\varepsilon - t| + 2\delta_\varepsilon d_\varepsilon(h_\varepsilon(1-c)^{-1} + 1)(1-\rho_\varepsilon)^{-1} + \qquad [10.12]$$

$$+ 2\delta_\varepsilon d_\varepsilon(h_{\varepsilon 0}c^{-1}d_\varepsilon^{-1} + 1)(1-\rho_{\varepsilon 0})^{-1} + 2\delta_\varepsilon d_\varepsilon \to 0 \text{ as } \varepsilon \to 0.$$

We now show that

$$\sup_{x\in X} |E_x\zeta_\varepsilon(t)^2 - t^2| \to 0 \text{ as } \varepsilon \to 0, \quad t > 0. \qquad [10.13]$$

Consider the Laplace transform

$$\varphi_\varepsilon(x,\lambda) = \int_0^\infty e^{-\lambda t} d_t E_x \zeta_\varepsilon(t) = \sum_{k=1}^\infty e^{-\lambda k b_\varepsilon} E_x f_\varepsilon(\eta_{\varepsilon k-1}),$$

$$\psi_\varepsilon(x,\lambda) = \int_0^\infty e^{-\lambda t} d_t E_x[\zeta_\varepsilon(t)]^2 =$$

$$= \sum_{k=1}^\infty e^{-\lambda k b_\varepsilon} E_x f_\varepsilon(\eta_{\varepsilon k-1})^2 + \sum_{k=1}^\infty \sum_{r=1}^{k-1} e^{-\lambda k b_\varepsilon} E_x f_\varepsilon(\eta_{\varepsilon k-1}) f_\varepsilon(\eta_{\varepsilon r-1}) =$$

$$= \psi'_\varepsilon(x,\lambda) + \psi''_\varepsilon(x,\lambda).$$

In a manner similar to equation [10.12], it can be shown that $\varphi_\varepsilon(x,\lambda) \to \lambda^{-1}$ as $\varepsilon \to 0$ uniformly for $x \in X$. By standard arguments connected with the "uniform version" of the continuity theorem for the Laplace transform, it is not difficult to show that equation [10.13] follows from the relation $\psi_\varepsilon(x,\lambda) \to 2\lambda^{-2}$ as $\varepsilon \to 0$ uniformly for $x \in X$. Obviously, $\psi'_\varepsilon(x,\lambda) \leq \delta_v e \varphi_\varepsilon(x,\lambda) \to 0$ as $\varepsilon \to 0$ uniformly for $x \in X$. For $\psi''_\varepsilon(x,\lambda)$, we have

$$\psi''_\varepsilon(x,\lambda) = 2\sum_{r=1}^\infty e^{-\lambda r b_\varepsilon} E_x f_\varepsilon(\eta_{\varepsilon r-1}) \sum_{m=1}^\infty e^{-\lambda m b_\varepsilon} f_\varepsilon(\eta_{\varepsilon r+m-1}) =$$

$$= 2\sum_{r=1}^\infty e^{-\lambda r b_\varepsilon} \int_X f_\varepsilon(y) P_\varepsilon^{(r-1)}(x,dy)\varphi_\varepsilon(y,\lambda),$$

which implies the estimate

$$|\psi''_\varepsilon(x,\lambda) - 2\lambda^{-1}\varphi_\varepsilon(x,\lambda)| \leq$$

$$\leq \left\{2\sup_{y\in X} |\varphi_\varepsilon(y,\lambda) - \lambda^{-1}|\right\} \sum_{r=1}^\infty e^{-\lambda r b_\varepsilon} \int_X f_\varepsilon(y) P_\varepsilon^{(r-1)}(x,dy) =$$

$$= \left\{2\sup_{y\in X} |\varphi_\varepsilon(y,\lambda) - \lambda^{-1}|\right\} \varphi_\varepsilon(x,\lambda).$$

Using the convergence of $\varphi_\varepsilon(y,\lambda)$ to λ^{-1} which is uniform for $x \in X$, we find that $\psi''_\varepsilon(x,\lambda) \to 2\lambda^{-2}$ as $\varepsilon \to 0$ uniformly for $x \in X$. The assertion of lemma 10.2 follows from equations [10.12] and [10.13]. □

REMARK 10.1.– *If conditions a) and b) are satisfied but the condition in lemma 10.2 is violated, i.e. there exists a sequence* $\varepsilon \to 0$ *such that* $b_{\varepsilon_n} \equiv 0$, *then*

$$\sup_{x\in X} E_x \sum_{k=1}^\infty f_{\varepsilon_n}(\eta_{\varepsilon_n k-1}) \to 0 \quad \textit{as } n \to \infty.$$

This follows from the fact that the estimate [10.12] (in which t must be equal to zero and $tb_{\varepsilon_n}^{-1}$ formally assumed to be $+\infty$ remains valid.

We will show that all the conditions of lemma 10.2 are obeyed by the Markov chains $\eta_{\varepsilon n}^R$ with state space (R, B_R') and transition probabilities $P\varepsilon(x, A)$ defined by equation [10.9], and by the functions $f\varepsilon(x) = -\log(1 - f_R(x, D_\varepsilon))$. To this end, we will use the following simple lemma, but omit the proof within.

LEMMA 10.3.– *For each $\varepsilon \geq 0$, let $\eta_{\varepsilon n}$ be a homogeneous Markov chain with state space $(X, \mathfrak{B})$, transition probabilities $P_\varepsilon(x, A)$, and let η_n be a cyclic exponentially ergodic Markov chain with state space $(X, \mathfrak{B})$, transition probabilities $P(x, A)$ and defining set $\{d, h_k, \rho_k, C_k, k = 0, ..., d\}$. If*

a) $\sup_{x,A} |P_\varepsilon(x, A) - P(x, A)| \to 0$ as $\varepsilon \to 0$, and

b) $P_\varepsilon(x, C_{k+1}) = 1$, $x \in C_k$, $k = 0, ..., d$, for all sufficiently small ε,

then $\varepsilon_0 > 0$ such that for $\varepsilon < \varepsilon_0$ the chains $\eta_{\varepsilon n}$ are cyclic exponentially ergodic with defining set $\{d, h_k, \rho_{\varepsilon k}, C_k, k = 0, ..., d\}$, where $\rho_{\varepsilon k} \to \rho_k$ as $\varepsilon \to 0$, $k = 0, ..., d$.

By definition of the transition probabilities of the chains $\eta_{\varepsilon n}^R$, and the chain η_n^R condition b) of lemma 10.3 holds for them. The fulfillment of condition a) of lemma 10.3 follows obviously from the fact that $R \in \mathfrak{L}_D$, and hence

$$\delta_{\varepsilon R} = \sup_{x,R} f_R(x, D_\varepsilon) \to 0 \quad \text{as } \varepsilon \to 0.$$

Since the Markov chain η_n^R is uniformly τ-recurrent, and the σ-algebra $\mathfrak{B}$ is separable, the chain η_n^R is cyclic exponentially ergodic. Applying lemma 10.3 to the chains $\eta_{\varepsilon n}^R$, and η_n^R, we conclude in particular that the chains $\eta_{\varepsilon n}^R$ are cyclic exponentially ergodic for all sufficiently small ε (without loss of generality, it may be assumed that this is true for all $\varepsilon > 0$), and so these chains satisfy condition a) of lemma 10.2. The fulfillment condition b) of lemma 10.2 for the function $f_\varepsilon(x) = -\log(1 - f_R(x, D_\varepsilon))$ follows from the fact that $\delta_{\varepsilon r} \to 0$ as $\varepsilon \to 0$. It remains to verify that condition c) of lemma 10.2 holds. In this case

$$b_\varepsilon = b_{\varepsilon R} = \int_R -\log(1 - f_R(x, D_\varepsilon))\pi_{\varepsilon R}(dx), \qquad [10.14]$$

where $\pi_{\varepsilon R}$ is the invariant probability measure of the chain $\eta_{\varepsilon n}^R$. Assume that there exists a sequence $\varepsilon_n \to 0$ such that $b_{\varepsilon_n} \equiv 0$. For any sequence $c_n \downarrow 0$ by virtue of equation [10.8]

$$P_x\{c_n\mu(R, D_{\varepsilon n}) > t\} = E_x \exp\{-\xi_\varepsilon(c_n^{-1}t)\} \geq E_x e^{-\xi_{\varepsilon_n}}. \qquad [10.15]$$

Here,

$$xi_{\varepsilon_n} = \sum_{k=1}^{\infty} - \log(1 - f_R(\eta_{\varepsilon_n k-1}, D_{\varepsilon_n})).$$

Since by virtue of remark 10.1

$$E_x \xi_{\varepsilon_n} \to 0 \quad \text{for } x \in R,$$

we have the convergence

$$e^{-\xi_{\varepsilon_n}} \xrightarrow{P_x} 1,$$

from which we find that

$$E_x e^{-\xi_{\varepsilon_n}} \to 1$$

by non-negativity of the random variables ξ_{ε_n}. This relation and equation [10.15] imply the convergence $c_n \mu(R, D_\varepsilon) \xrightarrow{P_x} \infty$. Since $\tau(n, R) \xrightarrow{P1_x} \infty$, the last two relations in obvious manner yield

$$c_n \tau(\mu(R, D_{\varepsilon_n}) - 1, R) \xrightarrow{P_x} \infty$$

which by virtue of the estimate [10.3] implies $c_n \tau(D_{\varepsilon_n}) \xrightarrow{P_x} \infty$. However, this last relation cannot be fulfilled for an arbitrary sequence $c_n \downarrow 0$ since $P_x\{\tau(D_{\varepsilon_n}) < \infty\} = 1$ by virtue of the enterability condition B; hence, a sequence $c_n \downarrow 0$ may always be selected such that

$$P_x\{\tau(D_{\varepsilon_n}) > c_n^{-1} \leq n^{-1} \quad \text{for } n = 1, 2, ...$$

Thus, all the conditions of lemma 10.2 are satisfied by the chains $\eta_{\varepsilon n}^R$ and functions $f_\varepsilon(x) = -\log(1 - f_R(x, D_\varepsilon))$. Application of the lemma yields

$$\sup_{x \in R} P_x\{|\xi(b_{\varepsilon R}^{-1} t) - t| > \delta\} \quad \text{as } \varepsilon \to 0, \ \delta > 0. \qquad [10.16]$$

Using equation [10.16], we have: for $\delta \leq 1$

$$\lim_{\varepsilon \to 0} \sup_{x \in R} \left| E_x \exp(-\xi_\varepsilon(b_{\varepsilon R}^{-1} t)) - e^{-t} \right| \leq \qquad [10.17]$$

$$\leq \lim_{\varepsilon \to 0} \sup_{x \in R} \Big(2P_x\{|\xi_\varepsilon(b_{\varepsilon R}^{-1} t) - t| > \delta\} + E_x |\exp(|\xi_\varepsilon(b_{\varepsilon R}^{-1} t) + t) - 1| \times$$

$$\times \chi(|\xi_\varepsilon(b_{\varepsilon R}^{-1} t) - t| \leq \delta) \Big) \leq e^{-t} \delta \to 0 \text{ as } \delta \to 0.$$

With the representation [10.8] taken into account, the uniform convergence in equation [10.5] for $x \in R$ follows from equation [10.17]. For $x \in X \setminus R$, we have: for $t > 0$

$$P_x\{b_{\varepsilon R}\mu(R, D_\varepsilon) > t\} = \qquad [10.18]$$

$$= \int_R P_x\{\tau(R) \le \tau(D_\varepsilon),\ \eta_{\tau(R)} \in dy\} P_y\{b_{\varepsilon R} \times (\mu(R, D_\varepsilon) - 1) > t\}$$

$$\sim e^{-t} P_x\{\tau(R) \le \tau(D_\varepsilon)\} \to e^{-t} \text{ as } \varepsilon \to 0.$$

Lemma 10.1, and with it the relation [10.7] (which establishes under conditions A–E the convergence of the distributions of the entry times $\tau(D_\varepsilon)$ under the normalization $\pi(R)b_{\varepsilon R}$ to exponential law with parameter 1 is completely proven. An explicit expression for normalizing factor $b_{\varepsilon R}$ is indicated in equation [10.14]. But it was shown there that $b_{\varepsilon R} \downarrow 0$ as $\varepsilon \to 0$. However, the normalizing factor $b_{\varepsilon R}$ differs from the normalizing functions $f_R(D_\varepsilon)$ shown in the assertion of theorem 10.1, and is considerably less suitable since its computation requires averaging with respect to the invariant measures $\pi_{\varepsilon R}$ of the "perturbed" Markov chains $\eta^R_{\varepsilon n}$ which depend on a parameter ε, whereas in computing $f_R(D_\varepsilon)$ the averaging is performed with respect to the invariant measure π of the original chain η_n. The proof of the first assertion of theorem 10.1 is completed by showing that $[\pi(R)]^{-1} f_R(D_\varepsilon) \sim b_{\varepsilon R}$.

Consider the random functionals

$$\mu_{\varepsilon n} = \min\big(k : k > \mu_{\varepsilon n-1},\ \chi_k(R, D_\varepsilon) = 1\big),\ \ n \ge 1,$$

$$\mu_{\varepsilon 0} = 0,\ \ a_{\varepsilon n} = b_{\varepsilon R}(\mu_{\varepsilon n} - \mu_{\varepsilon n-1}),\ \ n \ge 1,$$

and the renewal process

$$\nu_\varepsilon(t) = \max(n : a_{\varepsilon 1} + \ldots + a_{\varepsilon n} \le t),\ \ t \ge 0.$$

Let $J(t)$ ($t \ge 0$) denote the Poisson renewal process with parameter 1. Let us show that as $\varepsilon \to 0$

$$P_x\{\nu_\varepsilon(t_k) = m_k,\ k = 1, \ldots, n\} \to P\{J(t_k) = m_k,\ k = 1, \ldots, n\} \qquad [10.19]$$

uniformly for $x \in R$ for all $m_k = 0, 1, \ldots;\ k = 1, \ldots, n;\ n \ge 1$. To this end, it suffices to verify that

$$P_x\{a_{\varepsilon 1} > t_1, \ldots, a_{\varepsilon n} > t_n\} \to e^{-(t_1 + \ldots + t_n)} \text{ as } \varepsilon \to 0 \qquad [10.20]$$

uniformly for $x \in R$ for all $t_1, \ldots, t_n \ge 0$, $n = 1, 2, \ldots$ The times $\tau(\mu_{\varepsilon n}, R)$ are Markov times for the chain η_k, while the functionals $\mu_{\varepsilon n}$ have the form

$\theta_{\tau(\mu_{\varepsilon n-1},R)}\mu(R,D_\varepsilon)$ (where θ_n is the shift operator along a path). Therefore, by using the strong Markov property of the chain η_k, we have

$$P_x\{a_{\varepsilon k} > t_k,\ k=1,...,n\} = \qquad [10.21]$$

$$= \int_R P_x\{a_{\varepsilon k} > t_k,\ k=1,...,n-1,\ \eta_{\tau(\mu_{\varepsilon n-1},R)} \in dy\} P_y\{b_{\varepsilon R}\mu(R,D_\varepsilon) > t_n\},$$

which implies

$$\sup_{x\in R}\Big|P_x\{a_{\varepsilon k} > t_k,\ k=1,...,n\} - P_x\{a_{\varepsilon k} > t_k,\ k=1,...,n-1\}e^{-t_n}\Big| \to 0 \text{ as } \varepsilon \to 0,$$

since by virtue of lemma 10.1, the integrable function $P_\nu\{\cdot\}$ in equation [10.21] tends to e^{-t_n} as $\varepsilon \to 0$ uniformly for $y \in R$. Proceeding in turn with computations along the lines of relation [10.21], we obtain equation [10.20]. We now show that for any $\gamma > 0$

$$\lim_{\varepsilon\to 0} \sup_{x\in X} E_x \nu_\varepsilon(t)^\gamma < \infty. \qquad [10.22]$$

Choose some $h > 0$ and consider the random variables $a_{\varepsilon nh} = h\chi(a_{\varepsilon n > h}, n \geq 1$, and also the renewal process

$$\nu_{\varepsilon h}(t) = \max(n : a_{\varepsilon 1h} + ... + a_{\varepsilon nh} \leq t),\ \ t \geq 0.$$

Since $a_{\varepsilon nh} \leq a_{\varepsilon n}$,

$$P_x\{\nu_\varepsilon(t) \geq n\} \leq P_x\{\nu_{\varepsilon h}(t) \geq n\}. \qquad [10.23]$$

By definition,

$$P_x\{\nu_{\varepsilon h}(t) \geq n\} = P_x\{a_{\varepsilon 1h} + ... + a_{\varepsilon nh} \leq t\} = \qquad [10.24]$$

$$= \sum_{r_1<...<r_l} \sum_{l=0}^{[h^{-1}t]} P_x\{a_{\varepsilon r_j} > h,\ j=1,...,l,\ a_{\varepsilon k} \leq h,\ n \geq k \neq r_1,...,r_l\}$$

For convenience, we denote $e^{-h} = p$ and $1 - e^{-h} = q$. Let $0 < \delta < 1$. By virtue of lemma 10.1, there exists $\varepsilon_\delta > 0$ such that for $\varepsilon \leq \varepsilon_\delta$ we have

$$\sup_{x\in R}\Big|P_x\{b_{\varepsilon R}\mu(R,D_\varepsilon) > h\} - p\Big| = \qquad [10.25]$$

$$= \sup_{x\in R}\Big|P_x\{b_{\varepsilon R}\mu(R,D_\varepsilon) \leq h\} - q\Big| \leq \delta.$$

Using equation [10.25] and repeating calculations similar to equations [10.21] and [10.22], we obtain (for definiteness, we assume in the first iteration that $r_l < n$)

$$\begin{aligned} &P_x\{a_{\varepsilon r_j} > h,\ j = 1, ..., l,\ a_{\varepsilon k} \le h,\ n \ge k \ne r_1, ..., r_l\} = \\ &= \int_R P_x\{a_{\varepsilon r_j} > h,\ j = 1, ..., l,\ a_{\varepsilon k} \le h,\ n-1 \ge k \ne r_1, ..., r_l, \\ &\qquad \eta_{\tau(\mu_{\varepsilon n-1}, R)} \in dy\} P_y\{b_{\varepsilon R}\mu(R, D_\varepsilon) \le h\} \le \qquad [10.26] \\ &\le (q+\delta) P_x\{a_{\varepsilon r_j} > h,\ j = 1, ..., l,\ a_{\varepsilon k} \le h,\ n \ge k \ne r_1, ..., r_l\} \le \\ &\qquad \le ... \le (p+\delta)^l (q+\delta)^{n-l} \text{ for } \varepsilon \le \varepsilon_\delta. \end{aligned}$$

We point out that the estimate [10.26] for $\varepsilon \le \varepsilon_\delta$ acts simultaneously for all $0 \le l \le n$, $n = 1, 2, ...,$ $x \in R$. Continuing with equation [10.24] and taking equation [10.26] into account we have: for $\varepsilon \le \varepsilon_\delta$

$$\begin{aligned} P_x\{\nu_{\varepsilon h}(t) \ge n\} &\le \sum_{r_1 < ... < r_l} \sum_{l=0}^{[h^{-1}t]} \left(\frac{p+\delta}{1+2\delta}\right)^l \left(\frac{p+\delta}{1+2\delta}\right)^{n-l} = \\ &= (1+2\delta)^n P\{\widetilde{\nu}_h(t) \ge n\}, \quad n = 1, 2, ..., \ x \in R. \qquad [10.27] \end{aligned}$$

Here, we denote

$$\widetilde{\nu}_h(t) = \max(n : \ \beta_{1h} + ... + \beta_{nh} \le t), \quad t \ge 0$$

where the β_{nh} $(n = 1, 2, ...,)$ are independent random variables taking the values h and 0 with probabilities $p_\delta = (p+\delta)(1+2\delta)^{-1}$ and p_δ correspondingly. It is easy to find the one-dimensional distribution of $\widetilde{\nu}_h(t)$ explicitly, namely, the variable $\widetilde{\nu}_h(t)+1$ is distributed as a sum of $N_t = [h^{-1}t]$ independent random variables, geometrically distributed with parameter p. Therefore, by using equation [10.27], we have for $\varepsilon \le \varepsilon_\delta$

$$(1+2\delta)^n P\{\widetilde{\nu}_h(t) \ge n\} \le (1+2\delta)^n N_t (1-p_\delta)^{[n/N_t]}. \qquad [10.28]$$

Since $p_\delta \to p > 0$ as $\delta \to 0$, for any $\delta_t \in ((1-p)^{N_t^{-1}}, 1]$ a small δ can be chosen such that the expression on the right side in equation [10.28] is less than $N_t \sigma_t^n$ for each $n = 1, 2, ...,$ $x \in R$. Finally, by virtue of equations [10.23], [10.24], [10.26] and [10.27], we have: for $\varepsilon \le \varepsilon_\delta$

$$P_x\{\nu_v e(t) \ge n\} \le N_t \sigma_t^n, \quad n = 1, 2, ..., \ x \in R. \qquad [10.29]$$

Relation [10.22] follows from equation [10.24] in an obvious manner. Using equations [10.19] and [10.22] and standard calculations along the lines of the Lebesgue theorem in L_p, we can easily obtain the relation

$$E_x \nu_\varepsilon(t) \to EJ(t) = t \ \text{ as } \varepsilon \to 0 \qquad [10.30]$$

uniformly for $x \in R$ for each $t \geq 0$. We now use another representation for the renewal process $\nu_\varepsilon(t)$, as the stopped process

$$\nu_\varepsilon(t) = \sum_{n=1}^{[b_{\varepsilon R}^{-1}t]} \chi_n(R, D_\varepsilon), \quad t \geq 0. \qquad [10.31]$$

Representation [10.31] explicits the conditional expectation

$$E_x\nu_\varepsilon(t) = \sum_{n=1}^{[b_{\varepsilon R}^{-1}t]} \int_R P_R^{(n-1)}(x, dy) f_R(y, D_\varepsilon). \qquad [10.32]$$

Since the Markov chain is cyclic exponentially ergodic, the estimate [10.10], corresponding to the defining set $\{d = d_R, h_k = h_{kR}, \rho_k = \rho_{kR}, C_k = C_{kR}, k = 0, ..., d\}$, is valid for it. Applying this estimate, we have

$$\sup_{x\in R}\left|E_x\nu_\varepsilon(t) - [b_{\varepsilon R}^{-1}t]\int_R \pi_R(dy) f_R(y, D_\varepsilon)\right| \leq \qquad [10.33]$$

$$\leq \sup_{x\in R} \sum_{r<d^{-1}[b_{\varepsilon R}^{-1}t]} \left|\int_R \left(d^{-1}\sum_{k=0}^{d-1} P_R^{rd+k}(x, dy) - \pi_R(dy)\right) f_R(y, D_\varepsilon)\right| + 2\delta_{\varepsilon R} d \leq$$

$$\leq 2\delta\varepsilon Rd\left(\frac{1}{1-\rho}\left(\frac{h}{1-c}+1\right) + \frac{1}{1-\rho_0}\left(\frac{h_0}{cd}+1\right)+1\right) \to 0, \ \varepsilon \to 0,$$

where π_R is the invariant probability measure of the chain η_n^R, $\delta_{\varepsilon R} = \sup_{x\in R} f(x, D_\varepsilon)$, and $\rho = \rho_r$, $h = h_R$ are calculated from formula [10.10] with respect to ρ_{kR}, h_{kR}. From equations [10.30] and [10.33], considering that $0 < \pi_R < \infty$ for $R \in \mathfrak{L}_D$ and the measures π_R and π are related by $\pi_R(A) = \pi(A)[\pi(R)]^{-1}$, we have $[\pi(R)]^{-1} f_R(x, D_\varepsilon) \sim b_{\varepsilon R}$. Let us prove the second assertion of the theorem. Since $a_\varepsilon \to 0$, the relation $a_\varepsilon\tau(D_\varepsilon) \xrightarrow[weakly]{x} \xi$, where ξ is a random variable with distribution which does not have an atom at zero and holds if and only if $\tau(D_\varepsilon) \xrightarrow{P_x} \infty$. However, if there exist an x and a sequence $\varepsilon \to 0$ such that

$$P(x, D_{\varepsilon_n}) = P_x\{\tau(D_{\varepsilon_n}) = 1\} \to 0 \text{ then } \tau(D_{\varepsilon_n}) \xrightarrow{P_x} \infty.$$

Thus, condition E is fulfilled. As a result $f_R(x, D_\varepsilon) \downarrow 0$ and hence

$$f_R(x, D_\varepsilon)\tau(D_\varepsilon) \xrightarrow[weakly]{} L(1)$$

by virtue of the direct assertion I. If a number $a : 0 < a < \infty$ does not exist for which $a_\varepsilon \sim a f_R(x, D_\varepsilon)$, then there exists a sequence $\varepsilon_n \to 0$ such that

$a_{\varepsilon_n} f_R(x, D_\varepsilon)^{-1}$ tends to 0 or $+\infty$, or there exists a pair of sequences $\varepsilon_n^\pm \to 0$ such that $a_{\varepsilon_n^\pm} f_R(x, D_\varepsilon)^{-1}$, where $0 < a^- \neq a^+ < \infty$. In the first case

$$a_{\varepsilon_n} \tau(D_{\varepsilon_n}) = \left(a_{\varepsilon_n} f_R(x, D_{\varepsilon_n})^{-1}\right) \tau(D_{\varepsilon_n}) \xrightarrow{P_x} 0$$

necessarily, in the second

$$a_{\varepsilon_n} \tau(D_{\varepsilon_n}) \xrightarrow{P_x} \infty,$$

and in the third

$$a_{\varepsilon_n^\pm} \tau(D_{\varepsilon_n^\pm}) \xrightarrow[weakly]{x} L(1).$$

Any one of these relations contradicts relation [10.2] of assertion II.

Theorem 10.1 has been proven. □

REMARK 10.2.– *Theorem 10.1 is proven under the assumption that the class $\mathfrak{L}_D$ is non-empty.*

We will call a class $\mathfrak{M}$ of sets from $\mathfrak{B}$ a φ-dense class if for any S with $0 < \varphi(S) < \infty$ and $\delta > 0$ there exists a φ-positive set $S_\delta \subseteq S$ of $\mathfrak{M}$ such that $\varphi(S - S_\delta) \leq \delta$ and any φ-positive subset $S' \subseteq S_\delta$ also belongs to $\mathfrak{M}$.

Obviously, a φ-dense class is non-empty. The following lemma describes the structure of the class $\mathfrak{L}_D$.

LEMMA 10.4.– *Under conditions A, B, D and E, the class $\mathfrak{L}_D$ a φ-dense class.*

PROOF 10.2.– Denote the class of sets R with $0 < \varphi(R) < \infty$, for which the Markov chain η_n^R is uniformly φ-recurrent (with respect to the restriction of the measure φ to $\mathfrak{B} \cup R$). Under conditions A and B, the class $\mathfrak{L}$ is φ-dense [1], i.e. for arbitrary S with $0 < \varphi(S) < \infty$ and $\delta > 0$, a φ-positive set $R_0 \subseteq S$ can be found such that a) $\varphi(S \setminus R_0) \leq \delta/2$ and b) R_0 and any φ-positive $R \subseteq R_0$ are in $\mathfrak{L}$. The inclusion of events

$$\{\tau(D_\varepsilon) \leq \tau(R)\} = \bigcup_{n=1}^{\infty} \{\tau(n-1, R_0) < \tau(D_\varepsilon) \leq \tau(n, R_0)\}$$

$$\{\tau(D_\varepsilon) \leq \tau(R)\} \subseteq \bigcup_{n=1}^{N} \{\chi_n(R_0, D_\varepsilon) = 1\} \bigcup \{\tau(N, R_0) < \tau(R)\}$$

holds for any φ-positive $R \subseteq R_0$, which yields the estimate: for $x \in R_0$

$$R(x, D_\varepsilon) \leq \sum_{n=1}^{N} \int_{R_0} P_{R_0}^{-1}(x, dy) f_{R_0}(y, D_\varepsilon) + \\ + P_x\{\eta_k^{R_0} \notin R,\ k = 1, ..., N\}. \quad [10.34]$$

Since the chain $\eta_n^{R_0}$ is uniformly φ-recurrent and $\varphi(R) > 0$,

$$\sup_{x \in R_0} P_x\{\eta_n^{R_0} \notin R,\ n = 1, ..., N\} \to 0,\ N \to \infty \quad [10.35]$$

From equations [10.34] and [10.35], it follows that the following convergence

$$\sup_{x \in R_0} f_R(x, D_\varepsilon) \to 0 \ \text{as } \varepsilon \to 0 \quad [10.36]$$

takes place if for some φ-positive $R \subseteq R_0$

$$\Phi^{(n)}(x) = \int_{R_0} P_{R_0}^{(n-1)}(x, dy) f_{R_0}(y, D_\varepsilon) \to 0 \ \text{as } \varepsilon \to 0 \quad [10.37]$$

uniformly for $x \in R$, $n \geq 1$. Since $f_{R_0}(y, D_\varepsilon) \to 0$ as $\varepsilon \to 0$ for all $y \in R_0$, by Lebesgue's theorem $\Phi^{(n)}(x) \to 0$ as $\varepsilon \to 0$ for all $x \in R_0$, and hence by the Severini–Egoroff theorem for each $n = 1, 2, ...$ a φ-positive $R_n \subseteq R_0$ can be found such that

a) $\varphi(R_0 \setminus R_n) \leq 2^{-n}\delta'$, where $\delta' = 1/2 \min(\delta, \varphi(R_0))$, and
b) $\Phi^{(n)}(x) \to 0$ as $\varepsilon \to 0$ uniformly in $x \in R_n$.

Let us put $R = \bigcap_{n \geq 1} R_n$. By construction, equation [10.37] is fulfilled for the set R. Moreover, obviously $\varphi(R_0 \setminus R) \leq 2^{-n}\delta' = \delta'$. Therefore, $\varphi(S \setminus R) \leq \delta$, and hence $R \in \mathfrak{L}$ (as a φ-positive subset of R_0). □

REMARK 10.3.– *Let us dwell in somewhat more detail on the case where $X \in \mathfrak{L}_D$. In this situation*

$$\tau(D_\varepsilon) = \mu(R, D_\varepsilon) \ \textit{and} \ f_x(D_\varepsilon) = \int \pi(dx) P(x, D_\varepsilon) = \pi(D_\varepsilon).$$

Taking into account also that only the property of cyclic exponential ergodicity of the chain η_n^R was used in lemma 10.2, we can formulate as a consequence of lemma 10.1 the following statement.

THEOREM 10.2.– *Suppose a chain η_n be cyclic exponential ergodic and that condition D and the following condition hold:*

(sup E): $\quad \sup_{x \in X} P(x, D_\varepsilon) \to 0$ *as* $\varepsilon \to 0$.

Then,

$$\sup_{x \in X} |P_x\{\tau(D_\varepsilon)\pi(D_\varepsilon)\} - s^{-t}| \to 0 \ \ as\ \varepsilon \to 0,\ t \to 0.$$

The uniform convergence for $x \in X$ in theorem 10.2 is attained because of the considerable severity of ergodicity condition C and asymptotic remoteness condition E. For chains of random walk type, when the conditions of theorem 10.1 hold, but those of theorem 10.2 usually do not, there is no uniform convergence for $x \in X$ of the distributions of normalized $\tau(D_\varepsilon)$. In general, it is likewise not possible to simplify the normalizing function $f_R(D_\varepsilon)$ and replace it by $\pi(D_\varepsilon)$, or $E_\pi \tau(D_\varepsilon)$. There are examples in which the conditions of theorem 10.1 hold but under the normalizations $\pi(D_\varepsilon)$, or $E_\pi \tau(D_\varepsilon)$ the variable $\tau(D_\varepsilon)$ in general has no limit distribution.

EXAMPLE 10.1.– Let η_n, $n \geq 0$ be a random walk on integer half-line $X = \{0, 1, ...\}$ with jumps $i \to i+1$ and $i \to i-1$ with probabilities p, and $q = 1-p$ correspondingly for $i > 0$, and jumps $0 \to 1$ with probability 1.

The condition of φ-recurrence ($\varphi(A)$ is a number of points of the set X which are hitting the set A) is $0 < p \leq q < 1$. The condition of ergodicity is $0 < p < q < 1$. In this case, the stationary distribution is expressed as follows:

$$\pi_n = (q-p)(2pq)^{-1}(p/q)^n, \ \ n \geq 2,$$

$$\pi_1 = (q-p)/2q^2, \ \ \pi_0 = (q-p)/2q.$$

Let first $D_N = \{N, N+1, ...\}$ (here it is convenient to assume that $\varepsilon = N^{-1}$ and use as a series parameter N instead of ε).

In this case, the condition of asymptotic remoteness E is obviously satisfied, but the condition of uniform asymptotic remoteness sup E is not (see theorem 10.2).

It is convenient to choose $R = \{0\}$. In this case, the probabilities

$$f_R(0, D_N) = \frac{q-p}{p}\left(\left(\frac{q}{p}\right)^N - 1\right)^{-1}$$

can be considered as the probabilities that a Bernoulli random walk, beginning from point 1, hits point N before reaching point 0. So, the normalizing function, for which the hitting moments $\tau(D_N)$ have exponential distribution with parameter 1, has the following form:

$$a_N = \frac{(q-p)^2}{2pq}\left(\left(\frac{q}{p}\right)^N - 1\right)^{-1}.$$

The corresponding invariant measure is $\pi(D_N) = \frac{1}{2p}\left(\frac{p}{q}\right)^N$.

Therefore, when normalizing $\pi(D_N)$, the distribution of the random moment $\tau(D_N)$ is asymptotically exponential with paramenter $A = \frac{(q-p)^2}{p}$.

However, if we change the definition of areas D_N, considering $D_N = \{N, N+1, ...\}$ for $N = 2k$, and $D_N = \{N\}$ for $N = 2k+1$, then we obtain D

$$\pi(D_N) = \begin{cases} (1/2p)(p/q)^n, & \text{if } n \text{ is even,} \\ (q-p)/(2pq)(p/q)^n, & \text{if } n \text{ is odd.} \end{cases}$$

In this case, we have the following convergence:

$$\pi(D_{2k})^{-1} a_{2k} \to \frac{(q-p)^2}{p}, \quad \text{but} \quad \pi(D_{2k+1})^{-1} a_{2k+1} \to \frac{q(q-p)}{p}.$$

At the same time, the functional $\tau(D_N)$, as well as the normalizing function a_N, does not change with the initial state $i < N$, because the area $D_N = \{N, N+1, ...\}$ is reached by the random walk η_N only through the point N.

Therefore, when normalizing a_N, as in the first case, the hitting moments $\tau(D_N)$ will have an asymptotically exponential distribution with parameter 1, and when normalized $\pi(D_N)$, there is no limit distribution of $\tau(D_N)$.

We also note that in this example, the distribution functions $P_x\{a_N \tau(D_N) < \cdot\}$ weakly converge only for each x separately, and uniform convergence in x, obviously, does not take place.

EXAMPLE 10.2.– In some rather general cases, we can explicitly calculate the normalizing function.

Let η_n, $n \geq 0$ be a random walk on integer half-line $X = \{0, 1, ...\}$ with jumps $i \to i+1$ and $i \to i-1$ with probabilities p_i, and $q_i = 1 - p_i$ correspondingly for $i > 0$, and jumps $0 \to 1$ with probability 1.

The criterion for recurrence is the condition

$$H: \qquad \sum_k \frac{q_1 ... q_k}{p_1 ... p_k} = \infty.$$

The ergodicity criterion is the condition

$$I: \qquad \sum_k \frac{p_1 ... p_{k-1}}{q_1 ... q_k} < \infty.$$

Under condition I, there is a stationary probability distribution

$$\pi_0 = \left(1 + \sum_{k=1}^{\infty} \frac{p_1 ... p_{k-1}}{q_1 ... q_k}\right)^{-1},$$

$$\pi_n = \frac{p_1 ... p_{n-1}}{q_1 ... q_n} \pi_0, \quad n = 1, 2, ...$$

Let $D_N = \{N, N+1, ...\}$. We choose $R = \{0\}$. In this case, using the standard technique for solving difference equations, we have

$$f_R(0, D_N) = \left(\sum_{k=1}^{N} \frac{q_1 ... q_{k-1}}{p_1 ... p_{k-1}} \right)^{-1}.$$

The hitting moment $\tau(D_N)$, according to the limit theorem 10.1, has an exponential distribution with parameter 1 under normalization

$$a_N = \pi_0 f_R(0, D_N).$$

EXAMPLE 10.3.– This example illustrates an important fact observed under certain conditions for asymptotic large deviations of the Markov random evolutionary process. Namely, for regenerative processes, the normalization $a_{\varepsilon R} = \int_R \pi(dx) f_R(x, D_\varepsilon)$ is equivalent to the normalization $[E_\tau(D_\varepsilon)]^{-1}$: the inverse quantity of the average time to reach the region D_ε. Thus, the asymptotic behavior of the reaching time is determined by the asymptotic behavior of the hitting average time $E_\tau(D_\varepsilon)$. Its study is a non-trivial problem.

Consider a regenerative random walk on the half-line $x \geq 0$ with a delaying screen at $x = 0$, where a fairly simple formula for the asymptotics of the normalizing function (mean time to reach) is obtained.

Consider a lattice, upper-semicontinuous distribution with the following generating function:

$$p(s) = sq + \sum_{k=0}^{\infty} s^{-k} p_k, \quad \sum_{k=0}^{\infty} p_k = p = 1 - q > 0, \quad q > 0. \qquad [10.38]$$

Consider a Markov random walk with jump distribution

$$\begin{aligned} &P\{s_{n+1} = k - r \mid s_n = k\} = p_r, \quad -1 \leq r \leq k-1; \\ &P\{s_{n+1} = 0 \mid s_n = 0\} = 1 - P\{s_{n+1} = 1 \mid s_n = 0\} = p; \\ &P\{s_{n+1} = 0 \mid s_n = k\} = P_{k0} = \sum_{r=k}^{\infty} P_r. \end{aligned} \qquad [10.39]$$

The ergodicity of such an evolution is ensured by the condition

$$\sum_{k=0}^{\infty} k p_k - q = a > 0. \qquad [10.40]$$

It is easy to show that under condition [10.40] there exists a solution $s_0 > 1$ of the equation

$$p(s_0) = 1. \quad [10.41]$$

Let us enter τ_k^N – the number of jumps of the random walk [10.39] of reaching the level N with the beginning at the point k.

For the mean value $m_k^N = E\tau_k^N$, the following equation takes place:

$$m_k^N - qm_{k+1}^N - \sum_{r=0}^{k-1} P_r m_{k+r}^N - P_{k0} m_0^N = 1 \quad [10.42]$$

with additional condition

$$m_N^N = 0. \quad [10.43]$$

Let us redefine

$$m_{-k}^N = m_0^N, \quad k > 0. \quad [10.44]$$

Then, equations [10.42], taking into account equation [10.44], are reduced to the form

$$m_k^N - qm_{k+1}^N - \sum_{r=0}^{\infty} P_r m_{k-r}^N = 1. \quad [10.45]$$

Using the potential $\{R_n,\ n \geq 0\}$ of a semi-continuous random walk with generating function [10.38] (see Korolyuk 1975, Chapter 4), we are looking for a solution to the problem [10.43]–[10.45] in the form

$$m_k^N = cR_{k+1} + \sum_{n=1}^{k+1} R_n + m_0^N. \quad [10.46]$$

Hence, from equation [10.43], we have

$$m_N^N = cR_{N+1} - \sum_{n=1}^{N+1} R_n + m_0^N = 0, \quad [10.47]$$

$$m_0^N = -cR_{N+1} + \sum_{n=1}^{N+1} R_n. \quad [10.48]$$

Substituting equation into equation , we get

$$m_k^N = c(R_{k+1} - R_{N+1}) + \sum_{n=k+2}^{N+1} R_n. \qquad [10.49]$$

To determine the constant c, we use equation [10.42] for $k = 0$:

$$m_0^N - qm_1^N - pm_0^N = 1. \qquad [10.50]$$

From here,

$$m_0^N - m_1^N = 1/q. \qquad [10.51]$$

Notice that (see Korolyuk 1975, p. 87, formula (11))

$$R_1 = 1/q. \qquad [10.52]$$

From equations [10.49], [10.59] and [10.60], it follows that $c = 1$:

$$m_0^N = c(R_1 - R_{N+1}) + \sum_{n=1}^{N+1} R_n,$$

$$m_1^N = c(R_2 - R_{N+1}) + \sum_{n=3}^{N+1} R_n,$$

$$m_0^N - m_1^N = c(R_1 - R_2) + R_2 = c/q + R_2(1-c) = 1/q.$$

Therefore, from equation [10.49], we have

$$m_k^N = \sum_{n=k+1}^{N} R_n, \quad 0 \le k < N. \qquad [10.53]$$

The asymptotic representation of m_k^N is easy to obtain using the asymptotic representation of the potential (Korolyuk 1975, p. 92, formulas (13) and (15)):

$$R_n = RS_0^n - 1/a + V_n, \quad n \ge 0, \qquad [10.54]$$

where R (Cramer's constant) has the form

$$R = (S_0\rho'(S_0))^{-1}. \qquad [10.55]$$

The sequence V_n decreases as $n \to \infty$, while

$$\sum_{n=0}^{\infty} V_n = V < \infty. \qquad [10.56]$$

Substituting equation [10.62], taking into account equation [10.63], into equation [10.61], we find m_k^N:

$$m_k^N = \frac{S_0^N}{\rho'(S_0)}(1 - S_0^{-N+k}) - \frac{N-k}{a} + W_k^N, \qquad [10.57]$$

where $W_k^N = \sum_{n=k+1}^{N} V_n$. In particular, we have

$$\lim_{N\to\infty} S_0^{-N} m_k^N = \frac{1}{\rho'(S_0)}.$$

10.2. Asymptotically stopped Markov random evolutionary process

Markov random evolutionary processes are considered as sums of random variables defined on a Markov chain. A random evolution asymptotically stopped, meaning there is a procedure of random change of time, namely, the stop of random evolution at a random moment of time reaching an asymptotically receding region of the state space of the main Markov process.

As a typical example of a stopped random evolution, we can consider step sum processes defined on an ergodic Markov chain up to a normalized moment when the chain reaches an asymptotically receding region.

We will use the notation introduced at the beginning of Chapter 10 and conditions A–E.

Now, we will study the distribution of normalized functionals on Markov chains η_n, $n \geq 0$:

$$\xi_\varepsilon = \sum_{k=1}^{\tau(D_\varepsilon)} f(\eta_{k-1}),$$

where $f(x)$ is a measurable numeric function.

Conditions A and B ensure the existence of a unique, up to a constant factor, σ-finite invariant measure π for the chain η_n. Since it follows from conditions A and B that the chain η_n is π-recurrent, in what follows, without the loss of generality, we will assume that the invariant measure π appears as the measure φ in condition B.

In what follows, the designations $\xrightarrow{U}$, $\xrightarrow{J}$ will be used, denoting, respectively, the convergence of random processes in the topologies U and J on each finite interval.

In contrast to the classes $\mathfrak{L}$ and $\mathfrak{L}_D$ considered earlier, we will consider the classes of sets

$$\mathfrak{L}' = \{R : 0 < \pi(R) < \infty, \ \eta_n \text{ is exponentially ergodic Markov chain}\};$$
$$\mathfrak{L}'_D = \{R \in \mathfrak{L}' : \sup_{x \in R} f_R(x, D_\varepsilon) \to 0 \ \text{ as } \varepsilon \to 0\}.$$

Here, as before,

$$f_R(x, D_\varepsilon) = P_x\{\tau(D_\varepsilon) \leq \tau(R)\}.$$

DEFINITION 10.1.– *The class $\mathfrak{M}$ of measurable φ-positive sets is called weakly φ-dense if for an arbitrary S with $0 < S < \infty$ and $\delta > 0$, there are n: $S_1^\delta, ..., S_n^\delta \subseteq S$, $S_1^\delta, ..., S_n^\delta \in \mathfrak{M}$, such that $\varphi(S_i^\delta) > 0$ and $\varphi(S \setminus \cup_{i=1}^n S_i^\delta) \leq \delta$, and each $T \subseteq S_i^\delta$ with $\varphi(T) > 0$ also belongs to $\mathfrak{M}$.*

The structure of the class $\mathfrak{L}'_D$ describes the following:

LEMMA 10.5.– *Under conditions A, B, D, E, the class $\mathfrak{L}'_D$ is weakly π-dense.*

PROOF OF LEMMA 10.5.– The proof of lemma 10.5 is essentially contained in the proof of lemma 10.4. Indeed, if $S_\delta \in \mathfrak{L}_D$ is such that $S_\delta \subseteq S$, and $\pi(S \setminus S_\delta) \leq \delta$, then as sets S_δ^i we can choose the "cyclic components" of the state space S_δ uniformly along the π-return chain $\eta_n^{S_\delta}$. □

Note that lemma 10.5 implies, in particular, that the classes $\mathfrak{L}'$ and $\mathfrak{L}'_D$ are non-empty when its conditions are satisfied.

Let us introduce the functionals for $R \in \mathfrak{L}'$

$$\gamma_{kR} = \sum_{i=\tau(k-1,R)+1}^{\tau(k,R)} f(\eta_{i-1}), \quad \Delta_{kR} = \sum_{i=\tau(k-1,R)+1}^{\tau(k,R)} |f(\eta_{i-1})|,$$

and the normalizing function for $R \in \mathfrak{L}'_D$

$$a_{\varepsilon R} = \int_R \pi(dx) f_R(x, D_\varepsilon).$$

Recall the notation $\eta_n^R = \eta_{\tau(n+1,R)}$, π_R is invariant probabilistic measure of the chain η_n^R. It is connected with the measure π by the relation

$$\pi_R(A) = \pi(A)\pi(R)^{-1}, \quad A \subseteq R.$$

Hereinafter, $W(t)$ will denote the standard Wiener process, $L(a)$: a random variable, exponentially distributed with parameter a, $L = L(1)$.

THEOREM 10.3.– *Under conditions A, B, D, E and also the conditions:*

$F_1 : E_{\pi_R}|\gamma_{1R}| < \infty,$

$G_1 : tP_{\pi_R}\{\Delta_{1R} > t\delta\} \to 0, \ t \to \infty$ *for all* $\delta > 0.$

Then,

$$a_{\varepsilon R}\xi_\varepsilon \xrightarrow[weakly]{x} bL, \ \ \varepsilon \to 0, \ \ \forall x \in X,$$

where $b = \pi(R)E_{\pi_R}(\gamma_{1R})$.

REMARK 10.4.– *To fulfill the condition* G_1, *it is enough to require the following:*

$G'_1 : E_{\pi_R}\Delta_{1R} < \infty.$

THEOREM 10.4.– *Under conditions A, B, D, E and also the conditions:*

$F_2 : E_{\pi_R}\gamma_{1R} = 0, \quad E_{\pi_R}\gamma_{1R}^2 < \infty,$

$G_2 : tP_{\pi_R}\{\Delta_{1R} > \sqrt{t}\delta\} \to 0, \ t \to \infty$ *for all* $\delta > 0.$

Then,

$$\sqrt{a_{\varepsilon R}}\xi_\varepsilon \xrightarrow[weakly]{x} W(\sigma^2 L), \ \ \varepsilon \to 0, \ \ \forall x \in X,$$

where $W, \ L$ *are independent,*

$$\sigma^2 = \pi(R)\bigg(E_{\pi_R}(\gamma_{1R})^2 + 2\sum_{k>1} E_{\pi_R}(\gamma_{1R}\gamma_{kR})\bigg).$$

REMARK 10.5.– *To fulfill the condition* G_2, *it is enough to require the following:*

$G'_2 : E_{\pi_R}\Delta_{1R}^2 < \infty.$

REMARK 10.6.– *The constant* b *has the following representation:*

$$b = \pi_R \int_R \frac{\pi(dx)}{\pi(R)} \int_X E_x\nu(R, dy)f(y) = \int_X \pi(dy)f(y).$$

And also

$$E_{\pi_R}\Delta_{1R} = \int_X \pi(dy)|f(y)|.$$

PROOF OF THEOREM 10.3.– For asymptotically stopped Markov evolution ξ_ε, the following representation takes place:

$$\xi_\varepsilon = \sum_{k=1}^{\mu_\varepsilon - 1} \gamma_{kR} + \delta_\varepsilon, \qquad [10.58]$$

where $\mu_\varepsilon = \mu(R, D_\varepsilon)$ is the hitting time defined in equation [10.3], and

$$\delta_\varepsilon = \sum_{k=\tau(\mu_\varepsilon-1,R)+1}^{\tau(D_\varepsilon)} f(\eta_{k-1}).$$

Let us show that

$$a_\varepsilon \delta_\varepsilon \xrightarrow{P_x} 0 \quad \text{as } \varepsilon \to 0, \ x \in X. \qquad [10.59]$$

Notice that

$$P_x\{a_\varepsilon|\delta_\varepsilon| > \delta\} \le P_x\{a_\varepsilon \Delta_{\mu_\varepsilon R} > \delta\} =$$
$$= P_x\{\mu_\varepsilon > ta_\varepsilon^{-1}, a_\varepsilon \Delta_{\mu_\varepsilon R} > \delta\} + P_x\{\mu_\varepsilon \le ta_\varepsilon^{-1}, a_\varepsilon \Delta_{\mu_\varepsilon R} > \delta\} \le$$
$$\le P_x\{a_\varepsilon \mu_\varepsilon > t\} + P_x\{a_\varepsilon \max_{k \le ta_\varepsilon^{-1}} \Delta_{kR} > \delta\}.$$

By theorem 10.1 and the equivalence of normalizations

$$P_x\{a_\varepsilon \mu_\varepsilon > t\} \to \exp[(-\pi(R))^{-1}t] \quad \text{as } \varepsilon \to 0, \ x \in X. \qquad [10.60]$$

Consequently, the first term is arbitrarily small for enough big t. The second term

$$P_x\{a_\varepsilon \max_{k \le ta_\varepsilon^{-1}} \Delta_{kR} > \delta\} \to 0 \quad \text{as } \varepsilon \to 0. \qquad [10.61]$$

is an infinitesimal random variable due to condition G_1 and Doob's theorem on the convergence of a monotone bounded sequence.

Relations [10.58] and [10.59] imply that to prove lemma 10.5 it suffices to show that

$$a_\varepsilon \sum_{k=1}^{\mu_\varepsilon - 1} \gamma_{kR} \xrightarrow[weakly]{x} bL. \qquad [10.62]$$

To do this, we need to use theorem 3.2 (Sil'vestrov and Teugels 2004) on the weak convergence of a superposition of random functions.

Consider a two-dimensional sequence $\beta_{kR} = (\eta_k^R, \gamma_{kR})$. It forms a Markov renewal process, and since the leading component η_k^R is an exponentially ergodic Markov chain, then β_{kR} is also exponentially ergodic with an ergodicity factor $\widetilde{\rho_R}$.

For the Markov random evolutionary process β_{kR}, the law of large numbers is valid

$$\frac{1}{n} \sum_{k=1}^{[tn]} \gamma_{kR} \xrightarrow[weakly]{x} tE_{\pi_R}\gamma_{1R} \text{ as } n \to \infty, \ x \in X, \ t \ge 0. \qquad [10.63]$$

Due to the degeneracy of the limit distribution [10.63] and the relation [10.60], the joint convergence takes place

$$(a_\varepsilon \mu_\varepsilon,\ \xi_\varepsilon(t)) \xrightarrow[weakly]{x} (L((\pi(R)))^{-1},\ tE_{\pi_R}\gamma_{1R}) \quad \text{as} \quad \varepsilon \to 0,\ \ t \geq 0,$$

where

$$\xi_\varepsilon(t) = a_\varepsilon \sum_{k=1}^{[ta_\varepsilon^{-1}]} \gamma_{kR}.$$

Let us show the compactness of processes $\xi_\varepsilon(t)$ in the topology U. Let us represent $\xi_\varepsilon(t)$ as a difference of monotonous processes

$$\xi_\varepsilon(t) = \xi_\varepsilon^+(t) - \xi_\varepsilon^-(t),$$

where

$$\xi_\varepsilon^\pm(t) = a_\varepsilon \sum_{k=1}^{[ta_\varepsilon^{-1}]} \gamma_{kR}^\pm.$$

Since the sequence $\beta_{kR}^\pm = (\eta_k^R,\ \gamma_{kR}^\pm)$ forms a Markov renewal process, then for the same reasons as in equation [10.63],

$$\xi_\varepsilon^\pm(t) \xrightarrow[weakly]{x} tE_{\pi_R}\gamma_{1R}^\pm, \quad \text{as} \quad n \to \infty,\ \ x \in X,\ \ t \geq 0. \qquad [10.64]$$

Since the processes $\xi_\varepsilon^\pm(t)$ are monotone, and the corresponding processes in equation [10.64] are compact in the topology U, it follows that it is also compact in the topology U their difference, i.e.

$$\lim_{h\to 0} \overline{\lim_{\varepsilon \to 0}} P_x\{\Delta_u(\xi_\varepsilon(\cdot),\ h,\ T) > \delta\} = 0, \quad \forall \delta,\ T > 0.$$

It is obvious that the process $L((\pi(R)^{-1})$ is compact in the topology U.

The application of theorem 3.2 (Sil'vestrov and Teugels 2004) on the weak convergence of a superposition of random functions completes the proof of convergence [10.62].

Theorem 10.3 is proven. □

PROOF OF THEOREM 10.4.– Now, we will evaluate the residue δ_ε in the representation of equation [10.58] with the normalizing factor $\sqrt{a_\varepsilon}$:

$$\begin{aligned}
&P_x\{|\sqrt{a_\varepsilon}\delta_\varepsilon| > \delta\} \leq P_x\{\sqrt{a_\varepsilon}\Delta_{\mu_\varepsilon R} > \delta\} = \\
&= P_x\{\mu_\varepsilon > ta_\varepsilon^{-1},\ \sqrt{a_\varepsilon}\Delta_{\mu_\varepsilon R} > \delta\} + P_x\{\mu_\varepsilon \leq ta_\varepsilon^{-1},\ \sqrt{a_\varepsilon}\Delta_{\mu_\varepsilon R} > \delta\} \leq \\
&\leq P_x\{a_\varepsilon \mu_\varepsilon > t\} + P_x\{\sqrt{a_\varepsilon} \max_{k \leq ta_\varepsilon^{-1}} \Delta_{kR} > \delta\}.
\end{aligned}$$

By virtue of equation [10.60], the first term is arbitrarily small for sufficiently big t.

For the second term, the relation

$$P_x\{\sqrt{a_\varepsilon} \max_{k \le ta_\varepsilon^{-1}} \Delta_{kR} > \delta\} \to 0 \text{ as } \varepsilon \to 0, \ \forall t > 0, \quad x \in X. \qquad [10.65]$$

is shown literally in the same way as the ratio [10.61].

Consequently,

$$\sqrt{a_\varepsilon}\delta_\varepsilon \xrightarrow{P_x} 0 \text{ as } \varepsilon \to 0, \ \forall x \in X. \qquad [10.66]$$

As shown earlier, for all $x \in X$

$$J_\varepsilon(t) = \sum_{k=1}^{[ta_\varepsilon^{-1}]} \chi_k(R, D_\varepsilon) \xrightarrow{P_x} J(t/\pi(R)), \quad \text{as } \varepsilon \to 0, \ t \ge 0, \qquad [10.67]$$

where $J(t)$ is the standard Poisson process.

For random evolutionary processes of step sums

$$\gamma_\varepsilon(t) = \sqrt{a_\varepsilon} \sum_{k=1}^{[ta_\varepsilon^{-1}]} \gamma_{kR},$$

defined on the exponential ergodic Markov chain β_{kR} (the first term may be different from the others, but does not affect the validity of the assertion), the principle of invariance is valid, and therefore, for all $x \in X$

$$\gamma_\varepsilon(t) = \sqrt{a_\varepsilon} \sum_{k=1}^{[ta_\varepsilon^{-1}]} \gamma_{kR} \xrightarrow{P_x} W(t\sigma^2/\pi(R)), \quad \text{as } \varepsilon \to 0, \ t \ge 0. \qquad [10.68]$$

Let us now show that the joint convergence

$$\zeta_\varepsilon(t) = \left(J_\varepsilon(t), \ \gamma_\varepsilon(t)\right) \xrightarrow{P_\pi} \left(J(t/\pi(R)), \ W(t\sigma^2/\pi(R))\right), \ \varepsilon \to 0, \ t \in T^*, \qquad [10.69]$$

for some countable set T^* everywhere dense in $[0, \infty)$, for which $J(t/\pi(R))$ and $W(t\sigma^2/\pi(R))$ are independent.

To do this, we need an auxiliary assertion, which we formulate as a lemma.

Let η_n, $n \ge 0$ be a homogeneous exponentially ergodic Markov chain with the state space Y, B_Y, transition probabilities $Q(x, A)$ and invariant measure π,

$$\overline{\gamma_{k\varepsilon}} = (\gamma_{1\varepsilon}, ..., \gamma_{k\varepsilon}), \ k = 1, ..., n$$

be random vectors, conditionally independent with respect to the chain β_n , i.e.

$$P\{\overline{\gamma_{k\varepsilon}} < \overline{u_k} \mid \beta_k = x_k\} = \prod_{k=1}^{n} F_\varepsilon(\overline{u_k} \mid x_k, x_{k-1}). \qquad [10.70]$$

Remember the notations

$$P_x(A) = P\{\eta_1 \in A \mid \eta_0 = x\}, \quad P_\mu(A) = \int_X \mu(dx) P_x(A).$$

LEMMA 10.6.– *Let the following conditions be verified:*

a) for some $V_\varepsilon \to \infty$

$$\sum_{k=1}^{[V_\varepsilon]} \overline{\gamma_{\varepsilon k}} \xrightarrow{P_\pi} \overline{\gamma} \quad as \ \varepsilon \to 0;$$

b) for any arbitrary $x \in Y$

$$\overline{\gamma_{\varepsilon 1}} \xrightarrow{P_x} \overline{\gamma} \quad as \ \varepsilon \to 0.$$

Then, $\overline{\gamma}$ *has an infinitely divisible distribution and on some countable everywhere dense set* $T^* \subset [0,\infty)$ *such that*

$$\overline{\gamma_\varepsilon}(t) = \sum_{k=1}^{[tV_\varepsilon]} \overline{\gamma_{\varepsilon k}} \xrightarrow[weakly]{} \overline{\gamma}(t), \quad t \in T^*$$

where $\overline{\gamma}(t)$ *is a homogeneous, stochastically continuous process with independent increments such that* $\overline{\gamma}(1) \simeq \overline{\gamma}$.

PROOF OF LEMMA 10.6.– From condition b), it obviously follows that for arbitrary $n \in \mathbb{N}$, $x \in Y$

$$\sum_{k=1}^{n} \overline{\gamma_{\varepsilon k}} \xrightarrow{P_x} \quad \text{as } \varepsilon \to 0.$$

Consequently,

$$P_\pi\left\{\Big|\sum_{k=[V_\varepsilon/n]n+1}^{[V_\varepsilon]} \overline{\gamma_{\varepsilon k}}\Big| > \delta\right\} =$$

$$= \int_Y P_\pi\left\{\eta_{[V_\varepsilon/n]n} \in dy\right\} P_y\left\{\Big|\sum_{k=1}^{[V_\varepsilon]-[V_\varepsilon/n]n} \overline{\gamma_{\varepsilon k}}\Big| > \delta\right\} \leq$$

$$\leq \sum_{l=1}^{n} \int_Y \pi(dy) P_y\left\{|\sum_{k=1}^{l} \overline{\gamma_{\varepsilon k}}| > \delta/k\right\} \to 0 \quad \text{as } \varepsilon \to 0. \qquad [10.71]$$

Hence, it follows that

$$\sum_{k=[V_\varepsilon/n]n+1}^{[V_\varepsilon]} \overline{\gamma_{\varepsilon k}} \to 0 \quad \text{as } \varepsilon \to 0. \qquad [10.72]$$

Consequently,[1]

$$\Gamma_\varepsilon = \sum_{k=1}^{[V_\varepsilon]} \overline{\gamma_{\varepsilon k}} \overset{P_\pi}{\sim} \sum_{k=1}^{[V_\varepsilon/n]n} \overline{\gamma_{\varepsilon k}} = \Gamma_\varepsilon(n) \quad \text{as } \varepsilon \to 0. \qquad [10.73]$$

Obviously, $\Gamma_\varepsilon(n)$ can be broken down into two parts

$$\Gamma_\varepsilon(n) = \Gamma_\varepsilon^+(n) + \Gamma_\varepsilon^-(n) \qquad [10.74]$$

Here,

$$\Gamma_\varepsilon^\pm(n) = \sum_{k=1}^{n} \Gamma_{\varepsilon k}^\pm; \qquad \Gamma_{\varepsilon k}^+ = \sum_{i=(k-1)[V_\varepsilon/n]+[V_\varepsilon \delta_\varepsilon/n]}^{k[V_\varepsilon/n]} \overline{\gamma_{\varepsilon i}};$$

$$\Gamma_{\varepsilon k}^- = \sum_{i=(k-1)[V_\varepsilon/n]+1}^{(k-1)[V_\varepsilon/n]+[V_\varepsilon \delta_\varepsilon/n]} \overline{\gamma_{\varepsilon i}}; \qquad [10.75]$$

$$k = 1, ..., n; \;\; 0 < \delta_\varepsilon < 1, \;\; \delta_\varepsilon \to 0, \; \varepsilon \to 0, \;\; V_\varepsilon \delta_\varepsilon \to \infty.$$

From condition b), it follows that for some δ_ε, satisfying the conditions [10.75] and for arbitrary $\delta > 0$

$$P_\pi \left\{ \Gamma_\varepsilon^-(n) > \delta \right\} \le n P_\pi \left\{ \Gamma_{\varepsilon 1}^- > \delta/n \right\} \to 0, \quad \varepsilon \to 0. \qquad [10.76]$$

Since the chain β_n is exponentially ergodic, also the chain $(\beta_{n-1}, \beta_n, \overline{\gamma}_{\varepsilon n})$ is exponentially ergodic with defining parameters $\rho' = \rho'(\rho, h)$, $h' = h'(\rho, h)$ that depend only on the corresponding defining parameters (ρ, h) of the exponentially ergodic chain η_n and do not depend on ε. Therefore, applying Doob's estimate for the exponentially ergodic Markov chain β_n, we have

$$\sup_{y \in X} \left| E_y \exp\left(i\lambda \Gamma_{\varepsilon 1}^+\right) - E_\pi \exp\left(i\lambda \Gamma_{\varepsilon 1}^+\right) \right| \le \rho'^{\left[[\delta_\varepsilon V_\varepsilon/n] h'^{-1}\right]}. \qquad [10.77]$$

In addition, due to equation [10.76]

$$E_\pi \exp\left(i\lambda \Gamma_\varepsilon(1)\right) - E_\pi \exp\left(i\lambda \Gamma_{\varepsilon 1}^+\right) \to 0 \quad \text{as } \varepsilon \to 0. \qquad [10.78]$$

---

1 The symbol $\xi_\varepsilon \sim \eta_\varepsilon$ means that the random variables ξ_ε and η_ε if converge weakly, then simultaneously, and to the same limit.

For the characteristic function $\Gamma_{\varepsilon}^{+}(n)$, the following representation takes place:

$$E_{\pi} \exp\left(i\lambda\Gamma_{\varepsilon}^{+}(n)\right) =$$
$$= \int_{Y} E_{\pi} \exp\left(i\lambda\Gamma_{\varepsilon 1}^{+}(n-1)\right) \chi\left(\eta_{(n-1)[V_{\varepsilon}/n]} \in dy\right) E_{y} \exp\left(i\lambda\Gamma_{\varepsilon 1}^{+}\right). \tag{10.79}$$

Relations [10.77], [10.78] and [10.79] imply the convergence

$$E_{\pi} \exp\left(i\lambda\Gamma_{\varepsilon}^{+}(n)\right) - \left(E_{\pi} \exp\left(i\lambda\Gamma_{\varepsilon}(1)\right)\right)^{n} \to 0 \quad \text{as } \varepsilon \to 0. \tag{10.80}$$

On the other hand, by equation [10.76]

$$E_{\pi} \exp\left(i\lambda\Gamma_{\varepsilon}^{+}(n)\right) - E_{\pi} \exp\left(i\lambda\Gamma_{\varepsilon}(n)\right) \to 0 \quad \text{as } \varepsilon \to 0. \tag{10.81}$$

From the last two relations, we have

$$E_{\pi} \exp\left(i\lambda\Gamma_{\varepsilon}(n)\right) - \left(E_{\pi} \exp\left(i\lambda\Gamma_{\varepsilon}(1)\right)\right)^{n} \to 0 \quad \text{as } \varepsilon \to 0. \tag{10.82}$$

It follows from condition a) that the characteristic function on the left in equation [10.82] converges pointwisely to the limit characteristic function $\psi(\lambda)$ ($\psi(\lambda)$ is the characteristic function of the variable $\overline{\gamma}$). Therefore, due to equation [10.82], we have the fact of pointwise convergence of the function to some characteristic function $\varphi_n(t)$ such that $[\varphi_n(t)]^n = \psi(t)$. It follows that $\overline{\gamma}$ has an infinitely divisible distribution.

Reasoning similar to those given in the relations [10.77]–[10.82] shows that

$$\sum_{k=1}^{m[V_{\varepsilon}/n]} \overline{\gamma_{\varepsilon k}} \xrightarrow[weakly]{P_{\pi}} \overline{\gamma}_{n}^{(1)} + \ldots + \overline{\gamma}_{n}^{(m)}, \tag{10.83}$$

where $\overline{\gamma}_{n}^{(i)}$, $i = 1, \ldots, m$ are independent identically distributed random variables with characteristic function $\varphi_n(\lambda) = \sqrt[n]{\psi(\lambda)}$. And the reasoning given in equations [10.71] and [10.72] shows that

$$\sum_{k=1}^{m[V_{\varepsilon}/n]} \overline{\gamma_{\varepsilon k}} \overset{P_{\pi}}{\sim} \sum_{k=1}^{[mV_{\varepsilon}/n]} \overline{\gamma_{\varepsilon k}}. \tag{10.84}$$

Thus, we finally have

$$E_{\pi} \exp\left(i\lambda \sum_{k=1}^{[tV_{\varepsilon}]} \gamma_{\varepsilon k}\right) \to [\psi(\lambda)]^{t} \quad \text{as } \varepsilon \to 0, \tag{10.85}$$

for $t \in T^{*} = \mathbb{Q}$ – the set of rational numbers.

Carrying out reasoning similar to those given in the relations [10.71]–[10.72] and taking into account equations [10.77]–[10.82] , we have for $0 < t_0 < t_1 < ... < t_m$, $t_i \in T^*$

$$E_\pi \exp\left\{ i \sum_{l=1}^{m} \lambda_l \left(\sum_{k=1}^{[t_l V_\varepsilon]} \overline{\gamma}_{\varepsilon k} - \sum_{k=1}^{[t_{l-1} V_\varepsilon]} \overline{\gamma}_{\varepsilon k} \right) \right\} - $$
$$- \prod_{l=1}^{m} E_\pi \exp\left\{ i\lambda_l \left(\sum_{k=1}^{[t_l V_\varepsilon]-[t_{l-1} V_\varepsilon]} \overline{\gamma}_{\varepsilon k} \right) \right\} \to 0 \quad \text{as } \varepsilon \to 0. \qquad [10.86]$$

Taking into account equation [10.71], we have

$$E_\pi \exp\left\{ i\lambda_l \sum_{k=1}^{[t_l V_\varepsilon]-[t_{l-1} V_\varepsilon]} \overline{\gamma}_{\varepsilon k} \right\} - $$
$$- E_\pi \exp\left\{ i\lambda_l \sum_{k=1}^{[(t_l - t_{l-1}) V_\varepsilon]} \overline{\gamma}_{\varepsilon k} \right\} \to 0 \quad \text{as } \varepsilon \to 0. \qquad [10.87]$$

From equations [10.85]–[10.87], it follows the convergence, as $\varepsilon \to 0$:

$$E_\pi \exp\left\{ i \sum_{l=1}^{m} \lambda_l \left(\sum_{k=1}^{[t_l V_\varepsilon]} \overline{\gamma}_{\varepsilon k} - \sum_{k=1}^{[t_{l-1} V_\varepsilon]} \overline{\gamma}_{\varepsilon k} \right) \right\} \to \prod_{l=1}^{m} [\psi(\lambda_l)]^{t_l - t_{l-1}},$$

which is equivalent to the assertion of the lemma. Lemma 10.6 is proven. □

LEMMA 10.7.– *Let $\overline{\gamma}_{\varepsilon k} = (\overline{\gamma'}_{\varepsilon k}, \overline{\gamma''}_{\varepsilon k})$ be a random vector which components $\overline{\gamma'}_{\varepsilon k}$, $\overline{\gamma''}_{\varepsilon k}$ satisfy the conditions of lemma 10.6, and the corresponding limit vectors $\overline{\gamma'}$, $\overline{\gamma''}$ (which, by virtue of lemma 10.6, have infinitely divisible distributions) also have infinitely divisible distribution without a normal component and a normal multidimensional distribution, respectively.*

Then, for $\overline{\gamma}_{\varepsilon k}$, the conditions, and hence the statement of lemma 10.6, are satisfied, and $\overline{\gamma} = (\overline{\gamma'}, \overline{\gamma''})$, where $\overline{\gamma'}$ and $\overline{\gamma'}$ are independent.

PROOF OF LEMMA 10.7.– Since condition b) of lemma 10.6 is satisfied for $\overline{\gamma'}_{\varepsilon k}$,, $\overline{\gamma''}_{\varepsilon k}$, it is obvious that it is also satisfied for $\overline{\gamma}_{\varepsilon k}$.

Let us show that from any sequence $\varepsilon_k \to 0$, it is possible to choose a subsequence $\varepsilon_{n_r} \to 0$ such that

$$\sum_{k=1}^{[V_\varepsilon]} \overline{\gamma}_{\varepsilon_{n_r} k} \xrightarrow[weakly]{P_\pi} \overline{\gamma}. \qquad [10.88]$$

The convergence of

$$\sum_{k=1}^{[V_\varepsilon]} \overline{\gamma'}_{\varepsilon_n k} \quad \text{and} \quad \sum_{k=1}^{[V_\varepsilon]} \overline{\gamma''}_{\varepsilon_n k}$$

implies a weak compactness of the sequence of distributions of random variables $P_\pi \left\{ \sum_{k=1}^{[V_\varepsilon]} \overline{\gamma}_{\varepsilon_n k} < \cdot \right\}$. Therefore, we can choose a subsequence of indices $\varepsilon_{n_r} \to 0$ for which the following weak convergence takes place:

$$P_\pi \left\{ \sum_{k=1}^{[V_\varepsilon]} \overline{\gamma}_{\varepsilon_{n_r} k} < \cdot \right\} \xrightarrow[weakly]{} F(\cdot).$$

By lemma 10.6, the limit distribution $F(\cdot)$ is infinitely divisible, and by convergences

$$\sum_{k=1}^{[V_\varepsilon]} \overline{\gamma'}_{\varepsilon_{n_r} k} \xrightarrow[weakly]{P_\pi} \overline{\gamma'}, \qquad \sum_{k=1}^{[V_\varepsilon]} \overline{\gamma''}_{\varepsilon_{n_r} k} \xrightarrow[weakly]{P_\pi} \overline{\gamma''}$$

and the fact that for any infinitely divisible distribution the normal and jump components are independent, we have

$$\sum_{k=1}^{[V_\varepsilon]} \overline{\gamma}_{\varepsilon_{n_r} k} \xrightarrow[weakly]{P_\pi} \overline{\gamma} = (\overline{\gamma'}, \overline{\gamma''}),$$

where $\overline{\gamma'}, \overline{\gamma''}$ are independent, and the limit distribution of the random variable $\overline{\gamma}$ does not depend on the choice of subsequence. Therefore,

$$\sum_{k=1}^{[V_\varepsilon]} \overline{\gamma}_{\varepsilon_{n_r} k} \xrightarrow[weakly]{\pi} \overline{\gamma} = (\overline{\gamma'}, \overline{\gamma''}),$$

where $\overline{\gamma'}, \overline{\gamma''}$ are independent.

Lemma 10.7 is proven. □

Note now that from equation [10.67], it obviously follows that

$$J_\varepsilon(t) \xrightarrow[weakly]{\pi_R} J_0(t/\pi(R)), \quad \text{as } \varepsilon \to 0 \ \ t \geq 0,$$

and from equation [10.68] that:

$$\gamma_\varepsilon(t) \xrightarrow[weakly]{\pi_R} W(t\sigma^2/\pi(R)), \quad \text{as } \varepsilon \to 0 \quad t \geq 0.$$

From the last two relations, applying lemma 10.7, we have

$$(J_\varepsilon(1), \gamma_\varepsilon(1)) \xrightarrow[weakly]{\pi_R} (J_0(1/\pi(R)), W(\sigma^2/\pi(R))) \qquad [10.89]$$

where $J_0(1/\pi(R))$, $W(\sigma^2/\pi(R))$ are independent.

From equation [10.89] and lemma 10.6, it follows that

$$(J_\varepsilon(t), \gamma_\varepsilon(t)) \xrightarrow[weakly]{\pi_R} \left(J_0(t/\pi(R)), W(t\sigma^2/\pi(R))\right), \quad t \in T^*, \qquad [10.90]$$

where $J_0(t/\pi(R))$, $W(t\sigma^2/\pi(R))$ are independent.

Let us show that

$$(J_\varepsilon(t), \gamma_\varepsilon(t)) \xrightarrow[weakly]{x} \left(J_0(t/\pi(R)), W(t\sigma^2/\pi(R))\right), \quad t \in T^*, \qquad [10.91]$$

for any $x \in X$, where $J_0(t/\pi(R))$, $W(t\sigma^2/\pi(R))$ are independent.

Let us choose a variable $b_\varepsilon \downarrow 0$, as $\varepsilon \to 0$ such that $a_\varepsilon = o(b_\varepsilon)$. For arbitrary $0 < t_1 < ... < t_m$, $t_i \in T^*$, there exists $\varepsilon_0 > 0$ such that $b_\varepsilon^{-1} < t_1 a_\varepsilon^{-1}$ for $\varepsilon < \varepsilon_0$.

By virtue of equations [10.67] and [10.68], b_ε can be chosen such that

$$\left(\sum_{k=1}^{[tb_\varepsilon^{-1}]} \chi_{kR}, \sum_{k=1}^{[tb_\varepsilon^{-1}]} \gamma_{kR} \right) \xrightarrow[weakly]{P_x} 0, \quad t \geq 0, \quad x \in R. \qquad [10.92]$$

Taking into account the last relation, we have that for the distributions

$$P_x \left\{ \sum_{k=1}^{[t_j a_\varepsilon^{-1}]} \chi_{kR} = n_j, \sum_{k=1}^{[t_j a_\varepsilon^{-1}]} \gamma_{kR} = u_j, \quad j = 1, ..., m \right\}$$

and

$$P_x \left\{ \sum_{k=[b_\varepsilon^{-1}]+1}^{[t_j a_\varepsilon^{-1}]} \chi_{kR} = n_j, \sum_{k=[b_\varepsilon^{-1}]+1}^{[t_j a_\varepsilon^{-1}]} \gamma_{kR} = u_j, \quad j = 1, ..., m \right\}$$

weak limits exist simultaneously and coincide.

Due to Doob's inequality for an exponentially ergodic chain η_n^R, χ_{kR}, γ_{kR}, we have

$$\sup_{x \in R} \left| P_x \left\{ \sum_{k=[b_\varepsilon^{-1}]+1}^{[t_j a_\varepsilon^{-1}]} \chi_{kR} = n_j, \quad \sum_{k=[b_\varepsilon^{-1}]+1}^{[t_j a_\varepsilon^{-1}]} \gamma_{kR} = u_j, \quad j = 1, ..., m \right\} - \right.$$

$$\left. - P_{\pi_R} \left\{ \sum_{k=[b_\varepsilon^{-1}]+1}^{[t_j a_\varepsilon^{-1}]} \chi_{kR} = n_j, \quad \sum_{k=[b_\varepsilon^{-1}]+1}^{[t_j a_\varepsilon^{-1}]} \gamma_{kR} = u_j, \quad j = 1, ..., m \right\} \right| \leq$$

$$\leq {\rho'}_R^{[b_\varepsilon^{-1}/h'_R]} \to 0, \quad \text{as } \varepsilon \to 0,$$

where (ρ'_R, h'_R) is the defining parameters of the chain η_n^R, χ_{kR}, γ_{kR}.

Taking into account equation [10.90] and the last relation, we obviously obtain equation [10.91] for $x \in R$.

Now, we need to show that equation [10.91] also holds for $x \in \overline{R}$. Let us choose some $x \in \overline{R}$ and fix it. It is obvious that:

$$\zeta_\varepsilon(t) = \zeta_\varepsilon(a_\varepsilon \tau(R) \wedge t) + \zeta'_\varepsilon(t - a_\varepsilon \tau(R) \wedge t), \qquad [10.93]$$

where

$$\zeta'_\varepsilon(u) = \zeta_\varepsilon(u + a_\varepsilon \tau(R)) - \zeta_\varepsilon(a_\varepsilon \tau(R)).$$

It is obvious that

$$\zeta_\varepsilon(a_\varepsilon^{-1} \tau(R) \wedge t) \xrightarrow{P_x} 0, \quad \text{as} \quad \varepsilon \to 0, \quad \text{for all} \quad x \in \overline{R}. \qquad [10.94]$$

The process $\zeta'_\varepsilon(u)$ has the same finite-dimensional distributions as the process $\zeta_\varepsilon(u)$ also in the case when the initial distribution of η_n will be $p(A) = P_x\{\eta_{\tau_R} \in A\}$ (the distribution $p(\cdot)$ be localized on R).

From equation [10.91], it obviously follows that for an arbitrary normal distribution $p(\cdot)$ localized on R, we have

$$(J_\varepsilon(t), \gamma_\varepsilon(t)) \xrightarrow[weakly]{P_p} \left(J_0(t/\pi(R)), W(t\sigma^2/\pi(R))\right), \quad t \in T^*, \qquad [10.95]$$

where $J_0(t/\pi(R))$, $W(t\sigma^2/\pi(R))$ are independent.

It follows from equation [10.95] and the remark made above that for any $x \in \overline{R}$

$$\zeta'_\varepsilon(t) \xrightarrow[weakly]{P_x} \zeta_0(t), \quad t \in T^*$$

The second term on the right in equation [10.93] can be represented as a superposition of random functions

$$\zeta'_\varepsilon(t - a_\varepsilon \tau(R) \wedge t) = \zeta'_\varepsilon(\theta_\varepsilon(t)),$$

where

$$\theta_\varepsilon(t) = t - a_\varepsilon \tau(R) \wedge t.$$

For any $x \in \overline{R}$

$$\theta_\varepsilon(t) \xrightarrow{P_x} t \quad \text{as} \quad \varepsilon \to 0, \quad t \geq 0. \qquad [10.96]$$

It follows from equation [10.68] and the remarks made above that

$$\lim_{h\to 0} \overline{\lim_{\varepsilon \to 0}} P_p \left\{ \Delta_U(\gamma_\varepsilon(t),\, h,\, T) > \delta \right\} = 0$$

for arbitrary T, $\delta > 0$.

From relation [10.95], we have for arbitrary $t_1, ..., t_m > 0$

$$\alpha_\varepsilon(t) = (J_\varepsilon(t_1), ..., J_\varepsilon(t_m),\, \gamma_\varepsilon(t)) \xrightarrow[weakly]{P_p}$$

$$\xrightarrow[weakly]{P_p} \left(J_0(t_1/\pi(R)), ..., J_0(t_m/\pi(R)),\, W(f\sigma^2/\pi(R)) \right), \quad t \in T^*.$$

It is obvious that

$$\Delta_U(\alpha_\varepsilon(t),\, h,\, T) = \Delta_U(\gamma_\varepsilon(t),\, h,\, T).$$

It follows from the last three relations that for any initial distribution p localized on R

$$\alpha_\varepsilon(t) \xrightarrow{U} \alpha_0(t), \quad t \in T^*. \qquad [10.97]$$

Consequently, the weak convergence of the joint distributions of any U-continuous functionals defined on the process $\alpha_\varepsilon(t)$. In particular, for all t_i, $t'_i < t''_i \in T^*$, $i = 1, ..., m$

$$\left(J_\varepsilon(t_i),\, \sup_{t \in [t'_i, t''_i]} (\inf)\, \gamma_\varepsilon(t) \right) \xrightarrow[weakly]{P_p}$$

$$\xrightarrow[weakly]{P_p} \left(J_0(t_1/\pi(R)),\, \sup_{t \in [t'_i, t''_i]} (\inf)\, W(t\sigma^2/\pi(R)) \right). \qquad [10.98]$$

Since the processes $J_\varepsilon(t)$ are monotone, and in equation [10.96], the convergence to a degenerate law is verified, then from equations [10.98] and [10.96], we have for $t \geq 0$:

$$s\left(\theta_\varepsilon(t),\ \sup_{t\in[t_i',t_i'']}(\inf)J_\varepsilon(t),\ \sup_{t\in[t_i',t_i'']}(\inf)\gamma_\varepsilon(t)\right)\xrightarrow[weakly]{P_p}$$

$$\xrightarrow[weakly]{P_p}\left(t,\ \sup_{t\in[t_i',t_i'']}(\inf)J_0(t/\pi(R)),\ \sup_{t\in[t_i',t_i'']}(\inf)W(t\sigma^2/\pi(R))\right)$$

Moreover, since the limit process $\left(J_0(t/\pi(R)),\ W(t\sigma^2/\pi(R))\right)$ is stochastically continuous, t is a point of continuity of this process with probability 1.

Are all the conditions of the theorem 3.2 (Sil'vestrov and Teugels 2004) on the weak convergence of superpositions of random functions, applying which we obtain that for $x \in \overline{R}$

$$\zeta_\varepsilon'(t-\tau(R)a_\varepsilon \wedge t)\xrightarrow[weakly]{}\zeta_0(t),\quad t\in T^*.$$

Taking into account equations [10.93] and [10.94], we have

$$\zeta_\varepsilon'(t)\xrightarrow[weakly]{x}\zeta_0(t),\quad t\in T^*,\quad \forall x\in X. \qquad [10.99]$$

Note that for any $x \in X$, $u_i \in R_1$

$$P_x\{J_\varepsilon(t)=0,\ \gamma_\varepsilon(t_i)<u_i\}=P_x\{a_\varepsilon\mu_\varepsilon>t,\ \gamma_\varepsilon(t_i)<u_i\}\quad i=1,...,m. \qquad [10.100]$$

From equations [10.99] and [10.99], we have for arbitrary $u_i \in R_1$, $t, t_i \in T^*$, $i = 1, ..., m$

$$\begin{aligned}P_x\{a_\varepsilon\mu_\varepsilon>t,\ \gamma_\varepsilon(t_i)<u_i\}\to & P\{J_0(t/\pi(R)=0,\ W(\sigma^2t_i/\pi(R))<u_i\}=\\ &=\exp(t/\pi(R))P\{(W(\sigma^2t_i/\pi(R))<u_i\}.\end{aligned} \qquad [10.101]$$

Since T^* is dense everywhere, equation [10.101] is true for all $t \geq 0$.

Therefore, taking into account equation [10.60], we have for any $x \in X$

$$\left(a_\varepsilon\mu_\varepsilon,\ \sum_{k=1}^{[a_\varepsilon^{-1}t]}\gamma_{kR}\right)\xrightarrow[weakly]{x}\left(L(\pi(R))^{-1},\ W(\sigma^2t/\pi(R))\right),\quad t\in T^* \qquad [10.102]$$

where $L(\pi(R))^{-1}$ and $W(\sigma^2t/\pi(R))$ are independent.

It is obvious that $L(\pi(R))^{-1}$ is the point of continuity of the process $W(\sigma^2 t/\pi(R))$ with probability 1 (the process $W(\sigma^2 t/\pi(R))$ is continuous).

Because for $\gamma_\varepsilon(t)$ the invariance principle [10.68] is valid, the processes $\gamma_\varepsilon(t)$ are compact in topology U.

Thus, all conditions of the theorem 3.2 on the weak convergence of superpositions of random functions (Sil'vestrov and Teugels 2004) are satisfied, applying which in equation [10.58], taking into account equations [10.66], [10.60] and [10.68], we obtain

$$\sqrt{a_\varepsilon}\xi_\varepsilon \xrightarrow[weakly]{P_x} W(\sigma^2 L).$$

Theorem 2.2 is proven. □

10.3. Explicit representation for the normalizing function

Recall the definition of the normalizing function

$$a_{\varepsilon R} = \int_R \pi(dx) f_R(x, D_\varepsilon),$$

where

$$f_R(x, D_\varepsilon) = P_x\{\tau(D_\varepsilon) \leq \tau(R)\}$$

is the probability of reaching the "hard-to-reach set" D_ε before hitting the set R.

The purpose of this section is to clarify the conditions under which we have

$$a_{\varepsilon R} \sim \pi(D_\varepsilon). \qquad [10.103]$$

LEMMA 10.8.– *Let conditions A, B, D, E be satisfied, and there is a sequence of sets* K_N, $N = 1, 2, \ldots$ *for which*

a) $\pi(K_N) < \infty$, $N = 1, 2, \ldots$;

b) $\lim_{\varepsilon \to 0} \sup_{x \in K_N} P(x, D_\varepsilon)/\pi(D_\varepsilon) < \infty$, $N = 1, 2, \ldots$;

c) $\lim_{N \to \infty} \overline{\lim}_{\varepsilon \to 0} \int_{\overline{K}_N} P(x, D_\varepsilon)/\pi(D_\varepsilon)\pi(dx) = 0$.

Then for $R \in \mathfrak{L}'_D$ *the relation* [10.103] *is verified.*

PROOF OF LEMMA 10.8.– The probabilities $f_R(x, D_\varepsilon)$ satisfy the system of linear integral equations

$$f_R(x, D_\varepsilon) = P(x, D_\varepsilon) + \int_{\overline{R \cup D_\varepsilon}} P(x, dy) f_R(x, D_\varepsilon), \quad x \in X,$$

and can be represented as

$$f_R(x, D_\varepsilon) = P(x, D_\varepsilon) + \int_{\overline{R \cup D_\varepsilon}} \rho_x(dz, R \cup D_\varepsilon) P(z, D_\varepsilon) =$$
$$= P(x, D_\varepsilon) + \int_{\overline{R}} \rho_{x\varepsilon}(dz, R \cup D_\varepsilon).$$

Here,

$$\rho_x(A, B) = E_x \nu(A, B), \quad \rho_{x\varepsilon}(A, B) = E_x \nu(A \cup \overline{D}_\varepsilon, B),$$

where

$$\nu(A, B) = \sum_{k=1}^{\tau(B)} \chi_A(\eta_{k-1}).$$

Hence, we have

$$a_{\varepsilon R} = \int_R \pi(dx) f_R(x, D_\varepsilon) = \int_R \pi(dx) P(x, D_\varepsilon) +$$
$$+ \int_{\overline{R}} \rho^R_{\pi_\varepsilon}(dz, R \cup D_\varepsilon) P(z, D_\varepsilon). \quad [10.104]$$

Here,

$$\rho^s_p(A, B) = E_p \chi_s(\eta_0) \nu(A, B) = \int_s p(dx) \rho_x(A, B),$$
$$\rho^s_{p\varepsilon}(A, B) = \rho^s_p(A \cap \overline{D}^s_\varepsilon, B).$$

Since

$$\nu(A \cap \overline{D}_\varepsilon, R \cup D_\varepsilon) = \sum_{k=1}^{\tau(R) \wedge \tau(D_\varepsilon)} \chi_{A \cap \overline{D}_\varepsilon}(\eta_{k-1}) \leq \nu(A, R),$$

and by virtue of condition E

$$\nu(A \cap \overline{D}_\varepsilon, R \cup D_\varepsilon) \xrightarrow{P_p} \nu(A, R),$$

hence

$$\rho^R_{\pi\varepsilon}(A, R \cup D_\varepsilon) \leq \rho^R_\pi(A, R),$$

and by Lebesgue's theorem

$$\rho^R_{\pi\varepsilon}(A, R \cup D_\varepsilon) \to \rho^R_\pi(A, R). \quad [10.105]$$

Let us show that

$$R_\varepsilon = [\pi(D_\varepsilon)]^{-1} \left(\int_{\overline{R}} \pi(dz) P(z, D_\varepsilon) - \rho^R_{\pi\varepsilon}(dz, R \cup D_\varepsilon) P(z, D_\varepsilon) \right) \to 0 \qquad [10.106]$$

as $\varepsilon \to 0$.

Let us use the identity

$$\rho^R_\pi(A, R) = \int_R \pi(dx) E_x \nu(A, R) = \pi(R) \int_R \pi(dx) E_x \nu(A, R) = $$
$$= \pi(R)[\pi(R)]^{-1} \pi(A) = \pi(A).$$

The integral in the second part of the formula is an invariant measure for the chain η_n under conditions A, B, and by definition it takes the value 1 on R. As is well known, all invariant measures differ only by a constant factor.

So, we have

$$R_\varepsilon = \int_{\overline{R}} \left[\rho^R_\pi(dz, R) - \rho^R_{\pi\varepsilon}(dz, R) \right] P(z, D_\varepsilon)[\pi(D_\varepsilon)]^{-1} =$$
$$= \int_{\overline{R} \cap K_N} \left[\rho^R_\pi(dz, R) - \rho^R_{\pi\varepsilon}(dz, R) \right] P(z, D_\varepsilon)[\pi(D_\varepsilon)]^{-1} +$$
$$+ \int_{\overline{R} \cap \overline{K}_N} \left[\rho^R_\pi(dz, R) - \rho^R_{\pi\varepsilon}(dz, R) \right] P(z, D_\varepsilon)[\pi(D_\varepsilon)]^{-1} = R'_\varepsilon + R''_\varepsilon.$$

The term R'_ε tends to zero, as $\varepsilon \to 0$, due to conditions a) and b) and formula [10.105] for $N = 1, 2, \ldots$.

And the relation $R''_\varepsilon \to 0$ is proven by passing to the double limit

$$\lim_{N \to \infty} \overline{\lim_{\varepsilon \to 0}} R''_\varepsilon$$

using condition c).

Therefore, considering equations [10.104] and [10.106], we get

$$\frac{a_{\varepsilon R}}{\pi(D_\varepsilon)} = \frac{1}{\pi(D_\varepsilon)} \left(\int_R \pi(dx) P(x, D_\varepsilon) + \int_{\overline{R}} \pi(dx) P(x, D_\varepsilon) \right) + R_\varepsilon =$$
$$= 1 + R_\varepsilon \to 1, \quad \varepsilon \to 0.$$

Lemma 10.8 has been proven. □

11

Asymptotic Large Deviations for Semi-Markov Random Evolutionary Processes

11.1. Recurrent semi-Markov random evolutionary processes

As ever before, by the term "asymptotic large deviations", we mean the study of distribution a random time of entering a region with asymptotically decreasing probability of hitting it.

On some probability space $(\Omega, \mathfrak{F}, P)$, let there be defined:

(a) a random process $\xi(t)$, $t \geq 0$ with a state space $(X, \mathfrak{B})$, measurable relative to the pair of arguments (t, ω);

(b) $0 = a_0 < ... < a_n < ...$ a strictly monotonically increasing sequence with probability 1 of non-negative random variables a_n.

We will suppose that $\xi(t)$ has the "separability" property that the functionals $\tau(D) = \inf(s : s < t, \xi(s) \in D)$ are numerical non-negative (possibly, singular) random variables for any $D \in \mathfrak{B}$ and $t \geq 0$.

Let us also define the functionals:

$$\eta_n = \xi(a_n), \ n > 0,$$

and

$$\chi_{nD} = \chi(\tau_{\alpha_{n-1}}(D) \leq \alpha_n) = 1 - \chi(\xi(s) \notin D, \ \alpha_{n-1} < s \leq a_n), \ n \geq 1,$$

which are, due to the assumptions made above on the measurability and separability of the process $\xi(t)$, random variables with values in $(X, \mathfrak{B})$, and $\{0, 1\}$, $\mathfrak{F}_0$ respectively ($\mathfrak{F}_0 = \{\emptyset, \{0\}, \{1\}, \{0, 1\}\}$).

We will call $\xi(t)$ a semi-Markov random evolutionary process or random evolutionary process with semi-Markov switchings with switching instants a_n, if for any $D \in \mathfrak{B}$, the three-dimensional random sequence η_n, $\varkappa_n = \alpha_n - \alpha_{n-1}$, χ_{nD} (by definition $\varkappa_0 = \chi_{0D} = 0$ here) is a Markov renewal process, i.e. a homogeneous Markov chain with state space $Z = X \times [0, \infty) \times \{0, 1\}$; $\mathfrak{F}_z = \mathfrak{B} \times \mathfrak{F}_{[0,\infty)} \times \mathfrak{F}_0$ ($\mathfrak{F}_{[0,\infty)}$ is a Borel σ-algebra of subsets of $[0, \infty)$) where transition probabilities are the following:

$$P\left\{\eta_{n+1} \in A,\ \varkappa_{n+1} < t,\ \chi_{n+1D} = \frac{1 \pm 1}{2} \,\middle|\, \eta_n = x,\ \varkappa_n,\ \chi_{nD}\right\} =$$

$$= Q_D(x, A, t, \pm). \qquad [11.1]$$

Here and below, if no mention is made regarding for which of the parameters in it a relation is valid, it is assumed to hold for all admissible values of these parameters.

REMARK 11.1.– *The given definition of a semi-Markov random evolutionary process is especially rigged for investigating entry times $\tau_t(D)$ and is somewhat different from the general definition wherein equation* [11.1] *is replaced by the relation $P(A \mid \eta_n = x, B) = P(x, A)$, where A and B are the events from the appropriately defined σ-algebras of random events describing the "future" and the "past" of the process $\xi(t)$ with respect to the times a_n.*

When equation [11.1] holds, the sequence η_n, $n = 0, 1, \ldots$ is also a homogeneous Markov chain with state space $X, \mathfrak{B}$, and transition probabilities:

$$P(x, A) = Q_D(x, A, \infty, +) + Q_D(x, A, \infty, -).$$

It is called the embedded Markov chain for semi-Markov random evolutionary process $\xi(t)$. We will assume fulfillment of the following conditions that are satisfied by the embedded Markov chain η_n:

(A) the σ-algebra is separable;

(B) η_n is a Harris φ-recurrent chain.

When conditions A and B hold, the chain η_n has a unique (to within a constant factor) σ-finite invariant measure $\pi(\cdot)$.

Let $D = \langle D_\varepsilon, \varepsilon > 0\rangle$ be a series of the state-space domains that satisfy the following conditions:

(C) $\varphi(D_\varepsilon) > 0$ for $ve > 0$ (reachability condition of the domain D_ε).

(D) $Q_{D_\varepsilon}(x, X, \infty, -) \to 0$ as $\varepsilon \to 0$ for all $x \in X$ (the condition of asymptotic remoteness with respect to a semi-Markov random evolutionary process $\xi(t)$).

Condition D is necessary and sufficient in order that:

$$P_x\{\tau_0(D_\varepsilon) \geq \alpha_n\} \to 1 \text{ as } \varepsilon \to 0 \ for\ x \in X,\ n \geq 1.$$

Hereinafter:

$$P_x(A) = P\{A/\eta_0 = x\} \text{ and } E_x\xi = E\{\xi \,|\, \eta_0 = x\}$$

Since in the sequel we will impose on semi-Markov random evolutionary process $\xi(t)$, ergodicity conditions guarantee its regularity, i.e. fulfillment of the relation:

$$a_n \xrightarrow{P_x} \infty \text{ as } n \to \infty \text{ for all } x \in X.$$

For this purpose, the condition D will be necessary and sufficient in order that:

$$\tau_0(D_\varepsilon) \xrightarrow{P_x} \infty \text{ as } n \to \infty, \ x \in X, \, n \geq 1.$$

Let $\beta(R, D) = \min(n : \lambda_{nD} = 1)$ be the number of the cycle $(a_{n-1}, a_n]$ in which the first entry of the domain D_ε occurs and:

$$g_R(x, D_\varepsilon) = P_x\{\beta(R, D_\varepsilon) \leq \tau(R)\}.$$

Here and below:

$$\tau(R) = \min(n, \, n \geq 1, \, \eta_n \in R)$$

are the first entry times into R of the embedded Markov chain η_n (as opposed to the first entry times $\tau_0(R)$ for a semi-Markov random evolutionary process $\xi(t)$). Obviously, when the condition D holds, we have $g_R(x, D_\varepsilon) \to 0$ as $\varepsilon \to 0$ for all $x \in X$.

Now, we denote N_D the class of sets R with $0 < \varphi(R) < \infty$ such that:

(a) the embedded Markov chain considered at the times of successive entering in R (we will denote it by η_n^R) is uniformly φ-recurrent;

(b) $\sup_{x \in R} g_R(x, D_\varepsilon) \to 0$ as $\varepsilon \to 0$.

The structure of the class N_D is described by the next lemma (see Chapter 10, 10.4).

LEMMA 11.1.– *When conditions A, B, C and D hold, the class N_D is φ-dense. The role of normalizing functions for $\tau_0(D_\varepsilon)$ is played by the functions:*

$$g_R(D_\varepsilon) = \int_R \pi(dx) g_R(x, D_\varepsilon).$$

To formulate the limit theorem, we will also impose the ergodicity condition for a semi-Markov random evolutionary process $\xi(t)$:

$$\int_X E_x a_1 \pi(dx) = m_\pi < \infty.$$

The fact that $m_\pi > 0$ follows from the initial assumption on the positivity of the random variable a_1.

11.2. Asymptotic large deviations

The limit behavior of large deviations for semi-Markov random evolutionary process characterizes the following limit result.

THEOREM 11.1.– *Let conditions A, B, C and D hold:*

(I) if condition D holds, then:

$$g_R(x, D_\varepsilon) \downarrow 0 \quad \text{and } P_x\{m_\pi^{-1} g_R(x, D_\varepsilon)\tau_0(D_\varepsilon) > t\} \to e^{-t} \qquad [11.2]$$

$$\text{as } \varepsilon \to 0 \text{ for all } x \in X, \quad \text{for any } R \in N_D;$$

(II) if for some function a_ε, $0 < a_\varepsilon \to 0$, as $\varepsilon \to 0$, then:

$$P_x\{a_\varepsilon \tau_0(D_\varepsilon) < \cdot\} \xrightarrow[weakly]{} F(\cdot) \quad \text{as } \varepsilon \to 0 \text{ for all } x \in X. \qquad [11.3]$$

where F is a non-singular distribution function on $[0, \infty)$ continuous at zero, then the asymptotic remoteness condition D holds, $a_\varepsilon \sim a g_R(D_\varepsilon)$, for some constant $a > 0$ and F is the exponential distribution function with parameter $m_\pi^{-1} a^{-1}$.

REMARK 11.2.– *Theorem 11.1 and the lemma are generalizations of theorem 10.1 and lemma 10.4 of the Chapter 10, since in case $a_n \equiv n$ and $\xi(t) = \eta[t]$, $t \geq 0$, the considered semi-Markov random evolutionary process completely reduces to the case considered in Chapter 10, of a discrete-time homogeneous Markov chain.*

Conditions D and E here go over into conditions E and C of Chapter 10 respectively. The proof of lemma is completely analogous to that of lemma 10.4.

PROOF OF THEOREM 11.1.– The proof is basically analogous to that of theorem 10.1. Hence, we will only dwell on the points where it differs from that of theorem 10.1. For fixed $R \in N_D$, we introduce the functionals:

$$\tau(n, R) = \min(k : k > \tau(n-1, R), \ \eta_k \in R,$$

$$\varkappa_{nR} = a_{\tau(n+1,R)} - a_{\tau(n,R)}, \quad n \geq 0,$$

$$\psi_{nR}(D_\varepsilon) = 1 - \chi(\xi(s) \notin D_\varepsilon, \ a_{\tau(n-1,R)} < s \leq a_{\tau(n,R)} =$$

$$= 1 - \prod_{k=\tau(n-1,R)+1}^{\tau(n,R)} (1 - \chi_{kD_\varepsilon}), \quad n \geq 1,$$

$$\mu(R, D_\varepsilon) = \min(n : n \geq 1, \ \psi_{nR}(D_\varepsilon) = 1).$$

For $\tau_0(D_\varepsilon)$:

$$\varkappa_{0R} + \ldots + \varkappa_{\mu(R,D_\varepsilon)-2R} \leq \tau_0(D_\varepsilon) \leq \varkappa_{0R} + \ldots + \varkappa_{\mu(R,D_\varepsilon)-1R}. \qquad [11.4]$$

Let us show that for the sums of random variables $\varkappa_{kR}$, the strong law of large numbers holds:

$$\pi(R)m_{\pi}^{-1}n^{-1}\sum_{k=1}^{[nt]}\varkappa_{kR}\xrightarrow{P1_x}t,\ \text{ for all } x\in X. \qquad [11.5]$$

Together with the Markov chain $\eta_n^R = \eta_{\tau(n+1,R)}$, let us consider the three-dimensional random sequence:

$$\beta_n^R = (\eta_n^R, {}_{n+1}^R, \varkappa_{n+1}^R)$$

which is also a homogeneous Markov chain with state space:

$$R\times R\times\varkappa_{n+1}^R,\ \mathfrak{B}\cap R\times\mathfrak{B}\cap R\times\mathfrak{F}_{[0,\infty)},$$

and transition probabilities:

$$P\{\eta_{n+1}^R\in A,\ \eta_{n+2}^R\in B,\ \varkappa_{n+1}^R<t\,|\,\eta_n^R=x,\ \eta_{n+1}^R=y,\ \varkappa_n^R=s\}=$$
$$=\chi_A(y)Q_R(y,\ B\,t),$$

where:

$$Q_R(y,\ B,\ t)=P_y\{\eta_{\tau(R)}\in B,\ a_{\tau(R)}<t\}.$$

It is not difficult to prove that the uniform φ-recurrency of the chain η_n^R guarantees the uniform φ_R-recurrency of the chain β_n^R with respect to the measure given by the relation (on rectangles):

$$\varphi_R(A\times B\times[0,t))=\int_A\varphi(dx)Q_R(x,B,t),$$

while the unique invariant probability measure $\widetilde{\pi}_R$ of the chain β_n^R is given by the relation:

$$\widetilde{\pi}_R(A\times B\times[0,t))=\int_A\pi_R(dx)Q_R(x,B,t),$$

where π_R is the unique invariant probability measure of the chain η_n^R. By the uniform φ_R-recurrency of the chain β_n^R, the strong law of large numbers is valid for it, that is:

$$n^{-1}(f(\beta_1^R)+\ldots+f(\beta_n^R))\xrightarrow{P1_x}\int f(x,y,t)\widetilde{\pi}_R(dx,dy,dt)$$

as $n\to\infty$, $x\in R$ for any $\widetilde{\pi}_R$-integrable function f. Applying it for the function $f(x,y,t)=t$, we obtain:

$$P\left\{\lim_{n\to\infty}n^{-1}\sum_{k=1}^{n}\varkappa_{kR}=c_R\,|\,\eta_0^R=x\right\}=1,\ \ x\in R, \qquad [11.6]$$

where:

$$\begin{aligned}
c_R &= \int_R t\widetilde{\pi}_R(dx, dy, dt) = \int_R \pi_R(dx) E_x a_{\tau(R)} \\
&= \int_R \pi_R(dx) \sum_{n=1}^{\infty} E_x \chi(\tau(R) > n-1) \varkappa_n \\
&= \int_R \pi_R(dx) \sum_{n=1}^{\infty} \int_X P_x\{\tau(R) > n-1,\, \eta_{n-1} \in dy\} E_y \varkappa_1 \\
&= \int_X \int_R \pi_R(dx) E_x \nu(\tau(R), dy) E_y \varkappa_1 \\
&= \int_X \pi^R(dy) E_y \varkappa_1 = m_\pi R.
\end{aligned}$$

Here, the measure π^R is defined, for $x \in X$, as follows:

$$\begin{aligned}
&P_x\left\{ \lim_{n\to\infty} n^{-1} \sum_{k=1}^{n} \varkappa_{k-1R} = \pi(R)^{-1} m_\pi \right\} = \\
&= P_x\left\{ \lim_{n\to\infty} (n-1)(n(n-1))^{-1} \sum_{k=1}^{n-1} \varkappa_{kR} = \pi(R)^{-1} m_\pi \right\} = \\
&= \int_R P_x\{\eta_{\tau(R)} \in dy\} \times P_y\left\{ \lim_{n\to\infty} (n-1)^{-1} \sum_{k=1}^{n-1} \varkappa_{kR} = \pi(R)^{-1} m_\pi \right\} = 1,
\end{aligned}$$

which proves relation [11.5].

For $R \in N_D$, and some normalization $b_{\varepsilon R} \downarrow 0$, the proof of the limit relation:

$$P_x\{b_{\varepsilon R}\mu(R, D_\varepsilon) > t\} \to e^{-t} \text{ as } \varepsilon \to 0, \text{ for } x \in X, \qquad [11.7]$$

is conducted completely analogously to the proof of lemma 10.1. The only difference is that the transition probabilities of the corresponding ancillary Markov chains $\eta^R_{\varepsilon n}$ have more complex analogue of representation [10.9] in Chapter 10:

$$P_{\varepsilon R}(x, A) = P_x\{\eta_{\tau(R)} \in A,\, \tau(R) < \beta(R, D_\varepsilon)\}(1 - g_R(x, D_\varepsilon))^{-1}$$

Verification of the conditions for applicability to the chains $\eta^R_{\varepsilon n}$, and the functions:

$$f_\varepsilon(x) = -\log(1 - g_R(x, D_\varepsilon))$$

of lemma 10.2 are performed just as in Chapter 10.

As in Chapter 10, the normalizing function in equation [10.7] has the form:

$$b_{\varepsilon R} = \int_R \pi_{\varepsilon R}(dx) f_\varepsilon(x);$$

where $\pi_{\varepsilon R}$ is the invariant probability measure of the chain $\eta^R_{\varepsilon n}$.

The asymptotic representation $b_{\varepsilon R}$ is established analogously to the corresponding representation for $b_{\varepsilon R}$ in Chapter 10. Finally, we use theorem 10.1 on the weak limit of superpositions of random functions in order to go over from estimates [11.4] and relations [11.5] and [11.7] to relation [11.2] of theorem in exactly the same way as in Chapter 10 it is going over from estimates [10.3] and relations [10.4] and [10.5] to relation [10.1] of theorem 10.1.

The proof of the second assertion of theorem 11.1 is analogous to the proof of the second assertion of theorem 10.1. □

The next theorem substantially generalizes the "necessity" assertion II of theorem 11.1.

THEOREM 11.2.– *Let Conditions A, B, C and D hold. Then, if for some $R \in N_D$, we verify:*

$$0 < g_R(D_\varepsilon) \to 0 \quad and \quad P_x\{g_R(D_\varepsilon)\tau_0(D_\varepsilon) < \cdot\} \xrightarrow[weakly]{} F(\cdot) \quad as \quad \varepsilon \to 0,$$

for all $x \in X$, where F is a non-singular distribution function on $[0, \infty)$ continuous at O, then the conditions of asymptotic remoteness D and ergodicity E hold, and F has the exponential distribution with parameter m_π^{-1}.

PROOF 11.1.– The fulfillment of condition D was shown in proving the assertion of theorem 11.1 (the condition E was not used here).

Suppose that the condition E does not hold, i.e. $m_\pi = \infty$. Then, from equation [11.5], we have:

$$P_x\left\{\lim_{n\to\infty} n^{-1} \sum_{k=1}^{n} \varkappa_{k-1} = +\infty\right\} = 1, \quad x \in X. \qquad [11.8]$$

Since [11.8] holds, we have the convergence

$$\mu(R, D_\varepsilon) \xrightarrow{P_x} \infty \quad \text{as} \quad \varepsilon \to 0. \qquad [11.9]$$

From equations [11.7]–[11.9], we have the sum:

$$g_R(D_\varepsilon) \sum_{n=1}^{\mu(R,D_\varepsilon)-1} \varkappa_{n-1R} =$$

$$= g_R(D_\varepsilon)(\mu(R,D_\varepsilon)-1)(\mu(R,D_\varepsilon)-1)^{-1} \sum_{n=1}^{\mu(R,D_\varepsilon)-1} \varkappa_{n-1R}.$$

This converges, as $\varepsilon \to 0$, in probability to ∞ as the product of random variables weakly converging to a strictly positive random variable ξ, and random variables converging in probability to $+\infty$. By estimate [11.4], from the last relation, it follows that:

$$g_R(D_\varepsilon)\tau_0(D_\varepsilon) \xrightarrow{P_x} \infty \quad \text{as} \quad \varepsilon \to 0,$$

but this contradicts the assumption of theorem 11.2. □

REMARK 11.3.– *From theorem 11.2, it follows that under the order-"compatible" normalization $O(g_R(D_\varepsilon))$ indicated in theorem 11.1, the limit distribution for the entry times to asymptotically receding domains can exist under natural conditions only for ergodic random evolutionary process with semi-Markov switchings, and this distribution is necessarily exponential.*

EXAMPLE 11.1.– Piecewise deterministic semi-Markovian random evolution.

Consider a three-dimensional sequence of random variables $(\beta_n, \eta_n, \varkappa_n)$, $n \geq 0$, with the state space $X \times Y \times R_+, \mathfrak{B}_X \times \mathfrak{B}_Y \times \mathfrak{B}_+$, which represents a Markov recovery process with transition probabilities:

$$P\{\beta_{n+1} \in B, \eta_{n+1} \in A, \varkappa_{n+1} < t \,|\, \beta_n = y, \eta_n = x, \varkappa_n = s\} =$$

$$= \begin{cases} \displaystyle\int_0^t \lambda(x,y,s)\exp\left(-\int_0^s \lambda(x,y,u)du\right)\int_A P^1(x,y,s,dx^1)\mu(x^1,B)ds, \\ \hfill \text{if} \quad t \leq s(x,y), \\ \displaystyle\int_0^{s(x,y,)} \lambda(x,y,s)\exp\left(-\int_0^s \lambda(x,y,u)du\right)\int_A P^2(x,y,s,dx^1)\mu(x^1,B)ds + \\ \displaystyle + \left[1 - \int_0^{s(x,y,)} \lambda(x,y,s)\exp\left(-\int_0^s \lambda(x,y,u)du\right)ds\right] \times \\ \displaystyle \hfill \times \int_A P^1(x,y,dx^1)\mu(x^1,B)ds, \quad \text{if} \quad t > s(x,y). \end{cases}$$

Here:

– $s(x,y)$ is a function, jointly measurable by (x,y) which maps $X \times Y \to [0,+\infty)$;

– $\lambda(x,y,t)$ is a function, jointly measurable by (x,y,t) which maps $X \times Y \to [0,+\infty)$;

– $P^2(x,y,t,A)$ is a function, jointly measurable at a fixed A by the variables (x,y,t); at fixed (x,y,t) is a probabilistic measure on $\mathfrak{B}_Y$;

– $P^1(x,y,A)$ is a function, jointly measurable at a fixed A by the variables (x,y); at fixed (x,y) is a probabilistic measure on $\mathfrak{B}_Y$;

– $\mu(x,B)$ is a measurable function by x, and a probabilistic measure on $B \in \mathfrak{B}_X$.

Now, we define:

$$\xi_n(t) = f(\beta_{n-1}, \eta_{n-1}, t),$$

where $f(x,y,t)$ is a measurable function, jointly measurable by the variables (x,y,t) which maps $X \times Y \times R_+ \to Y$, and $f(x,y,0) = y$.

The sequence $\zeta_n = (\bar{\xi}_n, \eta_n, \varkappa_n), \bar{\xi}_n) = (\xi_n(t), t \geq 0)$ forms a Markov renewal process with transition probabilities:

$$Q(x,A,C,t) =$$

$$= \begin{cases} \displaystyle\int_Y \mu(x,dy)\chi(f(x,y,\cdot) \in A) \int_0^t \lambda(x,y,s) \exp\left(-\int_0^s \lambda(x,y,u)du\right) \times \\ \qquad \times P^2(x,y,s,C)ds, \qquad \text{if} \quad t \leq s(x,y); \\ \displaystyle\int_Y \mu(x,dy)\chi(f(x,y,\cdot) \in A) \times \left\{ \int_0^{s(x,y)} \lambda(x,y,s) \exp\left(-\int_0^s \lambda(x,y,u)du\right) \times \right. \\ \displaystyle \times P^2(x,y,s,C)ds + \left[1 - \int_0^{s(x,y)} \lambda(x,y,s)\exp(-\lambda(x,y,u)du)ds\right] \times \\ \qquad \left. \times P^1(x,y,C) \right\}, \qquad \text{if} \quad t > s(x,y), \end{cases}$$

for $A \in \mathfrak{B}_X$, $C \in \mathfrak{B}_Y$.

The semi-Markov random evolutionary process $\xi(t)$, constructed along the trajectories $\zeta(n)$, is called the semi-Markov random evolutionary process with piecewise deterministic trajectories.

This process evolves as follows. At the moment of time $t = \tau_n$ $(n \geq 0)$, the state of the control component η_{n+1} determines the distribution of the variable β_{n+1}:

$$\mu(x, B) = P(\beta_{n+1} \in B \,|\, \eta_{n+1} = x).$$

Random variables $\eta_{n+1} = x$, $\beta_{n+1} = y$ uniquely determine evolution of the process $\xi(t)$ along the trajectory of the deterministic function $f(x, y, t)$, and two situations are possible: either the Markov renewal cycle has a non-random duration $s(x, y)$, determined by the initial conditions of the cycle $\eta_{n+1} = x$, $\beta_{n+1} = y$, or at an instant $t < s(x, y)$ occurs random break of the cycle with intensity $\lambda(x, y, t)$.

$P^1(\cdot)$ and $P^2(\cdot)$ are the conditional distributions of the control component η_n in the first and second situations respectively.

The absence of cycles of zero duration is ensured by the condition:

$$s(x, y) > 0, \quad \forall x \in X,\ y \in Y,$$

and the absence of cycles of infinite duration – one of the conditions:

$$\int_0^\infty \lambda(x, y, s)ds = +\infty, \quad \text{or} \quad s(x, y) < \infty.$$

In this case, the probability:

$$P_x(D) = P_x\{0 \leq \tau_0(D) < \tau_1\} =$$
$$= \int_Y \mu(x, dy) \int_0^{s(x,y)} \lambda(x, y, s) \exp(-\lambda(x, y, u)du) \int_X P^2(x, y, s, dx^1) \times$$
$$\times\, \chi((f(x, y, u), x^1, u) \notin D,\ 0 \leq u < s)ds + \int_Y \mu(x, dy) \times$$
$$\times \left[1 - \int_0^{s(x,y)} \lambda(x, y, s) \exp(-\int_0^s \lambda(x, y, u)du)ds\right] \int_X P^2(x, y, s, dx^1) \times$$
$$\times\, \chi((f(x, y, u), x^1, u) \notin D,\ 0 \leq u < s(x, y)).$$

The well-known model of piecewise linear Markov processes is embedded in the scheme under consideration. In this scheme, each state x is assigned a state index $r(x)$ which is a measurable function that maps $X \to \mathbb{N} = \{0, 1, 2, ...\}$; an open area $\Gamma_x \subset R_r(x)$ and a velocity vector $\overline{V}_x \in R_r(x)$, which are a measurable function over x, and:

a) $Y = \cup_{n=0}^{\infty} R_n$;

b) $\mu(x, \Gamma_x) = 1$;

c) $s(x, y) = \inf(t :\ y + \overline{V}_x t \in \partial\Gamma_x)$;

d) $\lambda(x,y,s) = \lambda(x,y+\overline{V}_x)$;
e) $P^1(x,y,A) = p^1(x,y+s(x,y)\overline{V}_x,A)$;
f) $P^2(x,y,s,A) = p^2(x,y,s\overline{V}_x,A)$;
g) $f(x,y,t) = y+\overline{V}_x t$.

Here, it is assumed that if $r(x) \neq 0$, then also $\overline{V}_x \neq 0$.

If $r(x) = 0$, then $R_0 = \{0\}, \Gamma_0 = R_0, \overline{V}_x = 0, s(x,y) = +\infty$.

12

Heuristic Principles of Phase Merging in Reliability Analysis

In the developing of the methods of phase space merging in reliability theory for Markov and semi-Markov processes with the corresponding heuristic approach (Korolyuk and Turbin 1982; Koroliouk and Koroliuk 2021). A surprising property of such heuristic principles is that any results obtained with their use can be justified rigorously by means of the phase merging algorithms (Koroliouk and Limnios 2005). The stationary phase merging Markov process techniques represent a particular cluster analysis, based on asymptotic properties of semi-Markov systems and is useful for simplification of reliability analysis, as shown for a duplicated renewal system.

12.1. The duplicated renewal system

The basic model represents stochastic systems with two identical working devices and one repairing facility.

The description of such a duplicated renewal system is determined by the working times α_k, $k = 1, 2$ of devices with an arbitrary distribution function $F_k(t) = P(\alpha_k \leq t)$, and by the repairing times β_k, $k = 1, 2$ with the distribution function $G_k(t) = P(\beta_k \leq t)$.

The working times of the system up to the first failure $\tau_k, k = 1, 2$ are dependent on the type of the initial working components.

The Laplace transform functions of the working times of the system, that are:

$$\varphi_k(s) := Ee^{-s\tau_k} = \int_0^\infty e^{-st} d\Phi_k(t)\,, \quad k = 1, 2$$

may be obtained by using the stochastic relations (see Gnedenko (1964a, 1964b) and also Koroliouk and Koroliuk (2021)):

$$\begin{aligned} \tau_1 &\doteq \alpha_1 + I(\alpha_1 \geq \beta_2)\tau_2, \\ \tau_2 &\doteq \alpha_2 + I(\alpha_2 \geq \beta_1)\tau_1. \end{aligned} \qquad [12.1]$$

The equality $\doteq$ means that the left and the right parts are identically distributed.

The stochastic relations [12.1] mean that during the working times α_k, $k = 1, 2$, the failure of the system can occur under the condition $\alpha_k < \beta_{k'}$, $k = 1, 2$, $k' = 2, 1$ with probabilities:

$$q_k = \int_0^\infty \overline{G}_{k'}(t) dF_k(t)\ , \quad k = 1, 2\ , \quad k' = 2, 1.$$

Therefore, the relations [12.1] imply the following system of algebraic equations:

$$Q(s)\varphi(s) = \psi(s), \qquad [12.2]$$

where $\varphi(s) = (\varphi_1(s), \varphi_2(s))\ , \quad \psi(s) = (\psi_1(s), \psi_2(s))$,

$$\psi_1(s) := \int_0^\infty e^{-st}\overline{G}_1(t) dF_2(t)\ , \quad \psi_2(s) := \int_0^\infty e^{-st}\overline{G}_2(t) dF_1(t). \qquad [12.3]$$

The matrix Q is defined as follows:

$$Q(s) := \begin{bmatrix} 1 & -g_1(s) \\ -g_2(s) & 1 \end{bmatrix}, \qquad [12.4]$$

where:

$$g_1(s) := \int_0^\infty e^{-st} G_2(t) dF_1(t), g_2(s) := \int_0^\infty e^{-st} G_1(t) dF_2(t). \qquad [12.5]$$

12.2. The duplicated renewal system in the series scheme

In order to simplify the duplicated renewal system, described by the linear algebraic equations [12.2]–[12.5], let us introduce the series scheme with a small series parameter $\varepsilon \to 0$ ($\varepsilon > 0$), under the following asymptotical conditions:

$$C1: \qquad \psi_k^\varepsilon(s) = \varepsilon \int_0^\infty e^{-\varepsilon st}\overline{G}_{k'}(t) dF_k(t) = \varepsilon q_k + o(\varepsilon),$$

$$q_k := P\{\beta_{k'} > \alpha_k\}\ , \quad k = 1, 2\ ; \quad k' = 2, 1.$$

$$C2: \qquad 1 - f_k^\varepsilon(s) = \varepsilon s \int_0^\infty e^{-\varepsilon st}\overline{F}_k(t) dt = \varepsilon s a_k + o(\varepsilon),$$

$$a_k := E\alpha_k\ , \quad k = 1, 2.$$

The asymptotical conditions C1 and C2 mean that the probabilities of failure $q_k^\varepsilon := P\{\beta_{k'}^\varepsilon > \alpha_k^\varepsilon\}$ tend to zero together with the mean values $a_k^\varepsilon = E\alpha_k^\varepsilon$ such that the ratio $q_k^\varepsilon \lambda_k^\varepsilon = q_k^\varepsilon / a_k^\varepsilon$ tend to finite values $\Lambda_k = q_k \lambda_k$, $k = 1, 2$.

Then, the matrix of system [12.2] in the series scheme has the following asymptotic representation:

$$Q^\varepsilon(s) = Q_0 + \varepsilon Q_1(s) + o(\varepsilon), \qquad [12.6]$$

where:

$$Q_0 = \begin{bmatrix} 1 & -1 \\ -1 & 1 \end{bmatrix}, \quad Q_1 = \begin{bmatrix} 0 & q_1 + sa_1 \\ q_2 + sa_2 & 0 \end{bmatrix}. \qquad [12.7]$$

The singularity of the matrix Q_0 ($\det Q_0 = 0$) means that the phase merging algorithm (Koroliouk and Koroliuk 2021) may be applied to solve the singularly perturbed (truncated!) equation:

$$[Q_0 + \varepsilon Q_1(s)]\varphi^\varepsilon(s) = \psi^\varepsilon(s). \qquad [12.8]$$

According to the phase merging principles (see Korolyuk and Turbin (1982), Koroliouk and Koroliuk (2021) and Koroliouk and Limnios (2005)), the average (limit) result takes place in the following form:

$$\varphi_1^0(s) = \varphi_2^0(s) = q/(q + sa)\ , \ \ q = (q_1 + q_2)/2\ , \ \ a = (a_1 + a_2)/2. \qquad [12.9]$$

The time-to-failure limits of the duplicated renewal systems, under the asymptotical assumptions C1 and C2, have identical exponential distribution:

$$\lim_{\varepsilon \to 0} P\{\tau_k^\varepsilon > t\} = e^{-\Lambda t}\ , \ \ \Lambda = q/a. \qquad [12.10]$$

REMARK 12.1.– *Let us introduce the mean intensity of the working time $\lambda := 1/a$. Then, the intensity of the failure time is $\Lambda = q\lambda$. Therefore, the formula [12.10] represents the failure time of the duplicated system with the failure probability q and with intensity λ.*

12.3. Heuristic principles of the phase merging

The phase merging algorithms described in Koroliouk and Koroliuk (2021); Koroliouk and Limnios (2005) may be formulated as some *heuristic phase merging principles* in the reliability analysis of redundant renewal stochastic systems with N elements (see Koroliouk and Koroliuk (2021), Chapter 3).

(1) The lack of memory. The common working time of a system till the instant of failure τ is determined by exponential distribution:

$$P(\tau > t) = e^{-\Lambda t} t \geq 0. \qquad [12.11]$$

(2) The superposition of failures. The intensity of the system failure is determined by the sum of intensities of system failures in every renewal state:

$$\Lambda = \sum_{k=1}^{N} \Lambda_k \, , \quad \tau = \min_{1 \le n \le N} \tau_n. \qquad [12.12]$$

According to the principle (2), the failure of the system can occur in every renewal state as was explained in section 12.3 for duplicated systems.

(3) The independence of the elements failures. The system failures for every element are determined by the failure rule as follows:

$$1/E\tau_k = \Lambda_k = q_k \lambda_k, \qquad [12.13]$$

where q_k is the probability of failure for kth state, and λ_k is the stationary intensity of working time for k-th state.

The heuristic principles action can be illustrated by analysis of *the duplicated renewal system.* Namely, two working devices are described by independent working-repairing processes with given distribution functions of the working times α_k and the repairing times β_k:

$$F_k(t) = P(\alpha_k \le t) \, , \quad G_k(t) = P(\beta_k \le t) \, , \quad k = 1, 2. \qquad [12.14]$$

Such a classical example of the system is usually called "two lifts system" (Zubkov 1975; Szász 1977).

The heuristic principles of the phase merging technique are based on use of the limit renewal theorem (Feller 1966) for the stationary residual time α^* expressed as:

$$P(\alpha^* \le t) = \lambda \int_0^t \overline{F}(s) ds \, , \quad \lambda = 1/E\alpha.$$

According to the heuristic principles, the described above the failure intensity of two lift system is the following:

$$\Lambda = q_1 \lambda_1 + q_2 \lambda_2 \, , \quad \lambda_k = 1/E\alpha_k \, , \quad k = 1, 2. \qquad [12.15]$$

The failure probabilities $q_k, k = 1, 2$ are determined as follows:

$$q_1 = P(\alpha_2^* > \beta_1) \, , \quad q_2 = P(\alpha_1^* > \beta_2). \qquad [12.16]$$

Here, the stationary remaining working times α_k^*, $k = 1, 2$, have the following distribution functions:

$$P(\alpha_k^* \le t) = \lambda_k \int_0^t \overline{F}_k(s) ds \, , \quad k = 1, 2. \qquad [12.17]$$

Under the natural *assumption of the repairing relative brevity*:

$$E\beta_k \ll E\alpha_k \ , \ \ k = 1, 2, \tag{12.18}$$

the intensity of the system failure for the duplicated renewal system may be estimated as follows:

$$\Lambda \simeq [E[\alpha_2 \wedge \beta_1] + E[\alpha_1 \wedge \beta_2]]/E\alpha_1 E\alpha_2. \tag{12.19}$$

The phase merging algorithms in Koroliouk and Koroliuk (2021) are the basis which verifies the heuristic phase merging principles.

12.4. The duplicated renewal system without failure

The duplicated renewal system without failure ($\beta_k = 0, k = 1, 2$) is described by a superposition of two renewal processes given by sums:

$$S_n^{\pm} = \sum_{r=1}^{n} \alpha_r^{\pm}, \tag{12.20}$$

of jointly independent and identically distributed (by $r \geq 1$) random variables $\alpha_r^{\pm}$, $r \geq 1$. For simplicity, we denote the working times α_1 and α_2 as α^+ and α^-, correspondingly.

The duplicated renewal system without failure and with working times α_k^+, α_k^-, $k \geq 0$, means that the working device substitution is accompanied by its instantaneous repairing.

The phase merging principles provide the base model of the duplicated renewal system without failure as a Markov chain $\widehat{x}_n, n \geq 0$ on the phase space $E = \{+, -\}$, is given by the sojourn times:

$$\widehat{\theta}_n^{\pm} = \alpha_n^{\pm} \wedge \alpha_n^{\mp *} \ , \ \ n \geq 1. \tag{12.21}$$

The transition probabilities of the Markov chain $\widehat{x}_n, n \geq 0$ with the sojourn times [12.21] are calculated as follows:

$$q_{\pm} = P\{\widehat{x}_{n+1} = \mp | \widehat{x}_n = \pm\} = P(\alpha_n^{\pm} > \alpha_n^{\mp *}),$$

that is:

$$q_{\pm} = q\lambda_{\mp} \ , \ \ q = \int_0^{\infty} \overline{F}_+(t)\overline{F}_-(t)dt \ , \ \ \lambda_{\pm} = 1/E\alpha^{\pm}. \tag{12.22}$$

Its generating matrix has the following form:

$$Q = P - I = \begin{bmatrix} -q_+ & q_+ \\ q_- & -q_- \end{bmatrix}. \tag{12.23}$$

The stationary distribution of the Markov chain with the generating matrix [12.23] is given by:

$$\Pi = \begin{bmatrix} \rho_+ & \rho_- \\ \rho_+ & \rho_- \end{bmatrix}, \quad \rho_\pm = \lambda_\pm / \lambda, \quad \lambda = \lambda_+ + \lambda_-. \qquad [12.24]$$

Introduce the orthogonal matrix:

$$\overline{\Pi} := \Pi - I = \begin{bmatrix} -\rho_- & \rho_- \\ \rho_+ & -\rho_+ \end{bmatrix}. \qquad [12.25]$$

It is easy to note that the generating matrix [12.23] has the following representation:

$$Q = \lambda q \overline{\Pi}. \qquad [12.26]$$

Now, let us define the potential matrix R_0 as a solution of the following equation:

$$QR_0 = R_0 Q = \overline{\Pi}, \quad R_0 \Pi = \emptyset. \qquad [12.27]$$

It is easy to verify that:

$$R_0 = -(\lambda q)^{-1} \overline{\Pi}. \qquad [12.28]$$

Now, using the Markov chain, given by the generating matrix [12.26] and the potential matrix [12.28], we can analyze the asymptotic properties of the reward functional, defined on the duplicated renewal system with failure.

The limit working time of the system with failure gives us the following approximation estimate:

$$\begin{aligned} E\zeta_\pm &\simeq [\lambda_+ c_+ + \lambda_- c_-]/q, \\ c_\pm &:= E\gamma^\pm. \end{aligned} \qquad [12.29]$$

The real-valued random variables $\gamma_n^\pm := \gamma_n(\pm)$ are given by the distribution functions:

$$\Gamma_\pm(u) = P(\gamma^\pm \le u), \quad u \in R. \qquad [12.30]$$

The heuristic principles of the phase merging formulated in section 12.4 are based on limit theorems for semi-Markov processes with absorbing state.

References

Anderson, P.W. (1954). A mathematical model for the narrowing of spectral lines by exchange or motion. *J. Phys. Soc. Jpn.*, 9, 316–339.

Anisimov, V.V. (2008). *Switching Processes in Queueing Models*. ISTE Ltd, London and John Wiley & Sons, New York.

Barbu, V. (1976). *Nonlinear Semigroups and Differential Equations in Banach Spaces*. Noordhoff International Publishers, Leiden.

Bartlett, M. (1957). Some problems associated with random velocity. *Publ. Inst. Satist. Univ. Paris*, 6(3), 261–270.

Bartlett, M. (1978). A note on random walks at constant speed. *Adv. Appl. Prob.*, 10, 704–707.

Bateman, H. and Erdelyi, A. (1953a). *Higher Transcendental Functions*, Volume I. McGraw-Hill, New York.

Bateman, H. and Erdelyi, A. (1953b). *Higher Transcendental Functions*, Volume II. McGraw-Hill, New York.

Bateman, H. and Erdelyi, A. (1955). *Higher Transcendental Functions*, Volume III. McGraw-Hill, New York.

Borovskikh, Y.V. and Korolyuk, V.S. (1997). *Martingale Approximation*. VSP, Utrecht.

Cane, V. (1967). Random walks and physical processes. *Bull. Intern. Stat. Inst.*, 42, 622–640.

Cane, V. (1975). Diffusion models with relativity effects. In *Perspectives in Probability and Statistics*, Gani, J. (ed.). Applied Probability Trust, Sheffield.

Chung, K.L. (2012). *Markov Chains: With Stationary Transition Probabilities (Grundlehren der mathematischen Wissenschaften, V.104)*. Springer Science & Business Media, Berlin.

Cohen, S.N. and Elliott, R.J. (2015). *Stochastic Calculus and Applications*. Birkhauser, Basel.

Doob, L. (1962). *Stochastic Processes*. Wiley, New York.

Ethier, S.N. and Kurtz, T.G. (1986). *Markov Processes: Characterization and Convergence*. John Wiley & Sons, New York.

Feller, W. (1966). *An Introduction to Probability Theory and its Applications*, Volume 1. Wiley, New York.

Feller, W. (1971). *An Introduction to Probability Theory and its Applications*, Volume 2. Wiley, New York.

Foong, S.K. (1992). First-passage time, maximum diplacement, and Kac's soltion of the telegraph equation. *Phys. Rev.*, 46(2), 707–710.

Foong, S.K. and Kanno, S. (1994). Properties of the telegrapher's random process with or without a trap. *Stoch. Process. Appl.*, 53, 147–173.

Furstenberg, H. (1963). Noncomuting random products. *Trans. Am. Math. Soc.*, 108, 377–428.

Gnedenko, B.V. (1964a). On spare duplication. *Eng. Cybernet.*, 4, 3–12.

Gnedenko, B.V. (1964b). On duplication with renewal. *Eng. Cybernet.*, 5, 111–118.

Gnedenko, B.V. and Ushakov, I. (1995). *Probabilistic Reliability Engineering*. Wiley, New York.

Gnedenko, B.V., Belyaev, Y.K., Solovyev, A.D. (1969). *Mathematical Methods of Reliability Theory*. Academic Press, New York.

Goldstein, S. (1951). On diffusion by discontinious movements and the telegraph equation. *Quart. J. Mech. Appl. Math.*, 4, 129–156.

Gorostiza, L. (1972). A central limit theorem for a class of d-dimential random motions with constant speed. *Bull. Am. Math. Soc.*, 78, 575–577.

Gorostiza, L. (1973a). The central limit theorem for random motions of d-dimentional Euclidean space. *Ann. Prob.*, 1, 603–612.

Gorostiza, L. (1973b). An invariance principle for a class of d-dimentional polygonal random functions. *Trans. Am. Math. Soc.*, 177, 413–445.

Grenander, U. (1963). *Probabilities on Algebraic Structures*. Almquist and Wiksell, Stockholm and Qoteborg, Uppsala.

Griego, R. and Hersh, R. (1969). Random evolutions, Markov chains, and systems of partial differential equations. *Proc. Natl. Acad. Sci.*, 62, 305–308.

Griego, R. and Hersh, R. (1971). Theory of random evolutions with applications to partial differential equations. *Trans. Am. Math. Soc.*, 156, 405–418.

Hannan, E.J. (1965). Group representations and applied probability. *J. Appl. Probab.*, 2(1), 1–68.

Hersh, R. (1974). Random evolutions: Survey of results and problems. *Rocky Mount. J. Math.*, 4, 443–477.

Hersh, R. and Papanicolaou, G. (1972). Non-commuting random evolutions, and an operator-valued Feynman-Kac formula. *Comm. Pure Appl. Math.*, XXX, 337–367.

Hersh, R. and Pinsky, M. (1972). Random evolutions are asymptotically Gaussian. *Comm. Pure Appl. Math.*, XXV, 33–34.

Hida, T. (1980). *Brownian Motion*. Springer-Verlag, New York and Berlin.

Hille, E. (1948). *Functional Analysis and Semi Groups*. American Mathematical Society, Providence, RI.

Jacod, J. and Shiryaev, A.N. (1987). *Limit Theorems for Stochastic Processes*. Springer, Berlin/Heidelberg.

Jenssen, A. (1990). The distance between the Kac process and the Wiener process with applications to generelized telegraph equations. *J. Theor. Probab.*, 3, 349–360.

Kac, M. (1957). *Some Stochastic Problems in Physics and Mathematics*. Magnolia Petroleum Company, Field Research Laboratory, Dallas, TX.

Kac, M. (1974). A stochastic model related to the telegrapher's equation. *Rocky Mount. J. Math.*, 4, 497–509.

Kaplan, S. (1964). Differential equations in which the Poisson process plays a role. *Bull. Amer. Math. Soc.*, 70, 264–268.

Kisinski, J. (1974). On M. Kac's probabilistic formula for the solution of the telegraphist's equation. *Ann. Pol. Math.*, 29(3), 259–272.

Knight, F.B. (1981). *Essentials of Brownian Motion and Diffusion*. American Mathematical Society, Providence, RI.

Kolesnik, A.D. (2001). Weak convergence of a planar random evolution to the Wiener process. *J. Theoret. Probab.*, 14(2), 485–494.

Kolesnik, A.D. (2003). Weak convergence of the distributions of Markovian random evolutions in two and three dimensions. *Bul. Acad. Stiinte Repub. Mold. Mat.*, 3, 41–52.

Koroliouk, D.V. (2015a). Binary statistical experiments with persistent nonlinear regression. *Theor. Probab. Math. Statist., AMS*, 91, 71–80.

Koroliouk, D.V. (2015b). Two component binary statistical experiments with persistent linear regression. *Theor. Probab. Math. Statist., AMS*, 90, 103–114.

Koroliouk, D.V. (2016). Stationary statistical experiments and the optimal estimator for a predictable component. *J. Math. Sci.*, 214(2), 220–228. DOI: 10.1007/s10958-016-2770-9.

Koroliouk, D.V. and Koroliuk, V.S. (2021). Diffusion approximation of queueing systems and networks. In *Queueing Theory 1: Advanced Trends*. ISTE Ltd, London and John Wiley & Sons, New York. DOI: 10.1002/9781119755432.ch3.

Koroliouk, D.V. and Samoilenko, I.V. (2021). *Random Evolutionary Systems: Asymptotic Properties and Large Deviations*. ISTE Ltd, London and John Wiley & Sons, New York.

Koroliouk, D.V., Koroliuk, V.S., Rosato, N. (2014). Equilibrium process in biomedical data analysis: The Wright-Fisher model. *Cybernetics and System Analysis*, 50(2014), 890–897.

Koroliouk, D.V., Koroliuk, V.S., Nicolai, E., Bisegna, P., Stella, L., Rosato, N.A. (2016). A statistical model of macromolecules dynamics for Fluorescence Correlation Spectroscopy data analysis. *Stat. Optim. Inf. Comput.*, 4, 233–242.

Korolyuk, V.S. (1975). *Boundary Value Problems for Complex Poisson Processes*. Naukova Dumka, Kyiv.

Korolyuk, V.S. and Limnios, N. (2005). *Stochastic Systems in Merging Phase Space*. World Scientifc, Singapore.

Korolyuk, V.S. and Swishchuk, A.V. (1995a). *Semi-Markov Random Evolutions*. Kluwer Academic Publishing, Amsterdam.

Korolyuk, V.S. and Swishchuk, A.V. (1995b). *Evolution of Systems in Random Media*. CRC Press, Boca Raton, FL.

Korolyuk, V.S. and Turbin, A.F. (1982). *Markov Renewal Processes in Problems of Reliability of Systems* [in Russian]. Naukova Dumka, Kyiv.

Korolyuk, V.S. and Turbin, A.F. (1993). *Mathematical Foundations of the State Lumping of Large Systems*. Kluwer Academic Publishing, Amsterdam.

Limnios, N. and Samoilenko, I. (2013). Poisson approximation of processes with locally independent increments with Markov switching. *Teor. Imovir. ta Matem. Statyst.*, 89, 104–114.

Liptser, R.S. (1994). The Bogolyubov averaging principle for semimartingales. *Proceedings of the Steklov Institute of Mathematics*, 4, 1–12.

Liptser, R.S. and Shiryaev, A.N. (2001). *Statistics of Random Processes II. Applications*. Springer, Berlin and Heidelberg.

Loéve, M. (1977). *Probability Theory I*, 4th edition. Springer-Verlag, Berlin, Heidelberg and New York.

Loéve, M. (1978). *Probability Theory II*, 4th edition. Springer-Verlag, Berlin, Heidelberg and New York.

Masyutka, O., Moklyachuk, M., Sidei, M. (2019). Filtering of multidimensional stationary processes with missing observations. *Univers. J. Math. Appl.*, 2(1), 24–32.

Moklyachuk, M., Masyutka, O., Sidei, M. (2018). Minimax extrapolation of multidimensional stationary processes with missing observations. *Int. J. Math. Models Methods Appl. Sci.*, 12, 94–105.

Nevelson, M.B. and Hasminskii, R.Z. (1973). Stochastic approximation and recursive estimation. *Am. Math. Soc., Translations Math. Monogr.*, 47.

Orsingher, E. (1985). Hyperbolic equations arasing in random models. *Stoc. Proc. Appl.*, 21, 93–106.

Orsingher, E. (1986). A planar random motion governed by the two-dimentional telegraph equations. *J. Appl. Probab.*, 23, 385–397.

Orsingher, E. (1987a). Stochastic motions driven by wave equation. *Rend. Sem. Mat. Fis. di Milano*, LVII, 365–380.

Orsingher, E. (1987b). Probabilistic models connected with wave equation. *Bol. Un. Mat. Ital.*, 1B, 423–437.

Orsingher, E. (1987c). Stochastic motions on the 3-sphere governed by wave and heat equation. *J. Appl. Probab.*, 24, 315–327.

Orsingher, E. (1989). Random processes connected with third order equation. *Intern. Vilnius Conf. on Prob. Theory and Math. Stat., Abstr. Commun.*, Vilnius 2, 67–68.

Orsingher, E. (1990a). Probability law, flow function, maximum distribution of wave-governed random motions and their connections with Kirchoff's laws. *Stoc. Proc. Appl.*, 34, 49–66.

Orsingher, E. (1990b). Random motions governed by third-order equation. *Adv. Appl. Prob.*, 22, 915–928.

Orsingher, E. (2002). Bessel functions of third order and the distribution of cyclic planar motions with three directions. *Stoch. Stoch. Rep.*, 74(3–4), 617–631.

Orsingher, E. and Bassan, B. (1992). On a 2n-valued telegraph signal at the related integrated process. *Stoch. Stoch. Rep.*, 38, 159–173.

Orsingher, E. and Kolesnik, A.D. (1994). The explicit probability law of a planar random motion governed by a fourth order hyperbolic equation. *Serie A*, 6, 9.

Orsingher, E. and Sommella, A. (2004). Cyclic random motion in R^3 with four directions and finite velocity. *Stoch. Stoch. Rep.*, 76(2), 113–133.

Papanicolaou, G. (1971a). Motion of a particle in a random field. *J. Math. Phys.*, 12, 1494–1496.

Papanicolaou, G. (1971b). Wave propagation in a one-dimential random medium. *SIAM J. Appl. Math.*, 21, 13–18.

Papanicolaou, G. (1973). Stochastic equations and their applications. *Am. Math. Monthly*, 80, 526–544.

Papanicolaou, G. and Hersh, R. (1972). Some limit theorems for stochastic equations and applications. *Indiana U. Math. J.*, 21, 815–840.

Papanicolaou, G. and Kellek, J. (1971). Stochastic differential equations with applications to random harmonic oscillations and wave propagation in random media. *SIAM J. Appl. Math.*, 21, 287–305.

Pinsky, M. (1968). Differential equations with a small parameter and the central limit theorem for functions defined on a finite Markov chain. *Z. Wahrscheinlichkeitstheorie verw. Geb.*, 2, 101–111.

Pinsky, M. (1991). *Lectures on Random Evolutions*. World Scientific, Singapore.

Samoilenko, I.V. (2001). Markovian random evolution in $\mathbf{R}^n$. *Rand. Operat. and Stoc. Equat.*, 2, 139–160.

Samoilenko, I.V. (2012). Weak convergence of Markov random evolutions in a multidimensional space. *International Scholarly Research Network*, 509789. DOI: 10.5402/2012/509789.

Shiryaev, A.N. (2018). *Probability-2*. Springer, New York.

Shurenkov, V.M. (1984). On the theory of Markov renewal. *Theory Probab. Appl.*, 29, 247–265.

Sil'vestrov, D.S. (1972). Remarks on the limit of a composite random function. *Theory Prob. Appl.*, 17, 669–777.

Sil'vestrov, D.S. and Teugels, J.L. (2004). Limit theorems for mixed max-sum processes with renewal stopping. *Ann. Appl. Probab.*, 14(4), 1838–1868.

Skorokhod, A.V. (1989). *Asymptotic Methods in the Theory of Stochastic Differential Equations*. American Mathematical Society, Providence, RI.

Smith, W.L. (1958). Renewal theory and its ramifications. *J. Roy. Stat. Soc., Ser. B*, 20, 243–302.

Stroock, D.W. and Varadhan, S.R.S. (1979). *Multidimensional Diffusion Processes*. Springer-Verlag, Berlin.

Szász, D. (1977). A problem of two lifts. *Ann. Prob.*, 5(4), 550–559.

Turbin, A.F. and Kolesnik, A.D. (1992). Hyperbolic equations of the random evolutions in R^m. In *Probability Theory and Mathematical Statistics – Proceedings of the 6th Ussr-Japan Symposium*, Watanabe, S., Fukushima, M., Koroliouk, V.S., Shiryaev, A.N. (eds). World Scientific, Singapore.

Turbin, A.F. and Plotkin, D.J. (1991). Bessel equations of high order. *Asymptotic Methods in Problems of Random Evolutions* [in Russian], 112–121.

Tutubalin, V.N. (1965). On limit theorems for the product of random matrices. *Theory Probab. Appl.*, 10(1), 15–28.

Zubkov, A.M. (1975). On the rate of convergence of a renewal density. *Math. USSR-Sb.*, 27–1, 131–142.

Index

A, B

asymptotic
  diffusion environment, 125
  large deviations, 209, 212
Bernoulli distribution, 36, 146, 148
Bessel
  distribution, 32, 34, 38
  equation, 43, 44
  function, 37, 43, 74

C, D

complex-analytic initial conditions, 99
discrete stochastic basis, 126
double exponential distribution, 32, 34

E, F

embedded Markov chain, 125, 126
Erlang distribution, 8, 67, 98
exponential martingale, 132
fading
  Markov random evolutionary process, 78, 81, 84, 85, 89
  multidimensional homogeneous alternating process, 77
  telegraphic process, 77
filtered signal
  characterization of a, 141
filtering
  error, 164
  model, 159
  of discrete Markov diffusion, 161

G, H

γ-module of the vector, 32, 35, 36
group of matrices $GM_{S_{n+1}}(F_3)$, 29
heuristic principles, 223, 224, 226
hitting moment, 172, 186–188
hydrodynamic limit, 47, 67, 100
hyperbolic functions, 2
hyperparabolic
  equation(s), 39, 44–46, 54, 57, 64, 94

I, K

instantaneous energy spectrum, 79
Kolmogorov
  differential equations, 18, 21, 25, 26, 89
  inequality, 150
  integral equation, 58, 90
Kubo–Anderson process, 5, 6

M, N

Markov (*see also* embedded Markov chain *and* semi-Markov)
  non-symmetrical random evolutionary process, 119, 120
  process in asymptotic diffusion environment, 127

random evolutionary process, 6, 9–12, 14, 17, 23, 26, 46, 48, 53, 57, 64, 109, 110, 171, 188, 191, 194
symmetrical random evolutionary process, 110, 113, 119
multivariate alternating process, 12
normalizing function, 172, 186, 187, 192, 206, 211, 215

O, P

optimal filtration equation, 139
Ornstein–Uhlenbeck diffusion process, 125, 131
parameter estimation, 132
perturbing functions, 131
phase merging, 221, 223–226
Poisson distribution, 34–36
potential kernel, 128

R, S

random
change of time, 143, 147, 158
evolution in a random environment, 125
real-analytic conditions, 46, 47, 54, 57
reducibly invertible operator, 111
regular $n + 1$-hedron, 1
renewal system, 222–226
Schrödinger-type equation, 100
semi-Markov
random evolutioionary process, 210–212, 217
switchings, 210, 216
singular perturbation problem, 130
stochastic Doléans–Dade equation, 132, 133

T

telegraph equation, 46, 47, 57, 60, 64
telegraphic process, 9
theorem
of existence, 136
on normal correlation, 160, 162, 163
on stationarity, 160
transition probabilities, 171, 172, 175, 210, 213, 214, 216, 217
triangular distribution, 32, 33
truncated operator, 130